Placental–Fetal Growth Restriction

Placental–Fetal Growth Restriction

Edited by

Christoph Lees
Imperial College London

Gerard H. A. Visser
Department of Obstetrics and Gynaecology, University of Utrecht

Kurt Hecher
Department of Obstetrics and Fetal Medicine, University Medical Center, Hamburg

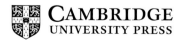

CAMBRIDGE
UNIVERSITY PRESS

CAMBRIDGE
UNIVERSITY PRESS

University Printing House, Cambridge CB2 8BS, United Kingdom

One Liberty Plaza, 20th Floor, New York, NY 10006, USA

477 Williamstown Road, Port Melbourne, VIC 3207, Australia

314–321, 3rd Floor, Plot 3, Splendor Forum, Jasola District Centre, New Delhi – 110025, India

79 Anson Road, #06-04/06, Singapore 079906

Cambridge University Press is part of the University of Cambridge.

It furthers the University's mission by disseminating knowledge in the pursuit of
education, learning, and research at the highest international levels of excellence.

www.cambridge.org
Information on this title: www.cambridge.org/9781107101395
DOI: 10.1017/9781316181898

First published 2018

Printed and bound in Great Britain by Clays Ltd, Elcograf S.p.A.

A catalogue record for this publication is available from the British Library.

Library of Congress Cataloging-in-Publication Data
Names: Lees, Christoph, editor. | Visser, Gerard Hille Adriaan, editor. | Hecher, Kurt, editor.
Title: Placental–fetal growth restriction / edited by Christoph Lees, Gerard H. A. Visser, Kurt Hecher.
Description: Cambridge, United Kingdom; New York, NY: Cambridge University Press, 2018. |
Includes bibliographical references and index.
Identifiers: LCCN 2017040151 | ISBN 9781107101395 (hardback)
Subjects: | MESH: Fetal Growth Retardation
Classification: LCC RG629.G76 | NLM WQ 211 | DDC 618.3/2–dc23
LC record available at https://lccn.loc.gov/2017040151

ISBN 978-1-107-10139-5 Hardback

....

Contents

Section 1 – Basic Principles

Section 2 – Maternal Cardiovascular Characteristics and the Placenta

Section 3 – Screening for Placental–Fetal Growth Restriction

Section 4 – Prophylaxis and Treatment

Section 5 – Characteristics of Fetal Growth Restriction

Section 6 – Management of Fetal Growth Restriction

Section 7 – Postnatal Aspects of Fetal Growth Restriction

Contributors

Birgit Arabin
Center for Mother and Child, Philipps University
Marburg, Marburg, Germany

Petra Arck
Department of Obstetrics and Fetal Medicine,
University Medical Center, Hamburg, Germany

C. M. Bilardo
Department of Obstetrics and Fetal Medicine,
University of Groningen, The Netherlands

K. E. Boers
Department of Obstetrics and Gynecology, Bronovo
Hospital, The Hague, The Netherlands

Christoph Brezinka
Department of Obstetrics and Gynecology,
University Hospital, Innsbruck, Austria

David J. Carr
Institute for Women's Health, University College
London, London, United Kingdom

Irene Cetin
Department of Obstetrics and Gynecology, Hospital
Luigi Sacco, University of Milan, Italy

Isabel Couck
Fetal Medicine Unit, University Hospitals Leuven,
Belgium

Fàtima Crispi
Barcelona Center for Maternal-Fetal and Neonatal
Medicine, University of Barcelona, Spain

Anna L. David
Institute for Women's Health, University College
London, London, United Kingdom

Jan Derks
Department of Obstetrics, University Medical Center
Utrecht, The Netherlands

Daniela Di Martino
IRCCS Fondazione Cà Granda, Ospedale Maggiore
Policlinico
Department of Woman, Child and Neonate
Milan, Italy

Werner Diehl
Department of Obstetrics and Fetal Medicine,
University Medical Centre, Hamburg-Eppendorf,
Germany

Johannes J. Duvekot
Department of Obstetrics, Erasmus
University Medical Center, Rotterdam,
The Netherlands

Enrico Ferrazzi
IRCCS Fondazione Cà Granda, Ospedale Maggiore
Policlinico
Department of Woman, Child and Neonate
Milan, Italy

Francesc Figueras
Department of Obstetrics and Fetal Medicine,
University of Barcelona, Spain

Tiziana Frusca
Department of Obstetrics and Gynaecology,
University of Parma, Parma, Italy

Rashmi Gandhi
UCL Elizabeth Garrett Anderson Institute for
Women's Health, University College London, United
Kingdom

J. W. Ganzevoort
Academic Medical Centre, Amsterdam, The Netherlands

Eduard Gratacós
Barcelona Center for Maternal-Fetal and Neonatal Medicine, University of Barcelona, Spain

Kurt Hecher
Department of Obstetrics and Fetal Medicine, University Medical Center, Hamburg-Eppendorf, Germany

Asma Khalil
Department of Fetal Medicine, St George's University of London, United Kingdom

Shirin Khanjani
Institute of Reproductive and Developmental Biology, Imperial College, London, United Kingdom

Steven Koenen
Department of Perinatology, University Medical Hospital Utrecht, Utrecht, The Netherlands

Anna Lawin-O'Brien
Department of Obstetrics and Fetal Medicine, the Whittington Hospital, United Kingdom

Christoph Lees
Centre for Fetal Care, Queen Charlotte's and Chelsea Hospital, Imperial College Healthcare NHS Trust, United Kingdom

Liesbeth Lewi
Fetal Medicine Unit, University Hospitals Leuven, Belgium

Silvia M. Lobmaier
Frauenklinik der Technischen Universität, München, Germany

Gemma Malin
Division of Child Health, Obstetrics and Gynaecology, School of Medicine, University of Nottingham, United Kingdom

Chiara Mandò
Department of Biomedical and Clinical Sciences Luigi Sacco, University of Milan, Italy

Neil Marlow
UCL Elizabeth Garrett Anderson Institute for Women's Health, University College London, London, United Kingdom

Pasquale Martinelli
Department of Obstetrics and Gynecology, University Federico II, Naples, Italy

Lesley McCowan
Department of Obstetrics and Gynaecology, Faculty of Medical and Health Sciences, University of Auckland, New Zealand

William Mifsud
Department of Developmental and Paediatric Pathology, Great Ormond Street Hospital and Institute of Child Health, UCL, London, United Kingdom

Raffaele Napolitano
Fetal Medicine Unit, Institute for Women's Health, University College London, United Kingdom

Gian Paolo Novelli
Department of Cardiology San Sebastiano Martire Hospital Frascati, Rome, Italy

Giovanna Oggé
Department of Surgical Sciences, Obstetrics and Gynecology Sant'Anna Hospital, University of Turin, Italy

Aris T. Papageorghiou
Department of Obstetrics, St George's Hospital, London, United Kingdom

Federico Prefumo
Department of Obstetrics and Gynaecology, University of Brescia, Brescia, Italy

Christopher W. G. Redman
Nuffield Department of Obstetrics and Gynaecology, John Radcliffe Hospital, Oxford, United Kingdom

Dietmar Schlembach
Vivantes Clinicum Neukölln, Clinic of Obstetrics, Berlin Germany

Karl-Theo M. Schneider
Perinatalmedizin München, University of Technology, Germany

Neil Sebire
Department of Developmental and Paediatric Pathology, Great Ormond Street Hospital and Institute of Child Health, UCL, London, United Kingdom

Rebecca N. Spencer
Institute for Women's Health, University College London, United Kingdom

Anne Cathrine Staff
Faculty of Medicine, University of Oslo, and Department of Obstetrics and Department of Gynaecology, Oslo University Hospital, Norway

Tamara Stampalija
Unit of Prenatal Diagnosis, Burlo Garofolo Pediatric Institute, Trieste, Italy

Basky Thilaganathan
Fetal Medicine Unit, St George's, University of London, United Kingdom

Jim G. Thornton
Division of Child Health, Obstetrics and Gynaecology, School of Medicine, University of Nottingham, United Kingdom

Tullia Todros
Department of Surgical Sciences, Obstetrics and Gynecology Sant'Anna Hospital, University of Turin, Italy

Rosemary Townsend
Department of Fetal Medicine, St George's University of London, United Kingdom

Sana Usman
Imperial College London, United Kingdom

Herbert Valensise
Department of Obstetrics and Gynaecology Policlinico Casilino, Tor Vergata University Rome, Italy

Blanka Vasak
Department of Obstetrics, University Medical Center, Utrecht, The Netherlands

Barbara Vasapollo
Department of Obstetrics and Gynaecology Policlinico Casilino, Tor Vergata University Rome, Italy

Gerard H. A. Visser
Department of Obstetrics, University Medical Center, Utrecht, The Netherlands

Hans Wolf
Academic Medical Centre, Amsterdam, The Netherlands

Foreword

The diagnosis of "small for gestational age" at birth affects at least 13 million neonates each year (based on 131 million births in one year, and the 10th percentile of birthweight for cutoff). A substantial number of these neonates are affected by fetal growth restriction, making these conditions common complications of pregnancy. Yet, there are fundamental, unresolved questions about virtually every aspect of these syndromes.

This book emerged from important discussions that the editors and many of the authors had when designing, analyzing, and interpreting the results of the Trial of Umbilical and Fetal Flow in Europe (TRUFFLE) Study, of which editors Christoph Lees, Gerry Visser, and Kurt Hecher were Principal Investigators and protagonists.

The conduct of the TRUFFLE Study challenged the team of investigators and advisors in virtually every area of the subject: fetal biometry, functional evaluation with Doppler velocimetry, cardiotocography, and timing and mode of delivery. The trial also raised questions about the fundamental pathophysiology of fetal growth and the role of uteroplacental ischemia in the genesis of fetal growth restriction.

The editors and authors bring unique expertise, experience, and wisdom to the treatment of this important subject. The authors review, with considerable depth, the rich body of recent literature. A major strength is the translational nature of the book, which bridges obstetrical practice, clinical research, and fundamental knowledge about the biology of growth and the placenta.

Fetal growth and placental biology have been subjects of interest throughout my career. During the last five years, major studies on longitudinal fetal biometry, maternal and fetal cardiovascular physiology and pathology, and placental pathophysiology have sparked intense dialogue, and this book could not have come at a better time.

Roberto Romero, M.D., D.Med.Sci. Chief, Perinatology Research Branch
Director, Division of Obstetrics and Maternal-Fetal Medicine Intramural Division, NICHD, NIH, DHHS Professor of Molecular Obstetrics and Genetics, Wayne State University Professor of Epidemiology and Biostatistics, Michigan State University Professor of Obstetrics and Gynecology, University of Michigan Editor-in-Chief for Obstetrics, *American Journal of Obstetrics & Gynecology*

Preface

The terms *fetal growth restriction* (FGR), *intrauterine growth restriction* (IUGR), *growth retardation*, and *small for gestational age* (SGA) have been used for many decades, but the definitions are not and have never been entirely satisfactory. That fetal growth restriction represents a failure of the fetus to achieve its optimal growth potential is unarguable, but there again to define growth restriction in this way is tautologous – and more importantly cannot be measured or diagnosed by divergence from a hypothetical trajectory. The term *SGA* cannot be used without defining the percentile at which the cut-off is defined: is it the 3rd, 5th, or 10th percentile?

Furthermore, *growth* and *size* are surely not the same – though they are frequently used synonymously. Growth implies velocity, change in size with time, and can be assessed only by longitudinal measurements. Does it matter if a fetus with the same estimated weight at 34 weeks is on the 3rd percentile showing entirely normal growth, or that its size has not changed in 2 weeks? Surely both are small – but which is more at risk of the complications of hypoxia/placental insufficiency? Then there is the live issue as to whether the size of a baby is determined by environmental and genetic factors, hence all should be "standardized" by customizing according to maternal characteristics, or whether a fetus – and baby – born to healthy parents should be the same size in Asia, as in Africa, as in Europe.

In this book, we discuss all these issues, the diagnostic criteria for FGR, its management, and its prognosis. The focus is on the most commonly encountered form of fetal growth restriction: namely that secondary to uteroplacental insufficiency. In using this term, we do not imply that the placenta per se causes fetal growth restriction, but there is little doubt that uteroplacental insufficiency is associated with it: hence the term *placental fetal growth restriction* (PFGR). PFGR implies a structurally and genetically normal baby that has the potential for a normal life ex-utero, but has very specific perinatal problems and risks associated with placental insufficiency.

Whether the problems of PFGR are primarily in the placenta – or associated with a more general maternal cardiovascular dysfunction – remains contested. Given these emerging theories, for the first time in our specialty, potential therapies exist for PFGR, all of which aim to maximize the uteroplacental circulation. But accurate prognostication relies on accurate diagnosis, and good outcome depends on attentive management. We consider the optimal management of these fetuses and the timing of delivery – which is probably the most crucial decision a perinatologist can make.

The idea of this book first arose from the TRUFFLE study of severe early-onset fetal growth restriction, reported in the *Lancet* in 2015. This group comprised 20 European centers that collaborated closely from 2002 to 2015. Many but not all chapter authors are TRUFFLE investigators whose careers and professional expertise are focused on fetal growth restriction; all authors are experts in their field. The aim of this book is to give a comprehensive overview of all aspects of PFGR, taking into account the latest research in the field and giving space to theories that may not yet have become "mainstream," but deserve further exposure.

Glossary and Commonly Used Abbreviations

22q11.2 deletion: includes DiGeorge and other syndromes such as craniofacial and velocardiofacial syndrome and is the most common microdeletion syndrome reported.

Abdominal circumference (AC)

Absent and reversed end-diastolic flows (AREDF)

Absent umbilical arterial diastolic flow (AEDF): occurs when 60–70% of the villous vascular tree is damaged

Achondrogenesis: an autosomal recessive condition, hence with a 25% risk of recurrence

A-Disintegrin and Metalloproteinase 12 (ADAM 12): a metalloproteinase highly expressed in placental tissue and known to be involved in placental development, as well as associated with a number of cancers and with fetuses being small for gestational age

Assisted reproduction techniques (ART)

Barker hypothesis: describes the inverse correlation between low birth weight and cardiovascular disease in adult life

Beta human chorionic gonadotrophin (b-hCG): hormone produced by the syncytiotrophoblast; low levels in the first trimester have been associated with adverse pregnancy outcomes

Brain-sparing effect

Cardiotocography (CTG): fetal heart rate assessment commonly used in the surveillance of fetuses compromised by fetal growth restriction

Cerebroplacental ratio (CPR)

Cornelia de Lange (also called Brachmann-de Lange Syndrome): an example of a multisystem malformation genetic syndrome associated with growth restriction. More than half can now be identified from genetic testing.

Cytomegalovirus (CMV): DNA virus of the herpes family and the most frequent cause of congenital infection

Doppler: a form of ultrasound used to assess blood flow velocity waveforms from which arterial impedance and blood flow velocity can be derived. Commonly referred to as uteroplacental Doppler (maternal circulation) and fetal Doppler

Down syndrome: named after John Langdon Down and also known as Trisomy 21, initially described the associated pattern of congenital abnormalities.

Ninety-five percent of cases are caused by non-disjunction of chromosome 21 during maternal meiosis, resulting in an extra chromosome 21.

Early-onset fetal growth restriction: usually results from severe placental insufficiency before 34 weeks' gestation, associated with preeclampsia, and constitutes a major cause of perinatal mortality and morbidity

Edward's syndrome (Trisomy 18): more than 99% of cases are of non-disjunction resulting in an additional chromosome 18. It is associated with high rates (70%) of intrauterine demise and a survival birth rate of only 5%, with 90% mortality within 6 months.

Estimated fetal weight (EFW)

Fetal growth restriction (FGR): the process where a fetus that has a certain growth potential based on genetic criteria is limited in its growth because of a pathological environmental influence

Fetal heart rate (FHR)

Gene therapy: the introduction of genetic material into a cell to produce a therapeutic effect

HELLP syndrome: Hemolysis, elevated liver enzymes, low platelet count

Intrauterine growth restriction (IUGR)

Intrauterine insemination (IUI)

In vitro fertilization (IVF)

Late-onset fetal growth restriction: fetuses associate a mild degree of placental insufficiency (not reflected by umbilical artery Doppler), are usually delivered near or at term, and present poorer perinatal and long-term results

Middle cerebral artery (MCA)

Myocardial performance index (MPI): considered a marker of global cardiac function and takes into account several systolic and diastolic time events

Osteogenesis imperfecta: a skeletal dysplasia of which there are several variants with different inheritance modes often recognized in the second trimester and associated with bowing and shortening of the limbs

Ovarian hyperstimulation syndrome (OHSS): a condition that presents with significantly enlarged ovaries and third-space fluid accumulation

Patau's syndrome (Trisomy 13): the least common autosomal trisomy to occur, affecting 1 in 12,500 births. The majority of cases are due to non-disjunction (75%), with the remaining due to Robertsonian translocation.

Phase-rectified signal averaging (PRSA): can eliminate artefacts and signal perturbations of bio-signals and extract areas of interest reflecting the autonomic nervous system by the "acceleration" and "deceleration capacity

Placental growth factor (PlGF): the most widely used serum marker low levels of which indicate placental dysfunction

Placental growth hormone (PGH): a product of the syncytiotrophoblast involved in regulating the maternal metabolic adaptation to pregnancy, associated with levels of IGF1 and trophoblast invasion

Placental protein 13 (PP13): a galectin expressed by the placenta and involved in placental implantation

Preeclampsia: a syndrome comprising new-onset hypertension and proteinuria in the second half of pregnancy, which was not present before pregnancy and does not persist afterward

Pregnancy-associated plasma protein A (PAPP-A): routinely measured as part of the first trimester aneuploidy screening; low levels have long been known to be associated with adverse pregnancy outcomes in euploid fetuses. PAPP-A is closely associated with placental mass.

Pregnancy-induced hypertension (PIH)

Reduced fetal movements (RFM)

Reversed end-diastolic flow (REDF): the most severe umbilical artery Doppler flow velocity waveform abnormality

Russell-Silver Syndrome: an imprinting disorder characterized by severe fetal growth restriction; the estimated incidence is 1 in 7,000

Short-term variation (STV): a method of heart rate analysis described by Dawes and Redman that can be used to detect fetuses at high risk of acidemia

Small for gestational age (SGA): a birth weight below the 10th centile

Thanatophoric dysplasia: a neonatally lethal condition caused most commonly by a new dominant mutation in fibroblast growth factor receptor gene 3 (FGFR3 gene) and associated with increased paternal age

Toxoplasmosis: A parasite infection that affects 3–4 in 10,000 pregnancies with the majority of infections presenting subclinically (85%) in the fetus and approximately 15% presenting with hydrocephalus, intracranial calcifications, and chorioretinitis

Triploidy: extremely rare condition usually lethal by 20 weeks due to a complete extra set of chromosomes (69), which can be of maternal or paternal origin and is not associated with advancing maternal age. Estimated incidence is 1 in 2,500–5,000 births.

Villitis of unknown etiology (VUE): characterized by chorionic villous infiltration by chronic inflammatory cells, particularly histiocytes, and to a lesser extent, lymphocytes, especially in basal/maternal floor villi, in the absence of a known, typically infective cause

Chapter

What Is Optimal Fetal Growth?

Blanka Vasak and Gerard H. A. Visser

Introduction

Normal fetal growth is usually defined as an estimated fetal weight between the 10th and 90th centiles based on population-specific birth weight centiles corrected for gestational age at delivery, parity, and fetal sex. So-called customized growth charts also correct for maternal ethnicity, weight, and length [1]. Such definitions are based on the fact that both impaired and excessive fetal growth result in an increased risk of perinatal morbidity and mortality. Indeed, in small for gestational age (SGA) fetuses, defined as a birth weight below the 10th centile, there is an increased risk of intrauterine fetal death across all gestational ages [2,3] compared with non-SGA fetuses, with the highest risk in infants with a birth weight below the 3rd centile [4]. Large for gestational age (> 90th centile, macrosomic) fetuses are at risk of labor complications and thus also of increased perinatal morbidity and mortality [5,6]. However, with a focus on too small or too big, it may be forgotten that the majority of perinatal (and especially antepartum) deaths occurs in fetuses with a "normal" weight. Moreover, the use of population-based fetal growth charts assumes that optimal size at birth for outcome is at the 50th centile.

In this chapter, optimal fetal growth/size for perinatal and long-term survival is reviewed in relation to birth weight centiles at birth. The clinical consequences are discussed.

Fetal Growth/Size and Short-Term Perinatal Survival

Several studies have been conducted on perinatal survival in relation to birth weight centiles. A study conducted in Newcastle in the United Kingdom using Z-scores for distribution of birth weight showed that the lowest stillbirth rate and infant mortality occurred in infants with a Z-score of +1, both between 1961–80 and 1981–2000, a period over which the overall stillbirth rate fell in that region of the UK from 23.4 to 4.7 per 1,000, respectively [7]. In a larger nationwide study in Norway, the lowest mortality was found for a birth weight Z-score between +1 and +2 [8]. Similar results were recently published from Australia [9] and Scotland [10]. In the latter study regarding 780,000 births, the lowest antenatal mortality occurred in fetuses with a birth weight in between the 90th and 97th centiles and in cases with unknown cause, antenatal hemorrhage, or maternal hypertensive disease. In cases of maternal diseases, including diabetes, the stillbirth rate was lowest in fetuses with a weight around the 20th centile. In the most recent study from The Netherlands, distribution of perinatal mortality according to birth weight centile and gestational age was studied in more than 1 million births from singleton pregnancies and non-malformed fetuses between 28 and 43 weeks gestation [11]. There were 5,075 (0.43%) perinatal deaths. The highest mortality occurred in infants with a birth weight below the 2.3rd centile (25.4/1,000 births), and the lowest mortality occurred in infants with birth weights between the 80th and 84th centiles (2.4/1,000 births), according to nationwide birth weight charts. Antenatal deaths were lowest with birth weights between the 90th and 95th centiles. Data were almost identical when analysis was restricted to infants born after 37 weeks or at 39–41 weeks only (Vasak et al.; Figure 1.1) [11]. In term gestations, 63% of perinatal deaths and 61% of antepartum deaths occurred in infants with a so-called normal weight between the 10th and 90th centiles. The majority of perinatal deaths occurred during the antepartum period (72%).

Data on cerebral palsy are also in line with the mortality figures; the lowest prevalence of cerebral palsy by Z-score of weight for gestation was found in infants with a Z-score of +1 [12].

These studies indicate that optimal fetal weight for intact perinatal survival occurs at a much higher

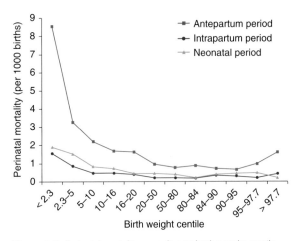

Figure 1.1 Perinatal mortality according to birth weight centile for babies delivered between 39 and 41 weeks' gestation in The Netherlands during 2002–8.

centile than the 50th centile. In fact, perinatal mortality of fetuses with a weight at the 50th centile is 34% higher than that of fetuses weighing in between the 80th and 84th centiles [11]. The lower "optimal weight" for intrapartum and neonatal survival (80th–84th centile), as compared to that of antepartum survival (90th–95th centile), may be explained by intrapartum complications in infants at the highest birth weight centiles. Regarding antepartum survival, it may be concluded that "the bigger the better" [8] and that most infants have a birth weight below optimal for perinatal survival, which seems illogical from an evolutionary perspective. However, mothers also have to survive, and the relatively small pelvis associated with bipedalism and the large human fetal head constitute major obstacles for uncomplicated childbirth. It may therefore well be that maternal factors restrain fetal growth that is below optimal for perinatal survival. In other words, a conflict takes place between mother and fetus, with a compromise as a result. Given the fact that during the whole existence of mankind women have looked after their offspring, such a compromise may have resulted in a net benefit for the infants at the end. In developing countries, this can nowadays still be seen in the poor survival of children whose mothers have died during or directly after childbirth [13,14]. These data also nicely fit with recent Doppler findings of blood flow redistribution to the fetal brain. In a large cohort of third trimester fetuses, it was shown that

the cerebro-placental ratio (CPR) increased progressively with increasing fetal weight centiles whereby signs of redistribution were only consistently absent in cases of an estimated fetal weight > 90th centile [15]. The association between CPR and weight centiles has recently been confirmed in another study [16].

Fetal Growth and Long-Term Survival

The high birth weight (centile) favorable for perinatal survival is also associated with reduced risk of later non-communicable disease. Studies on the Developmental Origins of Health and Disease (DOHaD) concept have shown that birth weight is inversely related in a graded manner to risk of later cardiovascular and cerebrovascular death [17–20] and to impaired glucose tolerance and Type 2 diabetes [21]. Thus, in historical studies in the UK, the lowest risks of adult cardiovascular disease (CVD) were found in infants weighing around 4 kg at birth, approximately the 90th centile at 40 weeks of gestation [17,19]. A high birth weight, indicative of absence of intrauterine growth restraint and resulting in a low perinatal mortality, therefore is also favorable for long-term health.

Clinical Implications

Early stillbirths are generally SGA [3]. So at early gestation, identification of SGA fetuses remains of utmost importance. After approximately 32 weeks of gestation, the majority of stillbirths concerns appropriate for gestation infants [3,11]. Identification of third trimester (SGA) infants remains important since mortality may be reduced when these fetuses have been identified as being small [22,23] (see Chapters 22 and 23 of this volume). However, identification of infants at risk of stillbirth who have a weight within the normal range may prove difficult. Factors to be assessed may include:

a) Maternal characteristics. In a study from Norway, it has been shown that being SGA increases the risk for stillbirth sevenfold [24]. Other independent risk factors for stillbirth were maternal age > 35 years (RR 4.1), maternal body mass index > 25 (RR 4.7), and maternal education < 10 years (RR 3.5). A combination of risk factors resulted in a dramatic increase in stillbirth risk. For instance, SGA in combination with maternal overweight resulted in an RR of 71 (univariate analysis). Confidence limits were large due to the relatively low number of inclusions (95% CI: 14–350), but these data indicate that a combination of risk factors may increase detection of fetuses at risk. Such a risk assessment might be made around 36–8 weeks, and if more than one of these variables is abnormal, delivery may be indicated. However, the latter policy has to be tested, preferably in a randomized controlled study.

b) Uterine artery pulsatility index (UtA-PI). An increased UtA-PI at 20 weeks of gestation has been found to be associated with an Odds ratio of 6.8 for third trimester stillbirth, after correction for maternal weight, body mass index, and smoking, with 50% of all stillbirth cases occurring in the 10% with an abnormal UtA-PI [25].

c) Cerebro-placental ratio (CPR). In preterm SGA fetuses, an increased PI in the umbilical artery identifies those at highest risk for perinatal death [26]. However, near term the diagnostic value of this tool is limited and significant changes are a late sign of impairment. However, subtle changes may be detected by using the ratio between middle cerebral artery and umbilical artery PI. In SGA term fetuses, it was found that a reduced CPR was associated with a poorer outcome than in cases with a normal ratio [27]. In a high-risk population of term fetuses, pH at delivery was lower in cases with an abnormal CPR, both in SGA and in normally grown fetuses [28]. This suggests that the CPR might be used to identify fetuses at risk of becoming hypoxemic, not only in SGA, but also in fetuses with a weight within the "normal" range. However, in a recent normal population of more than 6,000 fetuses assessed at around 36 weeks of gestation, no predictive value of the CPR was found regarding caesarean section for fetal distress, umbilical artery pH at birth, or Apgar score [16]. Reduced CPR immediately prior to delivery was associated with an increased risk of delivery by emergency caesarean section [29]. The value of the CPR in identifying the risks of intrauterine death or asphyxia in normally grown fetuses is therefore still uncertain.

d) Longitudinal fetal growth assessment. Single third trimester measurements of fetal growth have not been capable of identifying third trimester SGA reliably [30]. Detection of infants at risk with a weight within the normal range may only be possible by longitudinal growth assessment to identify decreasing growth velocity. Such studies are taking place at this moment.

e) Reduced fetal movements (RFM). RFM remain an important sign of fetal compromise, given the limited predictive values of the other assessment techniques. RFM have been associated with abnormal placental morphology [31]. A study from Norway has shown that structured information given to the mother at around 18 weeks of gestation on the importance of RFM may result in a more than 50% reduction of third trimester fetal deaths in nulliparous women [32].

f) Integrated risk assessment. Identification of fetuses at risk for intrauterine death is difficult. On the one hand SGA fetuses should be detected, and on the other hand the larger group of apparently normally grown fetuses at risk of dying in utero should be identified. This will require integrated risk models, including maternal characteristics (BMI, age, socioeconomic situation), Doppler measurements of the maternal and feto-placental circulation, fetal growth assessment, and measurement of biochemical markers of placental function. Most likely a contingent screening is required (e.g., to identify decreasing fetal growth velocity). Models must be first exhaustively tested in the population to which they will be applied, to obviate the risk of unnecessary intervention.

Conclusions

Optimal fetal growth for perinatal and long-term survival is a growth resulting in a birth weight in between the 80th and 90th centiles. This implies that the majority of infants will have a suboptimal fetal growth. Evolutionarily, this may be explained by a compromise between maternal survival, which will be lower in large fetuses, and fetal survival. In the third trimester of pregnancy, the majority of intrauterine deaths occurs in fetuses with a weight within the normal range. Identification of the fetuses at risk will be difficult and requires an integrated risk assessment including sequential measurements.

Key Points

- The majority of perinatal deaths occurs in fetuses with a weight within the normal range.
- Optimal fetal growth for perinatal and long-term survival is a growth resulting in a birth weight in between the 80th and 90th centiles.
- Identification of fetuses at risk, especially those with a weight within the normal range, remains difficult and requires an integrated risk assessment including sequential measurements.

References

1. Gardosi J, Chang A, Kalyan B, Sahota D, Symonds EM. Customised antenatal growth charts. *Lancet* 1992; 339(8788):283–7.

2. Pilliod RA, Cheng YW, Snowden JM, Doss AE, Caughey AB. The risk of intrauterine fetal death in the small-for-gestational-age fetus. *Am J Obstet Gynecol* 2012;207(4):318.e1, 318.e6.

3. Gardosi J, Madurasinghe V, Williams M, Malik A, Francis A. Maternal and fetal risk factors for stillbirth: Population based study. *BMJ* 2013;346:f108.

4. McIntire DD, Bloom SL, Casey BM, Leveno KJ. Birth weight in relation to morbidity and mortality among newborn infants. *N Engl J Med* 1999;340(16):1234–8.

5. Henriksen T. The macrosomic fetus: A challenge in current obstetrics. *Acta Obstet Gynecol Scand* 2008;87(2):134–45.

6. Zhang X, Decker A, Platt RW, Kramer MS. How big is too big? The perinatal consequences of fetal macrosomia. *Am J Obstet Gynecol* 2008;198(5):517.e1, 517.e6.

7. Glinianaia SV, Rankin J, Pearce MS, Parker L, Pless-Mulloli T. Stillbirth and infant mortality in singletons by cause of death, birthweight, gestational age and birthweight-for-gestation, Newcastle upon Tyne 1961–2000. *Paediatr Perinat Epidemiol* 2010;24(4):331–42.

8. Vangen S, Stoltenberg C, Skjaerven R, Magnus P, Harris JR, Stray-Pedersen B. The heavier the better? Birthweight and perinatal mortality in different ethnic groups. *Int J Epidemiol* 2002;31(3):654–60.

9. Francis JH, Permezel M, Davey MA. Perinatal mortality by birthweight centile. *Aust N Z J Obstet Gynaecol* 2014;54(4):354–9.

10. Moraitis AA, Wood AM, Fleming M, Smith GC. Birth weight percentile and the risk of term perinatal death. *Obstet Gynecol* 2014;124(2 Pt 1):274–83.

11. Vasak B, Koenen SV, Koster MP, Hukkelhoven CW, Franx A, Hanson MA, Visser GH. Human fetal growth is constrained below optimal for perinatal survival. *Ultrasound Obstet Gynecol* 2015;45(2):162–7.

12. Jarvis S, Glinianaia SV, Torrioli MG, et al. Cerebral palsy and intrauterine growth in single births: European collaborative study. *Lancet* 2003;362(9390):1106–11.

13. Houle B, Clark SJ, Kahn K, Tollman S, Yamin A. The impacts of maternal mortality and cause of death on children's risk of dying in rural South Africa: Evidence from a population based surveillance study (1992–2013). *Reprod Health* 2015;12 Suppl 1:S7,4755-12-S1-S7. Epub 2015 May 6.

14. Moucheraud C, Worku A, Molla M, Finlay JE, Leaning J, Yamin A. Consequences of maternal mortality on infant and child survival: A 25-year longitudinal analysis in Butajira Ethiopia (1987–2011). *Reprod Health* 2015;12 Suppl 1:S4,4755-12-S1-S4. Epub 2015 May 6.

15. Morales-Rosello J, Khalil A, Morlando M, Papageorghiou A, Bhide A, Thilaganathan B. Changes in fetal Doppler indices as a marker of failure to reach growth potential at term. *Ultrasound Obstet Gynecol* 2014;43(3):303–10.

16. Akolekar R, Syngelaki A, Gallo DM, Poon LC, Nicolaides KH. Umbilical and fetal middle cerebral artery Doppler at 35–37 weeks' gestation in the prediction of adverse perinatal outcome. *Ultrasound Obstet Gynecol* 2015;46(1):82–92.

17. Barker DJ, Winter PD, Osmond C, Margetts B, Simmonds SJ. Weight in infancy and death from ischaemic heart disease. *Lancet* 1989;2(8663):577–80.

18. Barker DJ. Fetal origins of coronary heart disease. *BMJ* 1995;311(6998):171–4.

19. Lawlor DA, Ronalds G, Clark H, Smith GD, Leon DA. Birth weight is inversely associated with incident coronary heart disease and stroke among individuals born in the 1950s: Findings from the Aberdeen Children of the 1950s prospective cohort study. *Circulation* 2005;112(10):1414–18.

20. Osmond C, Kajantie E, Forsen TJ, Eriksson JG, Barker DJ. Infant growth and stroke in adult life: The Helsinki birth cohort study. *Stroke* 2007;38(2):264–70.

21. Hales CN, Barker DJ, Clark PM, Cox LJ, Fall C, Osmond C, Winter PD. Fetal and infant growth and impaired glucose tolerance at age 64. *BMJ* 1991;303(6809):1019–22.

22. Gardosi J, Francis A. Adverse pregnancy outcome and association with small for gestational age birthweight by customized and population-based percentiles. *Am J Obstet Gynecol* 2009;201(1):28.e1,28.e8.

23. Boers KE, Vijgen SM, Bijlenga D, et al. Induction versus expectant monitoring for intrauterine growth restriction at term: Randomised equivalence trial (DIGITAT). *BMJ* 2010;341:c7087. doi:10.1136/bmj.c7087.

24. Froen JF, Gardosi JO, Thurmann A, Francis A, Stray-Pedersen B. Restricted fetal growth in sudden intrauterine unexplained death. *Acta Obstet Gynecol Scand* 2004;83(9):801–7.

25. Singh T, Leslie K, Bhide A, D'Antonio F, Thilaganathan B. Role of second-trimester uterine artery Doppler in assessing stillbirth risk. *Obstet Gynecol* 2012;119(2 Pt 1):256–61.

26. Alfirevic Z, Stampalija T, Gyte GM. Fetal and umbilical Doppler ultrasound in high-risk pregnancies. *Cochrane Database Syst Rev* 2013; 11:CD007529.

27. Cruz-Martinez R, Figueras F, Hernandez-Andrade E, Oros D, Gratacos E. Fetal brain Doppler to predict cesarean delivery for nonreassuring fetal status in term small-for-gestational-age fetuses. *Obstet Gynecol* 2011;117(3):618–26.

28. Morales-Rosello J, Khalil A, Morlando M, Bhide A, Papageorghiou A, Thilaganathan B. Poor neonatal acid-base status in term fetuses with low cerebroplacental ratio. *Ultrasound Obstet Gynecol* 2015;45(2):156–61.

29. Prior T, Mullins E, Bennett P, Kumar S. Prediction of intrapartum fetal compromise using the cerebroumbilical ratio: A prospective observational study. *Am J Obstet Gynecol* 2013;208(2):124.e1,124.e6.

30. Bricker L, Medley N, Pratt JJ. Routine ultrasound in late pregnancy (after 24 weeks' gestation). *Cochrane Database Syst Rev* 2015;6:CD001451.

31. Warrander LK, Batra G, Bernatavicius G, et al. Maternal perception of reduced fetal movements is associated with altered placental structure and function. *PLoS One* 2012;7(4):e34851.

32. Saastad E, Tveit JV, Flenady V, Stray-Pedersen B, Fretts RC, Bordahl PE, Froen JF. Implementation of uniform information on fetal movement in a Norwegian population reduced delayed reporting of decreased fetal movement and stillbirths in primiparous women – a clinical quality improvement. *BMC Res Notes* 2010;3(1):2, doi: 10.1186/1756-0500-3-2.

Definition of Fetal Growth Restriction and Uteroplacental Insufficiency

J. W. Ganzevoort and Basky Thilaganathan

Introduction

To understand any discussion, it is of paramount importance to be consistent in defining the discussed subject. This is a particular problem when dealing with impaired fetal growth. Even though the measurement of fetal size has significant challenges of its own, comparing this measurement to previously observed variation in a population provides a comparison to a reference standard that is measurable and agreed upon. However, "smallness" or being small for gestational age (SGA) in itself is not the item of interest, but rather "pathological smallness of uteroplacental origin" – otherwise termed fetal *growth restriction* (FGR). FGR is a functional problem of unmet fetal need, and the definition should include descriptions of pathological functional processes.

FGR is a descriptive term for a pathological process and not easily defined. FGR can be described as the process where a fetus that has a certain growth potential based on genetic criteria is limited in its growth because of a pathological environmental influence. It is distinct from the term *small for gestational age* (SGA). SGA is much easier to define because it is a statistical deviation from a population reference standard.

As such, many studies erroneously assume that SGA is synonymous with FGR. Because overlap between the two subgroups is significant, this is a tempting strategy that does still come up with results. However, this assumption may attenuate or even obscure important associations or identify spurious associations that may be misleading. In this chapter, the pathophysiology of FGR is shortly discussed and FGR is defined by functional parameters and compared to definitions of SGA.

Pathophysiology of Uteroplacental Insufficiency

The classical pathophysiological concept of FGR is that of poor placentation. In early pregnancy, the uterine spiral arteries are invaded by the developing endovascular trophoblast, resulting in uteroplacental blood circulation. In adequate placentation, the uterine spiral arteries are remodeled into dilated inelastic tubes without maternal vasomotor control. This is a process that probably occurs between 8–18 weeks of pregnancy [1]. The physiological consequence of vascular remodeling is that a low-resistance unit is accomplished that allows liberal blood flow. If this process is imperfect, the disturbed remodeling will not change the high-resistance unit adequately, leading to the maintenance of high uteroplacental vascular resistance. This can be measured in early pregnancy, by Doppler measurements of the upstream uterine artery. High pulsatility indices already in the first trimester reflect an increased risk for clinical disorders related to poor placentation: fetal growth restriction and preeclampsia [2,3].

The pathophysiological pathways for this defective placentation process are plentiful and none is completely explanatory in itself. Immunological factors, endogenous vascular factors, and thrombogenic factors have been shown to have consistent relationships with the process and the clinical phenotype [1]. Most of these theories were derived from work restricted to cases of preeclampsia. Since most of the pathophysiology on the placental level is shared between hypertensive disorders of pregnancy and FGR, some of this knowledge can be extended into the field of FGR.

Poor placentation is particularly associated with early-onset phenotype of both preeclampsia and FGR. Before 34 weeks' gestation, most women presenting with maternal hypertensive disorders will also have FGR – and both conditions share comparable placental pathology [4]. At later gestations, this association becomes less obvious – at or near term, neonates from mothers with preeclampsia are usually not growth-restricted [5]. Thus, both late FGR and late preeclampsia require another explanation. For this, some hypothesize a secondary placental cause based on the evidence that slowing of placental growth in term pregnancy is more prominent in the largest placentas [1]. This finding suggests that placental growth has a physical limit, depending on size and not gestational age. At term, the placenta apparently becomes more "crowded," compromising intervillous perfusion and predisposing to dysfunction – leading to a similar process as in early-onset FGR and preeclampsia. For the maternal phenotype, the most likely etiology is maternal constitutional susceptibility, among which are (cardio)vascular dysfunction [6,7] and an excessive immunological response [8]. These findings, negating early placentation disorders as an explanation for late FGR and late preeclampsia, are consistent with the finding that the placental pathology in term FGR and preeclampsia is not very discriminative between cases and normal controls [9]. Since term fetuses have less placental reserve capacity, the interval between onset of the disease and subsequent adverse outcome is shorter. Both hypotheses explain why late-onset FGR is less easy to predict and harder to distinguish from pregnancies with normal growth.

In conclusion, it is likely that there are two main routes to FGR based on placental dysfunction or insufficiency. The first is the classic concept of defective placentation leading to early-onset overt FGR, which is easily diagnosed because of abnormal fetal size and related biophysical/biochemical parameters. The second concept is that of a maturational process leading to placental hypoperfusion and late-onset FGR that is difficult to diagnose because size and accompanying parameters may not be severely abnormal. Combinations of the two can also occur, explaining intermediate phenotypes.

Definition of SGA

SGA is a defined statistical deviation from the population standard. Antenatal measurement variation for fetal, maternal, or observer reasons does introduce some uncertainty, but the comparison with a reference standard is a rather uniform practice. Reference ranges (as opposed to standards) are population curves constructed from observed fetal dimensions on ultrasound and birth weights. These ranges are usually normally distributed, because the majority of cases do not have pathological growth. However some skewing may occur, particularly at lower gestational ages and at the lower margin of the curve, where pathological growth is more common. When

the charts are constructed prospectively using strict criteria to define an "optimal" population, then "optimal" reference standards are created, such as in the recent Intergrowth-project [10].

In obstetric populations, centiles usually describe the position of a fetus/newborn within the curve. Within a perfectly normally distributed population, this has large commonalities with the more statistically correct standard deviation scores (SD or z-scores) where the position is expressed as the number of standard deviations the fetus/newborn is from the mean. An alternative option, less statistically correct but with some clinical and statistical advantages, is the weight ratio – the ratio between the observed weight and the median weight for the gestational age (multiples of the median or MoMs).

Defining SGA is a dichotomization within the chosen curve. In most studies, the 10th and 90th centiles are chosen as the cut-off, defining those below the 10th centile as SGA. Other commonly used cut-offs are the 5th centile or the 2.3rd centile. With lowering of the chosen cut-off, the concentration of pathology within the defined group increases. However, because there are no thresholds to distinguish normal growth from pathological growth, no specific cut-off will define a totally abnormal or normal population correctly [11].

Definition of FGR

The definition of FGR is more difficult because the gold standard is not defined. Thus, all attempts focus on defining the process where a fetus with a certain genetic growth potential is limited in its growth because of a pathological environmental influence. This pathological influence is frequently termed *uteroplacental insufficiency* to express that the limitation is located in the transfer of nutrients and waste substances across the placenta. Thus, it is abnormal placental function that needs to be defined accurately in FGR. There are several candidates of measurable parameters to signal impaired placental function and abnormal fetal growth. These parameters have different statistical time relationships with the occurrence of fetal distress (Figure 2.1) [12].

Abnormal Umbilical Artery Doppler Indices

An abundance of studies has demonstrated the relationship between uteroplacental insufficiency and the consequent increased impedance in the uteroplacental vessels and in the umbilical artery. These changes are strongly associated with hypoxemia and poor perinatal outcomes, and the associations can be described in a temporal fashion [13–15]. Among the earliest phenomenon in early-onset FGR are abnormal umbilical artery flow velocity waveforms as measured with

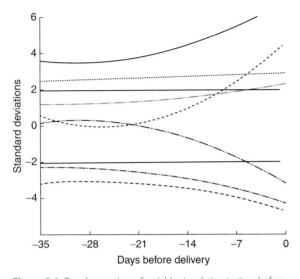

Figure 2.1 Trends over time of variables in relation to time before delivery and reference ranges (±2 SD) for Group 1 (fetuses delivered before or at 32 weeks of gestation). ___, umbilical artery; _ _ _, ductus venosus; ___, aorta; _.._, inferior vena cava; ___, short-term variation; _._, middle cerebral artery; _ _, amniotic fluid index.
Source: Reproduce Figure 3 with permission from Hecher et al. [12].

Doppler ultrasound [12,16]. It is described quantitatively by increased pulsatility index and qualitatively by absent or reversed end-diastolic (ARED) flow. Its occurrence is specific for very early-onset fetal growth restriction and not for term or late preterm growth restriction. This phenomenon is the tip of the iceberg with respect to the fetal hemodynamic status, because an estimated 70% of the placental vascular bed is obliterated or dysfunctional before ARED flow is seen. Thus, in later gestational ages, umbilical artery waveforms do not typically become abnormal before fetal distress occurs, because fetuses have less placental reserve and fetal distress will already have become apparent. Other Doppler studies that may indicate increased impedance of the fetal central vasculature include the aortic isthmus and the descending aorta [17].

Signs of Redistribution in the Fetal Circulation

An early response to placental insufficiency is redistribution of blood flow in the fetal circulation. Blood flow is selectively redirected to myocardium, adrenal glands, and the brain. The last phenomenon is called "brain-sparing effect" and is particularly available for measurement [18,19]. The effect is also measurable in term pregnancies [20]. Other organs may be selectively deprived of blood flow. Among these are

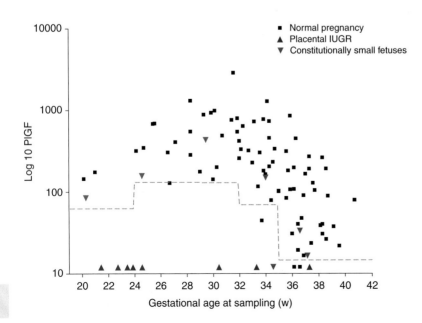

Figure 2.2 PIGF concentrations in the circulation of women with placental IUGR/FGR fetuses, constitutionally small fetuses, and normal pregnancies at the time of sampling. Constitutionally small fetuses (red triangles) and normal pregnancy controls (black squares) had increased PIGF levels compared with placental IUGR/FGR cases (blue triangles). The gray dashed black line represent the fifth percentile PIGF concentration cutoff according to the product insert. The y-axis is log transformed. Two blue triangles overlap at 33+2 weeks' gestation because of the sampling of these women occurring at the same gestational age.
IUGR, intrauterine growth restriction; PIGF, placental growth factor.
Figure reproduced with permission from Benton et al. [23].

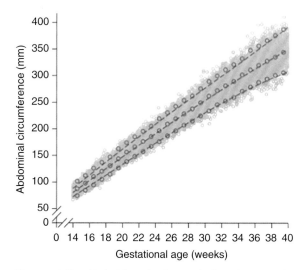

Figure 2.3 Fitted 3rd, 50th, and 97th smoothed centile curves of fetal measurements.
Fitted 3rd (bottom dashes line), 50th (middle dashed line), and 97th (top dashed line) smoothed centile curves for fetal abdominal circumference measured by ultrasound according to gestational age. Open red circles show empirical values for each week of gestation and open grey show actual observations.

the renal arteries – explaining the phenomenon of oligohydramnios.

Venous Doppler Changes

Other changes, usually later in the temporal sequence of deterioration of placental function, are in the fetal venous circulation. Both abnormal ductus venous measurements and pulsations in the umbilical vein are related to fetal hypoxemia and adverse perinatal outcomes [12,15,21].

Uterine Artery

Uteroplacental insufficiency is also signified by increased impedance in the uteroplacental vessels. In physiological pregnancy, the uterine arteries demonstrate a transition from a unit of high resistance to very low resistance. The opening of the spiral arteries into low-resistance units causes the upstream resistance of the uterine artery to decrease to levels where the notching of the uterine artery disappears around 24 weeks. If this does not occur sufficiently, the notching continues to be measurable, and/or the pulsatility index remains high. This situation significantly increases the risk for placental dysfunction later in

pregnancy in both low- and high-risk populations. As a predictor this phenomenon does not distinguish between various placentally mediated disorders such as preeclampsia, placental abruption and stillbirth, but it may help in the diagnosis of FGR.

Type of Growth Measurements

Asymmetrical measurements of growth in the antenatal period may hint at the diagnosis of FGR. The brain-sparing effect causes the measurements that signify brain growth (biparietal diameter, head circumference) to be less affected than the measurements of the other organs (abdominal circumference, femur length). Particularly the abdominal growth is heavily influenced by liver size, which is the predominant location of fetal energy storage. In energy-deprived situations, the liver will consequently grow less fast and the abdominal circumference will be typically smaller in the curve than the cerebral measurements. Another suggestive finding is when consecutive measurements of the fetus show the measurements as "crossing centiles." This may signal FGR even when the measurements are not officially SGA, or even below the median for gestation. Such an approach, by definition, may be the optimal method for identifying suboptimal fetal growth. However, there are significant resource implications to routinely undertaking serial growth scans in all pregnancies, and the clinical interpretation of when crossing centiles becomes clinically relevant is yet to be determined.

PlGF

Placental dysfunction is reflected in several serum markers, the most predominant of which is Placental Growth Factor (PlGF). It has strong associations with early-onset hypertensive disorders of pregnancy and its clinical manifestations [22]. There are increasing suggestions it may have significant benefit in identifying FGR fetuses [23–25], although the effect is diluted significantly if SGA rather than FGR is chosen as the endpoint [26].

Decreased Fetal Activity

When placental insufficiency deteriorates to the extent where the fetus experiences hypoxemia, a decline in fetal activity can occur [27]. This is a phenomenon that the mother can recognize and is as such an important monitoring tool.

Maternal Manifestations – Hypertensive Disorders of Pregnancy

Especially in earlier gestational ages [5,28], hypertensive disorders of pregnancy have a very high prevalence of FGR. Up to 94% are SGA, and those above the 10th centile may also be FGR [29]. The association is reciprocal [30].

Fetal Distress during Uterine Contractions

One of the defining revealing symptoms of fetuses that are growth-restricted is the incapacity to cope with the challenges of uterine contractions in overt labor or subclinical contractions. In previous times, subclinical contractions were elicited by oxytocin administration to test the fetus's reserve. This was termed the *stress test*, as opposed to the *non-stress test*, the current form of cardiotocography.

Postpartum Neonatal Morbidity

Neonatal jaundice, disordered glucose metabolism, and insufficient temperature regulation are forms of maladaptation to the extra-uterine milieu. These transitional problems are associated with FGR and can also be used as differentiators between FGR and SGA.

Absence of an Alternative Diagnosis

Clinicians, when confronted with a fetus/newborn that is SGA, must consider different causes of smallness. These are uncertain dating of pregnancy, fetal viral infections, congenital anomalies, and constitutional smallness. The absence of additional ultrasound findings of a viral infection or congenital anomaly in an appropriately dated pregnancy leaves the clinician with the scenario of pure SGA/FGR.

Together, the aforementioned signs may help form a diagnosis of FGR. It may be stated that if there are several signs associated with uteroplacental insufficiency and signs of other diagnoses are absent, the case for FGR may be made. In a recent consensus procedure, a more apt definition was agreed upon that encompasses some of these functional parameters [31]. This may, however, still leave ample room for diagnostic doubt, especially in later gestations where measurements are less sensitive and specific.

Differences between SGA and FGR

It is increasingly apparent that not all FGR babies are SGA, and vice versa. The clinical significance of this distinction is important because children with a pathological process are at risk for severe adverse outcomes, whereas this is probably not the case for constitutionally small children.

There is considerable overlap between the two populations, since many fetuses with significant growth restriction will also be statistically deviant from the norm population, and the further deviant a fetus/infant is from the population norm, the bigger the chance it is caused by a pathological process [11]. Because of the easier identification, most studies on FGR identify their patients on a statistical basis (for instance, birth weight or estimated fetal weight) and as such define an SGA population. As a result, most studies on FGR are undermined by the inclusion of physiological SGA pregnancies.

The likeness between the two populations and the distinct differences pose significant clinical problems and scientific challenges. First, there is the group of fetuses/newborns who are SGA but not FGR. Especially near the cut-off values chosen, many of the SGA children/fetuses will actually not be FGR. This has significant consequences. In clinical management, once identified, fetuses in this group will be subjected to more intensive surveillance and consequently more (unnecessary) interventions and adverse effects from these interventions. In the interpretation of findings from studies, the conflation of FGR with SGA may mask significant associations or identify associations that in fact are not important for FGR [26].

Second, there is the group of fetuses/newborns who are not SGA, but still FGR. There are strong arguments to suggest that fetuses with optimal intrauterine growth within a population are those eventually born as above average. In a Dutch registry study, the highest perinatal mortality occurred in the lowest birth weight percentiles, decreasing with every decile even beyond the median birth weight in the population [32]. The nadir was at the 80th–84th percentile, suggesting that this is the optimal birth weight for children. This implies that the majority of fetuses may be subjected to some form of growth restriction. This is further substantiated by the findings from the Intergrowth study [33]. In eight populations across the globe, optimal growth curves were established in a non-deprived subset of the population. The findings were that population curves were remarkably alike and that the curves were significantly shifted toward higher birth weights in comparison with unselected populations [34]. This suggestion of widespread fetal growth restriction may have evolutionary reasons that improve overall survival, but reinforce the idea that even though fetuses may not be a statistical outlier (yet), they may be growth-restricted to some extent, and thus at increased risk for adverse perinatal outcomes. For instance, a fetus may have an estimated fetal weight according to the 20th centile for gestational age, but may have had a genetic predisposition to become 80th centile. These fetuses may not be picked up by our current methods, unless we observe abnormal growth patterns of fetuses who are moving through the curves on consecutive scans. This is particularly true in term FGR, where absolute growth is often not as compromised as in early-onset FGR: the first being "difficult to diagnose, easy to treat" and the second being "easy to diagnose, difficult to treat."

The gestation-dependent diagnostic difficulty in defining and diagnosing impaired fetal growth is interesting. As outlined earlier in this chapter, the underlying disorder in FGR is placental insufficiency. This is a relative disorder that may manifest because of impaired placental development, excessive fetal demands, or a combination of both. At different gestations, the underlying factor may vary and the presentation will vary accordingly. For instance, early placental failure at mid-gestation due to impaired placental development results in a long latency between onset and eventual fetal demise because of the low metabolic demands of a mid-gestational fetus. During this protracted period, the fetus has the time to "fail to thrive" much like a malnourished infant and manifest SGA as a cardinal feature of FGR secondary to placental failure. Also, most of the mentioned criteria for FGR become apparent due to the fetus's ability to deal with an extremely poorly functioning placenta. In contrast, the inability of a term placenta to meet the metabolic demands of a thus far normally grown fetus would allow only a short interval between the placental insult and fetal demise because of the relatively high metabolic needs of a term fetus. Therefore, late placental failure may occur in normally sized fetuses that do not tend to present with SGA or any of the other FGR-features secondary to placental failure. This also explains the finding that the majority of so called unexplained stillbirths at term are not SGA, yet still exhibit signs of hypoxemia of placental origin.

Conclusion

FGR and SGA have considerable overlap. SGA is easily measured as a statistical phenomenon and with the availability of a gold standard. However, SGA is not the denominator of interest, because it does not intrinsically identify abnormality. FGR, which is a functional problem resulting from placental insufficiency, should be described by measurable parameters that identify pathological functional processes that have statistical and pathophysiological associations with adverse outcomes of interest. These parameters were discussed in this chapter. Future studies and discussions on this subject should aim at identifying study populations with FGR rather than SGA, preferably with a consensus working definition. This will allow clinical management that focuses on the correct identification of fetuses and newborns at risk of adverse outcomes.

Key Points

- FGR secondary to placental insufficiency, not SGA, is the disorder of interest associated with adverse pregnancy outcomes.

- SGA is often incorrectly used as a proxy for FGR: it is often a physiological finding, only a common feature of early-onset preterm FGR, and an infrequent finding in term FGR.

- The definition of FGR should ideally include clinical, imaging, and biochemical functional parameters of placental insufficiency and fetal hypoxemia, rather than use "smallness" as a defining feature.

References

1. Redman CW, Sargent IL, Staff AC. IFPA Senior Award Lecture: Making sense of preeclampsia – two placental causes of preeclampsia? *Placenta* 2014;35 Suppl:S20–5.

2. Poon LC, Syngelaki A, Akolekar R, Lai J, Nicolaides KH. Combined screening for preeclampsia and small for gestational age at 11–13 weeks. *Fetal Diagn Ther* 2013;33(1):16–27.

3. Akolekar R, Syngelaki A, Poon L, Wright D, Nicolaides KH. Competing risks model in

early screening for preeclampsia by biophysical and biochemical markers. *Fetal Diagn Ther* 2013;33(1):8–15.

4. Ganzevoort W, Rep A, Bonsel GJ, De Vries JI, Wolf H, for the Pi. Dynamics and incidence patterns of maternal complications in early onset hypertension of pregnancy. *BJOG* 2007;114(6):741–50.

5. Rasmussen S, Irgens LM. Fetal growth and body proportion in preeclampsia. *Obstet Gynecol* 2003;101(3):575–83.

6. Melchiorre K, Sharma R, Thilaganathan B. Cardiovascular implications in preeclampsia: An overview. *Circulation* 2014;130(8):703–14.

7. Roberts JM, Cooper DW. Pathogenesis and genetics of pre-eclampsia. *Lancet* 2001;357(9249):53–6.

8. Redman CW, Sacks GP, Sargent IL. Preeclampsia: An excessive maternal inflammatory response to pregnancy. *Am J Obstet Gynecol* 1999;180(2 Pt 1):499–506.

9. Pathak S, Lees CC, Hackett G, Jessop F, Sebire NJ. Frequency and clinical significance of placental histological lesions in an unselected population at or near term. *Virchows Arch* 2011;459(6):565–72.

10. Kloosterman GJ. On intrauterine growth – the significance of prenatal care. *Int J Gynaecol Obstet* 1970;8(6 part 2):895–912.

11. Unterscheider J, Daly S, Geary MP, Kennelly MM, McAuliffe FM, O'Donoghue K, et al. Optimizing the definition of intrauterine growth restriction: The multicenter prospective PORTO Study. *Am J Obstet Gynecol* 2013;208(4):290 e1–6.

12. Hecher K, Bilardo CM, Stigter RH, Ville Y, Hackeloer BJ, Kok HJ, et al. Monitoring of fetuses with intrauterine growth restriction: A longitudinal study. *Ultrasound Obstet Gynecol* 2001;18(6):564–70.

13. Oros D, Figueras F, Cruz-Martinez R, Meler E, Munmany M, Gratacos E. Longitudinal changes in uterine, umbilical and fetal cerebral Doppler indices in late-onset small-for-gestational age fetuses. *Ultrasound Obstet Gynecol* 2011;37(2):191–5.

14. Ferrazzi E, Bozzo M, Rigano S, Bellotti M, Morabito A, Pardi G, et al. Temporal sequence of abnormal Doppler changes in the peripheral and central circulatory systems of the severely growth-restricted fetus. *Ultrasound Obstet Gynecol* 2002;19(2):140–6.

15. Baschat AA, Cosmi E, Bilardo CM, Wolf H, Berg C, Rigano S, et al. Predictors of neonatal outcome in early-onset placental dysfunction. *Obstet Gynecol* 2007;109(2 Pt 1):253–61.

16. Baschat AA, Gembruch U, Harman CR. The sequence of changes in Doppler and biophysical parameters as

17. Del Rio M, Martinez JM, Figueras F, Bennasar M, Olivella A, Palacio M, et al. Doppler assessment of the aortic isthmus and perinatal outcome in preterm fetuses with severe intrauterine growth restriction. *Ultrasound Obstet Gynecol* 2008;31(1):41–7.

18. Cruz-Martinez R, Figueras F, Hernandez-Andrade E, Oros D, Gratacos E. Fetal brain Doppler to predict cesarean delivery for nonreassuring fetal status in term small-for-gestational-age fetuses. *Obstet Gynecol* 2011;117(3):618–26.

19. Flood K, Unterscheider J, Daly S, Geary MP, Kennelly MM, McAuliffe FM, et al. The role of brain sparing in the prediction of adverse outcomes in intrauterine growth restriction: Results of the multicenter PORTO Study. *Am J Obstet Gynecol* 2014;211(3):288 e1–5.

20. Morales-Rosello J, Khalil A, Morlando M, Papageorghiou A, Bhide A, Thilaganathan B. Changes in fetal Doppler indices as a marker of failure to reach growth potential at term. *Ultrasound Obstet Gynecol* 2014;43(3):303–10.

21. Bilardo CM, Wolf H, Stigter RH, Ville Y, Baez E, Visser GH, et al. Relationship between monitoring parameters and perinatal outcome in severe, early intrauterine growth restriction. *Ultrasound Obstet Gynecol* 2004;23(2):119–25.

22. Chappell LC, Duckworth S, Seed PT, Griffin M, Myers J, Mackillop L, et al. Diagnostic accuracy of placental growth factor in women with suspected preeclampsia: A prospective multicenter study. *Circulation* 2013;128(19):2121–31.

23. Benton SJ, Hu Y, Xie F, Kupfer K, Lee SW, Magee LA, et al. Can placental growth factor in maternal circulation identify fetuses with placental intrauterine growth restriction? *Am J Obstet Gynecol* 2012;206(2):163 e1–7.

24. Calabrese S, Cardellicchio M, Mazzocco M, Taricco E, Martinelli A, Cetin I. Placental growth factor (PLGF) maternal circulating levels in normal pregnancies and in pregnancies at risk of developing placental insufficiency complications. *Reprod Sci* 2012;19(3):211A–2A.

25. Chaiworapongsa T, Romero R, Korzeniewski SJ, Kusanovic JP, Soto E, Hernandez-Andrade E, et al. Prediction of stillbirth and late-onset preeclampsia. *Reprod Sci* 2012;19(3):90A–1A.

26. Griffin M, Seed P, Webster L, Tarft H, Chappell L, Shennan A. Placental growth factor (PLGF) and ultrasound parameters for predicting the small for gestational age infant (SGA) in suspected small for gestational age: Pelican FGR study. *J Matern Fetal Neonatal Med* 2014;27:121–2.

27. Arduini D, Rizzo G, Caforio L, Boccolini MR, Romanini C, Mancuso S. Behavioural state transitions in healthy and growth retarded fetuses. *Early Hum Dev* 1989;19(3):155–65.

28. Groom KM, North RA, Poppe KK, Sadler L, McCowan LM. The association between customised small for gestational age infants and pre-eclampsia or gestational hypertension varies with gestation at delivery. *BJOG* 2007;114(4):478–84.

29. Ganzevoort W, Rep A, Bonsel GJ, Fetter WP, Van Sonderen L, De Vries JI, et al. A randomised controlled trial comparing two temporising management strategies, one with and one without plasma volume expansion, for severe and early onset pre-eclampsia. *BJOG* 2005;112(10):1358–68.

30. Dektas B, Sibai B, Habli M. Pregnancies complicated with fetal growth restriction (FGR) are associated with a high rate of subsequent development of preeclampsia? *Am J Obstet Gynecol* 2013;208(1):S179–S80.

31. Gordijn SJ, Beune IM, Thilaganathan B, Papageorghiou A, Baschat AA, Baker PN, et al. Consensus definition of fetal growth restriction: a Delphi procedure. *Ultrasound Obstet Gynecol* 2016;48(3):333–9.

32. Vasak B, Koenen SV, Koster MP, Hukkelhoven CW, Franx A, Hanson MA, et al. Human fetal growth is constrained below optimal for perinatal survival. *Ultrasound Obstet Gynecol* 2014.

33. Villar J, Papageorghiou AT, Pang R, Ohuma EO, Ismail LC, Barros FC, et al. The likeness of fetal growth and newborn size across non-isolated populations in the INTERGROWTH-21 Project: The Fetal Growth Longitudinal Study and Newborn Cross-Sectional Study. *Lancet Diabetes Endocrinol* 2014.

34. Papageorghiou AT, Ohuma EO, Altman DG, Todros T, Cheikh Ismail L, Lambert A, et al. International standards for fetal growth based on serial ultrasound measurements: the Fetal Growth Longitudinal Study of the INTERGROWTH-21st Project. *Lancet* 2014;384(9946):869–79.

Differential Diagnosis of Fetal Growth Restriction

Sana Usman, Anna Lawin-O'Brien, and Christoph Lees

The Initial Diagnosis

History

Fetal growth and birth weight are determined not only by a genetic basis, but also from placental and maternal factors extrinsic to the fetus. Thus, it is imperative at the first consultation to take a detailed history (Figure 3.1) from the patient and partner, including family history if available. In this context, of importance are smoking, exposure to viral infections (working with children, veterinary work), previous pregnancy history, hypertension, or other maternal illnesses. The father's history may be relevant, for example, in autosomal-dominant conditions such as Russell-Silver Syndrome, and Advanced paternal age is of significance if skeletal dysplasias are considered as a differential of growth restriction.

The conventional definition of fetal growth restriction (FGR) referred to in this chapter uses an estimated fetal weight (EFW) or abdominal circumference (AC) below the 10th percentile in the presence of abnormal umbilical artery Doppler [1] (see Chapter 3).

The diagnosis of true FGR is furthermore supported by the observation of reduced growth velocity over serial scans with fetal biometry crossing percentiles indicating fetal deviation from its original genetic growth potential. FGR is classically caused by uteroplacental impairment, confirmed by typical abnormal functional parameters such as increased uterine artery Doppler PI with notching and reduced amniotic fluid.

However, especially at the initial suspicion of FGR, the underlying cause of the growth impairment is not always obvious. A number of differential diagnoses should be taken into consideration and systematically excluded to ensure the management of the pregnancy is determined by the actual underlying cause of fetal "smallness" (Table 3.1). Identifying the cause of

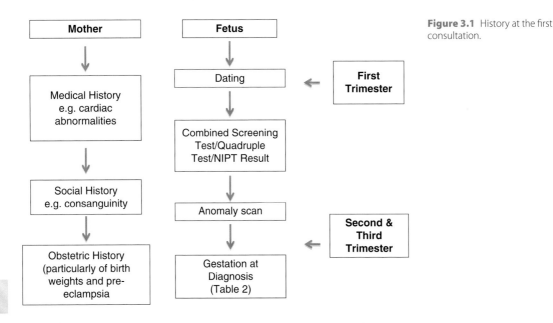

Figure 3.1 History at the first consultation.

growth restriction allows appropriate parental counseling and enables informed parental decision making. This is particularly important in cases of growth restriction caused by structural malformations or aneuploidy. Management of the pregnancy according to the specific cause of FGR safeguards optimal timing of delivery and improves fetal prognosis. Moreover, the possible coexistence of more than one cause of FGR should be anticipated and taken into consideration for an individualized care plan. When ultrasound examination suggests fetal growth restriction (FGR), the investigation for causality and management depends on the gestation (Table 3.2) and other features on ultrasound (Table 3.3). The diagnosis of placental fetal growth restriction is particularly crucial as the correct management and timing of delivery can alter outcome and improve prognosis.

This chapter focuses on the differential diagnosis of the fetus that is small for gestational age, including those that have true growth restriction primarily caused by *abnormal placentation*. It will consider the *constitutional small-for-gestational-age fetus* (SGA), which, while still at risk of increased perinatal morbidity, faces an overall better prognosis while also being a variant of normal. Rarely, an *isolated structural malformation* can lead to growth restriction and warrants involvement of paediatric surgical expertise for management guidance and treatment planning.

If a *chromosomal or genetic condition* is considered, this is important for diagnosis, dependent on parental wishes, with invasive testing or tests after birth. Subsequent management may include further support and advice for care after birth (including palliation) or termination of pregnancy.

If *infection* is suspected due to maternal history and/or ultrasound features, this will allow more focused counseling with the option of termination if the fetus is severely affected, and, in some infections, treatment may improve fetal prognosis.

Table 3.1 Differential diagnoses of FGR

Uteroplacental impairment (FGR)

Small for gestational age (SGA)

Isolated structural malformations

Genetic-chromosomal cause

Infection (TORCH)

Table 3.2 Likely cause of growth restriction per trimester

Trimester of diagnosis	First	Second	Third
Likely cause of growth restriction	Genetic/chromosomal	Genetic/chromosomal Uteroplacental growth restriction Infection	Uteroplacental growth restriction Genetic Infection

Table 3.3 SGA and its associations

	Uteroplacental Fetal Growth Restriction	Structural	Chromosomal/genetic	Infection
General	Oligohydramnios Placental calcification	Congenital heart disease E.g., Tetralogy of Fallot	Abnormal limb position Nuchal thickening	Hydrops Fetalis
Central Nervous System		Neural tube defects	Ventriculomegaly Agenesis of the corpus callosum Dandy-Walker Malformation	Ventriculomegaly calcification
Cardiovascular system	Relative cardiomegaly Thickened interventricular septum and right-sided heart dominance		Atrio-ventricular septal defect Ventricular septal defect Tetralogy of Fallot	Pericardial effusion Poor cardiac contractility
Gastrointestinal system	Echogenic bowel	Abdominal wall defects e.g., Gastroschisis, exomphalos	Echogenic bowel	Hepatomegaly Echogenicity and calcification of the liver

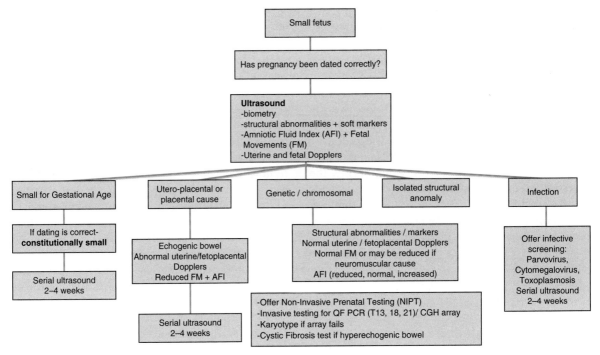

Figure 3.2 Investigation flow chart for FGR.

The time of diagnosis and hence the onset of growth restriction, early or late in pregnancy, is an important factor in determining the differential diagnoses of FGR. Early-onset severe FGR may be diagnosed from 20 weeks' gestation onward and is usually associated with substantial perinatal mortality, neonatal morbidity, prematurity, and long-term postnatal disease (see Chapter 22). Diagnoses may, apart from uteroplacental impairment (FGR), include the constitutionally small-for-gestational-age (SGA) fetus, placental damage, genetic-chromosomal cause, infection, and, rarely, structural abnormalities (Figure 3.2).

Fetal "smallness" diagnosed in later gestation is much more common (see Chapter 23) and is usually associated with lower mortality compared to early-onset growth restriction, but still faces significant perinatal morbidity and the risk of late stillbirth. Differential diagnoses of causes here include primarily SGA, the constitutionally small baby, and, less often, a true late presentation of FGR fetus with uteroplacental insufficiency of a milder phenotype (Figure 3.3). Rarely fetal congenital malformation, genetic-chromosomal causes, or infections are the cause of late-onset FGR.

Structural abnormalities may be either associated with or cause FGR through different mechanisms depending on the type of abnormality; for example, a fetal heart defect may limit perfusion to the rest of the fetal body; an abdominal wall defect with herniated viscera leads to the abdominal circumference appearing smaller than expected.

Constitutionally Small-for-Gestational-Age (SGA) Fetuses

The term *small for gestational age* (SGA) describes those fetuses that are small and normal. Usually the 10th percentile is chosen as the arbitrary cut-off for abdominal circumference or estimated fetal weight, defining those below the 10th percentile as SGA. They represent a population of mostly (70%) constitutionally small babies with normal growth trajectory [2] and without underlying pathology (normal uteroplacental Doppler; Figure 3.3 and Table 3.4). Smallness may be associated with maternal ethnicity, parity, or BMI [3].

The percentiles used to plot fetal growth are derived from reference ranges constructed from observed fetal dimensions on ultrasound. These percentile charts have been criticized as they may not reflect heterogeneous populations nor allow for ethnic differences in growth. Different strategies have

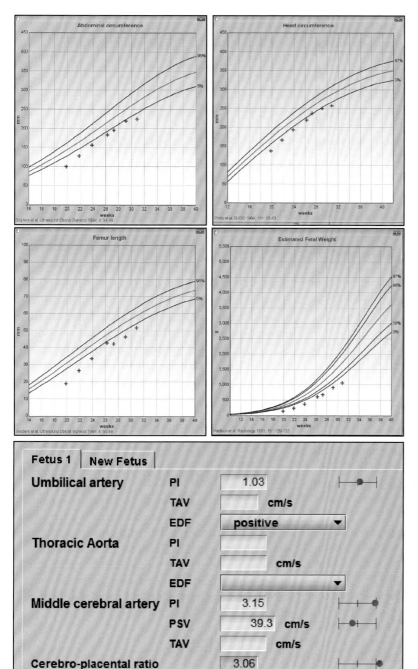

Figure 3.3 Growth charts and fetal arterial Doppler patterns typically observed in the constitutional SGA fetus. Note the growth along the percentiles and normal Doppler values.

been invented to improve percentile charts: In the recent "Intergrowth 21" project, data were prospectively collected to create new descriptive percentile charts of normal fetal growth. Here the growth measurements have been collected in eight geographically diverse but "optimally" healthy populations [4]. While describing fetal growth in a healthy population of similar characteristics (weight, height, etc.), it is not clear how these data relate to "normal" populations.

Reflecting that different maternal characteristics influencing growth may not necessarily represent pathological growth, customized growth charts have been created to respect ethnic diversity and individual

17

Table 3.4 USS features of SGA fetus

First Trimester Screening	Anatomy	Amniotic Fluid Volume	Uteroplacental Doppler	Growth along Percentiles
Low risk	Normal	Normal	Normal	Forward Symmetrical

growth potential [5]. The "Gestation Network" (www.gestation.net), for example, provides tools for assessment of fetal growth by defining each pregnancy's growth potential with a "Gestation-Related Optimal Weight" (GROW) software. The validity of this approach remains to be proven.

Naturally, the diagnosis of an SGA fetus can be concluded only after longitudinal assessment of growth. Nevertheless, it has to be remembered that as there are no definite thresholds to distinguish normal growth from pathological and restricted growth, no specific cut-off will define a totally abnormal or normal population correctly [6].

Placental Fetal Growth Restriction

Typically, a fetus growth restricted secondary to placental insufficiency is said to exhibit an asymmetrical pattern of growth restriction, but mixed patterns of fetal growth are possible. In very early FGR, symmetrical fetal growth is frequently seen, for example, with all parameters below the 3rd percentile. The defining characteristic in addition to fetal growth is raised umbilical and/or uterine artery Doppler impedance (Figure 3.4 and Table 3.5).

In early preterm FGR, that is generally considered to be less than 32/40, progressive abnormalities in the ductus venosus Doppler are used to time delivery [1,16] (unless the CTG becomes abnormal, in which case delivery is mandated), as it is shown to have a better association with subsequent neurodevelopmental outcome than that based on umbilical Doppler abnormality alone [17,18]. Beyond this gestation, a combination of CTG, umbilical artery, and middle cerebral artery Doppler is normally used for timing of delivery.

After 34 weeks, major aberrations in umbilical artery flow velocity waveforms are rare due in part to the high flow through the umbilical circulation. Absent umbilical arterial diastolic flow (AEDF) occurs when 60–70% of the villous vascular tree is damaged [19], eventually leading to reversed end-diastolic flow (REDF), hence this is highly unusual.

Isolated Structural Malformations

One quarter of all infants with congenital structural malformations will have FGR, and there is increased risk of FGR with increasing number of malformations [20] (Table 3.6).

Cardiac Anomalies

In the "The Baltimore-Washington Infant Study," fetuses with cardiac anomalies were found to be approximately 100–200g lighter than unaffected babies at the same gestation [21,22]. The causation between growth restriction and cardiac abnormalities is unclear, but proposed mechanisms include embryos with intrinsic growth disturbances may be at increased risk of developmental errors during cardiogenesis [23]. Alternatively, fetal circulatory patterns in the presence of specific cardiovascular malformations may be incompatible with optimal fetal growth [24].

Abdominal Wall Defects

Seventy percent of fetuses affected by gastroschisis are growth restricted [25]; the exact cause is unknown. It is simplistic to assume that fetal growth is restricted simply because of the reduced AC from herniated abdominal viscera. The mechanism could be due to underlying hypoxia [26] evidenced by raised umbilical artery pulsatility index, but could also be due to increased protein loss from the exposed viscera [27].

Neural Tube Defects

A fetus affected with a neural tube defect is 2.6 times more likely to also be born with a birthweight <10th percentile (aOR 2.6, 95% confidence interval [CI] 1.8 to 3.9) [28].

Chromosomal Aberrations

There is a strong association between FGR, chromosome aberrations, and congenital malformations that significantly increases perinatal morbidity [29].

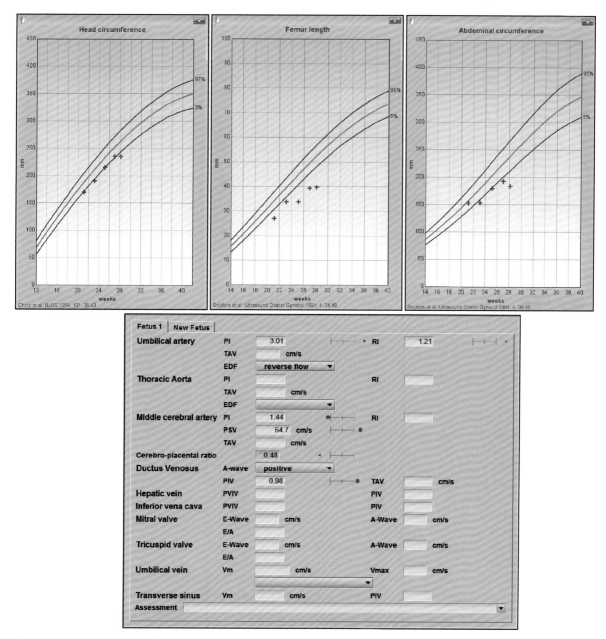

Figure 3.4 Growth charts for HC, FL, and AC typically observed in placental fetal growth restriction, with the Doppler parameters shown at the final scan.

Abnormal fetal karyotype is responsible for approximately 20% of all FGR fetuses, and the percentage is substantially higher if growth failure is detected before 26 weeks' gestation [30]. Confined placental mosaicism is more common in placentas of FGR fetuses compared with those from appropriately grown fetuses [31].

Trisomy 21

Trisomy 21, also known as Down syndrome, named after John Langdon Down, initially described the associated pattern of congenital abnormalities. The incidence increases with advancing maternal age; 95% of cases are caused by non-disjunction of chromosome 21 during maternal meiosis, resulting in an

Table 3.5 USS features of placental fetal growth restriction

First Trimester Screening	Anatomy	Amniotic Fluid Volume	Doppler (in order of severity)	Growth along Centiles
Low PAPP-A [7,8] Low b-hcg [9]	Echogenic bowel	Oligohydramnios	**Uterine Artery**: Notches, may be unilateral or bilateral [10,11]. Raised impedance (pulsatility index: PI). Can be used as a screening tool **Umbilical Artery**: Raised PI >95th centile Absent or Reversed End-Diastolic Flow [12,13] **Middle Cerebral Artery**: reduced PI <5th percentile [14] **Ductus Venosus**: Deepening in the "a" wave toward baseline or reversed "a" wave reflects a decrease in forward flow during atrial systole [15]	Small AC (asymmetrical) But can be symmetrical Short long bones may be the initial sign in the third trimester.

Table 3.6 USS features of genetic syndromes

First Trimester Screening	Anatomy	Amniotic Fluid Volume	Fetal-Placental Doppler	Growth along Percentiles
May be normal or high risk on nuchal translucency and/or biochemistry	May be normal, specific or non-specific abnormalities	Normal or increased	Often normal	Symmetrical reduction in growth

extra chromosome 21, and the remaining 5% are due to Robertsonian translocation or mosaicism with a recurrence risk of 1% and 25%, respectively.

Fifty percent of affected fetuses do not show any evidence of minor or major abnormalities on scan. The major abnormalities associated with this condition in the other half are cardiac (50%) and gastrointestinal (30%). Cardiac abnormalities include atrioventricular septal defects and ventricular septal defects. Gastrointestinal abnormalities include duodenal atresia and esophageal atresia. Short femur and humerus can be seen. Soft markers are often observed at USS and are used to modify pre-invasive risk analysis of Down syndrome diagnosis. These include hypoplasia of the nasal bone, right aberrant subclavian artery, and thickened nuchal fold.

The severity of the condition in terms of neurodevelopmental and motor delay can vary greatly from mild mental and motor delay to severe neurodevelopmental and motor delay. It was traditionally thought that Down syndrome babies were affected with fetal growth restriction [32], however, a recent paper by Morris and colleagues suggests that babies affected by T21 have similar growth potentials until 38 weeks of pregnancy [33], thus it is appropriate to use the UK-WHO birth weight charts up to this point. Thereafter birth weight is below that of unaffected babies (on average 159–304g for boys, 86–239g for girls), and thus it should be plotted on the UK Down syndrome growth chart.

Trisomy 18

Trisomy 18 is also known as Edwards syndrome. More than 99% of cases are of non-disjunction resulting in an additional chromosome 18. Very rarely, it can be the result of gonadal mosaicism, which explains the 1% empirical risk of recurrence. It is associated with high rates (70%) of intrauterine demise and a survival birth rate of only 5%, with 90% mortality within 6 months.

A wide range of anomalies may be seen on ultrasound and include cardiac, central nervous system, gastrointestinal, and urinary tract abnormalities. Early-onset symmetrical FGR is observed (Figure 3.5), and soft markers such as enlarged nuchal translucency and choroid plexus cysts may also be seen. In 2003, of a series of 38 patients with T18, 63% of fetuses exhibited fetal growth restriction [34].

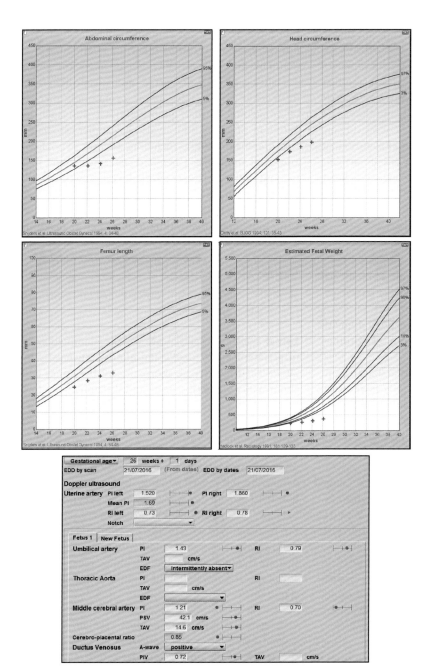

Figure 3.5 Growth and Doppler findings typically seen in a Trisomy 18 fetus. Note FGR in this fetus with abnormal uterine and middle cerebral artery Doppler. The neonate survived for 3 days after birth.

Trisomy 13, also known as Pataus syndrome, is the least common autosomal trisomy to occur, affecting 1 in 12,500 births. The majority of cases are again due to non-disjunction (75%), with the remaining due to Robertsonian translocation. Only 2.5% of fetuses will reach term, and 3% survive at 6 months of life. Early-onset FGR is observed typically in the first trimester [35], but FGR is not a specific feature of T13 (unlike T18), only affecting 10% of the cases [36].

Major congenital abnormalities involving the cardiac, urinary tract, and central nervous system with craniofacial abnormalities are particularly evident (cleft, microphthalmia). Enlarged nuchal translucency is often how initial diagnosis occurs in the first trimester.

Triploidy is extremely rare, with an incidence of 1 in 2,500–5,000 births. It is due to a complete extra set of chromosomes (69), which can be of maternal or paternal origin and is not associated with advancing maternal age. The majority of triploidy is due to 69XXY with the remaining mainly due to 69XXX and only a few due to 69XYY. The majority miscarry in the first trimester, but of those that do survive, early-onset FGR is seen (often extremely asymmetrical), and thus most cases result in an intrauterine death by 20 weeks or survival of only a few hours after birth. Other features that may be seen on ultrasound include CNS abnormalities such as Dandy-Walker variant, congenital heart disease, syndactyly, and molar changes in the placenta accompanied with high b-hcg (diandric-paternal origin) or low hCG (digynaenic-maternal origin).

Genetic Causes

Russell-Silver Syndrome, with an estimated incidence of 1 in 7,000 [37], is an imprinting disorder characterized by severe FGR. Half of all patients exhibit DNA hypomethylation at the *H19/IGF2* imprinted domain; 10% have maternal uniparental disomy of chromosome 7 [38].

Typical facial appearances are frontal bossing and triangular-shaped face with marked body asymmetry as the head circumference is maintained [39]. Café au lait spots and fifth-finger clinodactyly may also be seen, and postnatally patients can exhibit speech and neurodevelopmental delay [40].

Cornelia de Lange (also called Brachmann-de Lange Syndrome) is an example of a multisystem malformation syndrome associated with growth restriction. In 50–60% of cases, a mutation is found in the NIPBL gene located at 5p13.2 encoding components of the cohesin complex [41]. The remaining 5–10% of cases are x-linked mutations related to the cohesin complex but found on other chromosomes. On ultrasound, FGR is seen with polyhydramnios. Upper limb abnormalities can be detected, including oligosyndactyly and radial aplasia. The typical facial appearances are often diagnosed postnatally, but with the help of 3D imaging may now be possible to visualize in utero. These include anteverted nares with a long philtrum, prognathism, micrognathia, and prefrontal edema. This condition can also be associated with congenital diaphragmatic hernia and heart disease. Postnatally, these babies have a poor outcome with severe neurodevelopmental delay and failure to thrive.

22q11.2 deletion, which includes DiGeorge and other syndromes such as craniofacial and velocardiofacial syndrome, is the most common microdeletion syndrome reported. It can be inherited as an autosomal dominant trait, but can also arise de novo. The major causative gene is TBX1, part of the T-box protein family of genes. These babies are most commonly affected by congenital cardiac abnormalities (75%) such as Tetralogy of Fallot, but can also have other associated sonographic findings, including thymic hypoplasia and renal anomalies. Chen and colleagues found that in 3 out of the 27 fetuses affected with growth restriction but normal karyotype, 22q11 microdeletion was detected (11%) [42]. FGR in this cohort is associated with poor prognosis leading to intrauterine death or early postnatal death [43].

Skeletal Dysplasia

Skeletal dysplasias are broadly classified into two main forms; lethal and nonlethal.

Lethal skeletal dysplasias are usually identified early in gestation by 16 weeks and almost universally by 20 weeks. The extreme shortening of the bones and abnormality of the ribs, head, and skeleton means that there is very rarely a diagnostic confusion with early-onset fetal growth restriction (Table 3.7). These are, however, described briefly:

Thanatophoric dysplasia is a condition that is lethal neonatally. It is caused by a new dominant mutation in fibroblast growth factor receptor gene 3 (FGFR3 gene) [44] and associated with increased paternal age. It can be diagnosed with invasive testing. There are two main subtypes. Type I classically shows curved femurs that are thought to look like telephone receivers [45], and Type II shows straight femurs and a cloverleaf skull [46].

Osteogenesis imperfecta is often recognized in the second trimester and is associated with bowing and shortening of the limbs. Decreased mineralization of the bones may be seen with decreased skull echogenicity. In type II, which causes the majority of defects, it is due to a defect in the synthesis of collagen type 1. This is a very severe form and usually results in perinatal lethality, whereas fetuses affected with Type III often survive.

The recurrence risk is quoted to be as high as 5% to 7% if secondary to collagen type 1 defects occur due to the high incidence of gonadal mosaicism. Non-invasive prenatal diagnosis (NIPD) is an option in

Table 3.7 Comparison of ultrasound features of skeletal dysplasias with fetal growth restriction

Ultrasound Features	Anatomy	Amniotic Fluid Volume	Uterine/Umbilical Artery Doppler	Growth along Percentiles
Skeletal dysplasia	Small chest circumference Abnormal mineralization of the long bones Angulation Fractures	Increased	Normal	Particularly short long bones, including humerus
Fetal growth restriction	Bone structure appears normal Initially in the third trimester, FL<3rd centile may be the first feature	Decreased	Abnormal	Asymmetrical growth restriction: may present with isolated reduced femur length

a subsequent pregnancy if mutation in the previous fetus is identified in collagen 1.

Achondrogenesis is an autosomal recessive condition with a 25% risk of recurrence. Two types exist. Type 1 is due to a defect in the *SLC26A2* recessive gene that causes severe bone shortening. Type 2 causes severe micromelia with poor mineralization of the long bones, spiky metaphyseal spurs, and absent vertebral bodies; this is due to a new dominant mutation in collagen type 2.

A less common diagnosis that must be considered is campomelic dysplasia, with an incidence of 0.05 to 1.6 per 10,000 live births. This distinct skeletal dysplasia is characterized by bowing of the long bones of the lower extremity, phenotypic sex reversal, flat face, micrognathia, and cleft palate, as well as associated renal and cardiac abnormalities. It is caused by a mutation in the SOX 9 gene, essential transcription factor in chondrogenesis found on chromosome 17.

Nonlethal

The nonlethal forms of skeletal dysplasia are usually diagnosed in the second or third trimester. Achondroplasia is the most common form. It is an autosomal dominant condition with a high new mutation rate of approximately 80%. The majority of cases are due to one of two mutations in the *FGFR3* gene (>98%) and rarely present before 24 weeks. It is associated with increased paternal age. Recurrence risk is extremely small at <1%. On ultrasound, typically rhizomelic short limbs are seen with short fingers known as the trident hand. There is relative macrocephaly with frontal bossing and a depressed nasal bridge. A normal trunk is observed with a wide angle at the

proximal femur. Polyhydramnios is often observed (Figure 3.6).

Investigations: Invasive testing is offered with an amniocentesis usually in the third trimester, but NIPD is also highly reliable.

SHOX deficiency may also present in the second or third trimester with short long bones and no other abnormalities.

Specific History: Three-generation family history should be gathered, including previous pregnancy losses/parental ages/short stature.

Examination: Examine parents, especially height and proportion.

Infections

These are particularly difficult to diagnose as patients often have ultrasound features suggestive of infection before any clinical suspicions or tests are carried out (Table 3.8). A late MRI around 30–32 weeks is often useful if cranial abnormality is suspected on ultrasound [47]. A traditional TORCH screen represents testing for CMV, toxoplasmosis, and parvovirus and checking rubella immunity on booking bloods.

Cytomegalovirus (CMV)

CMV is a DNA virus of the herpes family. It is the most frequent cause of congenital infection, affecting 0.3–2.4% of all births in the UK, and in the majority of cases is due to primary infection [48], CMV is the most common cause of sensorineural hearing loss and neurodevelopmental delay. There is approximately a 50% seronegativity in developed countries.

Table 3.8 Ultrasound features of congenital infection

First Trimester Screening	Anatomy	Amniotic Fluid Volume	Doppler	Growth along Percentiles
Normal	*General:* Hydrops fetalis (Parvovirus B19) Anemia Myocarditis *Eyes:* Cataracts *Cranial:* Brain lesions, including calcifications Periventricular brain cysts Ventriculomegaly *Abdominal:* Hepato-spleno megaly Calcifications Echogenic bowel	Oligohydramnios		Can be reduced along all centiles

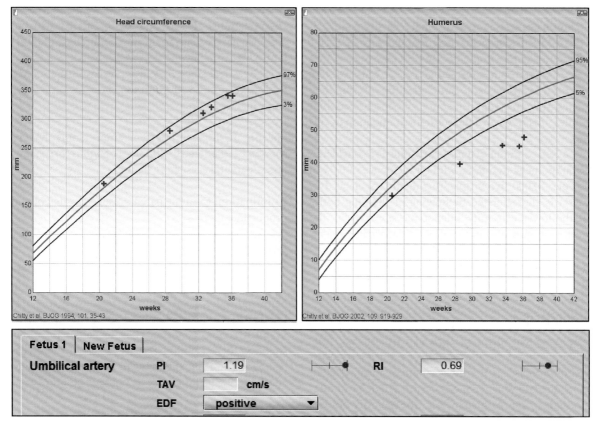

Figure 3.6 Head circumference and humerus growth and normal Doppler studies observed in a fetus with achondroplasia. Note that the humerus is (just) within the normal range at 20 weeks and has fallen well below at 28 weeks.

When infection does occur, most women are asymptomatic, but some may suffer subtle symptoms. Secondary infection can occur, which is thought to be either a reactivation or infection with a different strain. If non-primary infection occurs, although the vertical transmission rate is lower, it can still cause severe congenital infection (1% to 2.2%) [41] (Table 3.9).

Table 3.9 Transmission rate of toxoplasmosis and cytomegalovirus infection [49]

Infection	Toxoplasmosis	Cytomegalovirus
Transmission rate		
First Trimester	15%	34.8%
Second Trimester	30%	42%
Third Trimester	60%	58.6%

Transmission: Transmission is by close contact and through bodily fluids: urine, saliva, cervical secretions, blood, breast milk. Vertical transmission is thought to occur through infected leucocytes that cross the placental barrier. Children can continue to shed the virus for months and years afterward.

Symptoms: low-grade fever, arthralgia

Signs: moderate lymphadenopathy

Investigations: Abnormal liver function tests may be detected. IgM may persist in maternal blood for up to 1 year after a primary infection. Thus, anti-IgG avidity tests can provide more information. A high avidity result suggests a past infection. A primary infection has IgM antibodies as well as low IgG avidity. If high IgG avidity is present as well as positive IgM, it normally denotes reinfection.

Ultrasound scan: Microcephaly, ventriculomegaly, hepatosplenomegaly

Management: Serial ultrasound scans are offered every 2–4 weeks. Offer amniocentesis for PCR above 21 weeks' gestation or if less than this, 6 weeks after maternal seroconversion in order for it to be excreted in fetal urine [50]. The value of the results of quantitative PCR for CMV in amniotic fluid as a prognostic indicator of symptomatic congenital infection is controversial. Some authors have found that a high CMV viral load in amniotic fluid is associated with a high risk of symptomatic infection in the fetus [51,52]. Others have failed to demonstrate such an association [53,54]. There is also a proposed association between the viral load in amniotic fluid and the gestational age at the time of amniocentesis [53]. If fetal infection is confirmed, there is a 10% risk of delivering a symptomatic newborn.

In a phase 2, randomized, placebo-controlled, double-blind study in 123 women, hyperimmune globulin did not significantly modify the course of primary CMV infection during pregnancy [55]. The role of maternal valaciclovir has been studied in confirmed symptomatic fetal CMV infection in 21 fetuses. Good placental transfer occurred with therapeutic concentrations both in the maternal and fetal compartment, and this resulted in proven reduction in viral load in the fetal blood. This is turn improved outcomes compared to the untreated group [56]. However, a randomized controlled trial has not been performed in ongoing pregnancies to study this affect in larger numbers. Although in neonates improvement in outcomes has been found, especially with longer duration of treatment [57].

Counselling: Risk of sequelae in confirmed fetal infection is highest in the first trimester; however, if ultrasound and MRI features are normal, the risk of sequelae is significantly reduced [58]. If fetal brain ultrasound is normal, this predicts a normal early neuropsychological outcome in fetuses with congenital CMV infection [59,60]. In contrast, neonatal outcome did not correlate with suspected abnormal white matter on fetal MR imaging [59].

Postnatally, 30–40% of neonates show signs of infection, but most are asymptomatic (85–90%). Of the 10–15% that are symptomatic at birth, usually presenting with seizures, up to one-third of babies will die with 90% of survivors experiencing severe neurological problems [61].

Toxoplasmosis

Toxoplasmosis affects 3–4 in 10,000 pregnancies with the majority of infections presenting subclinically (85%) in the fetus and approximately 15% presenting with hydrocephalus, intracranial calcifications, and chorioretinitis.

Transmission: Fetuses infected in early pregnancy are much more likely to show clinical signs of infection (Figure 3.7). These effects counterbalance, and women who seroconverted at 24–30 weeks' gestation

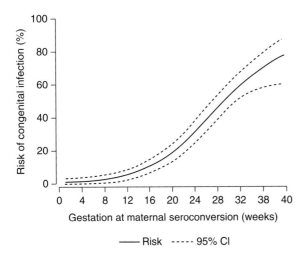

Figure 3.7 Risk of congenital toxoplasmosis infection by gestation at maternal seroconversion. With permission from the *Lancet* [62].

carried the highest risk (10%) of having a congenitally infected child with early clinical signs at risk of long-term complications (Table 3.9).

Symptoms: low-grade fever, malaise, headache.

Signs: Cervical lymphadenopathy. Very rarely, a mother can develop encephalitis, myocarditis, hepatitis, or pneumoniae.

Investigations

IgM can persist for up to 18 months after infection. Avidity testing of IgG antibodies can help to assess fetal risk.

Amniocentesis can be offered >4 weeks from infection and a PCR can generally be performed from amniotic fluid after 18 weeks with a sensitivity of between 64–99%. In 2004, Romand showed the relationship between high parasite concentrations and severe outcome [63].

Ultrasound scans: Scans are performed serially to assess for signs of ventriculomegaly, microcephaly, calcification, cataracts, echogenic bowel, and ascites. Ventriculomegaly with multiple echo-dense nodules is characteristic of severe fetal toxoplasmosis and carries a poor prognosis [64].

Management: If there is any suspicion, spiramycin can be commenced at 2–3g/day as soon as possible.

If positive amniocentesis occurs or if >32 weeks pregnant, pyrimethamine 50mg/day and sulphadiazine

3g/day with folinic acid 50mg weekly is advised. The detrimental effects of potential teratogenicity are no longer of concern in the third trimester; however, there is still a risk of bone marrow toxicity, thus a weekly full blood count is advised.

Counseling: Cohort studies have shown that prenatal treatment is effective if started within 4 weeks of intracranial lesions (OR=0.28), but not after 4 weeks. Prenatal treatment reduces serious neurological sequelae or death by 75%, although these data are only available from small studies. There is no evidence for change in outcome in ocular lesions. There is no evidence that pyrimethamine-sulphonamide is more effective than spiramycin.

Berrebi in 2010 assessed the long-term outcomes of children with congenital toxoplasmosis [65] and found that 26% of confirmed congenital toxoplasmosis patients had chorioretinitis, mainly diagnosed before the age of 5 and infrequently severe.

Rubella

Rubella is part of the togaviridae family, but since the 1970s, immunity has been formed as a result of the childhood MMR vaccination program. In 2006, Public Health England decided to end rubella (German measles) susceptibility screening in pregnancy in England as the number of women affected by rubella in pregnancy had dramatically decreased from the 1970s and rubella was now classified as eliminated in the UK by the World Health Organization. In the past decade, fewer than five cases per year of rubella have been reported to the Health Protection Agency in the UK [66]. Within the UK, however, mothers born abroad, particularly in sub-Saharan Africa and South Asia, were more likely to be seronegative than UK-born mothers, with adjusted odds ratios of 4.2 (95% CI 3.1–5.6) and 5.0 (3.8–6.5), respectively [67]. As such, it is still a recognized problem in African and Asian countries because a childhood vaccination program including the MMR vaccine is not in place. It has been estimated that more than 100,000 cases of congenital rubella syndrome (CRS) occur in developing countries each year [68].

Transmission: If the infection is acquired in the first trimester, the risk of transmission is up to 80% with most risk of multiple defects in the first 8 weeks. In the first trimester, of those infected, 85% develop severe infections and malformations. The risk of transmission decreases after 12 weeks, but then rises again in the third trimester to 60%.

Symptoms: Mothers may present with a rash, arthralgia, cough, or headache.

Signs: Maculopapular rash or conjunctivitis.

Investigation: Rubella antibody status should be checked from maternal screening bloods. If initial bloods were negative, positive IgM will indicate current infection. A second blood test should then be prepared 7–10 days later, which will demonstrate increased IgG levels. If no screening blood test is available, the IgG avidity test will give you an idea of the timescale of events with high avidity if infection is older than 6 months and low if within the past 3 months.

The viral DNA can be checked on the amniotic fluid with PCR after 20 weeks' gestation and 8 weeks after maternal infection.

Ultrasound: The features seen on ultrasound will very much depend on the gestation in which the infection was acquired.

In first trimester rubella infection, major congenital abnormalities can be seen, whereas in later gestation, subtle signs of congenital infection only may be seen.

These major congenital anomalies include microcephaly, ventriculomegaly, pulmonary artery stenosis, or atresia. Later in the pregnancy, features include growth restriction and echogenic bowel.

Management: Termination of pregnancy is offered to parents if infection has occurred in the first trimester due to the poor outcome.

Key Points

- Fetal growth restriction implies reduced fetal size with evidence of functional uteroplacental impairment.
- *Small for gestational age* refers to a fetus whose measurements are small (commonly less than the 10th percentile), but where there are no signs of fetal pathology or uteroplacental impairment.
- FGR and SGA can be difficult to differentiate, but as the biometry percentile cut-off used to define the conditions is lowered, the incidence of pathological FGR rises and of constitutional SGA falls.

- The most common cause of FGR is uteroplacental impairment; less common causes are chromosomal or genetic conditions, congenital infection, and structural abnormality.
- Elucidating the cause antenatally allows management to be targeted at the condition and timing of delivery and for postnatal investigation to be optimized.

References

1. Lees C, Marlow N, Arabin B, Bilardo CM, Brezinka C, Derks JB, Duvekot J, Frusca T, Diemert A, Ferrazzi E, Ganzevoort W, Hecher K, Martinelli P, Ostermayer E, Papageorghiou AT, Schlembach D, Schneider KTM, Thilaganathan B, Todros T, Van Wassenaer Leemhuis A, Valcamonico A, Visser GHA, Wolf H. Perinatal morbidity and mortality in early-onset fetal growth restriction: Cohort outcomes of the trial of randomized umbilical and fetal flow in Europe (TRUFFLE). *Ultrasound Obstet Gynecol* 2013;42(4):400–8. doi:10.1002/uog.13190.

2. Mongelli M, Gardosi J. Fetal growth velocity. *Lancet* 1999;353(9170):2156. doi:10.1016/S0140-6736(05)75590-2.

3. Lin CC, Santolaya-Forgas J. Current concepts of fetal growth restriction: Part I. Causes, classification, and pathophysiology.*Obstet Gynecol* 1998;92(6):1044–55.

4. Papageorghiou AT, Ohuma EO, Altman DG, Todros T. International Fetal and Newborn Growth Consortium for the 21st Century (INTERGROWTH-21st). International standards for fetal growth based on serial ultrasound measurements: the Fetal Growth Longitudinal Study of the INTERGROWTH-21st Project. *Lancet* 2014 Sep 6;384(9946):869–79. doi: 10.1016/S0140-6736(14)61490-2.

5. Gardosi J, Figueras F, Clausson B, Francis A. The customised growth potential: An international research tool to study the epidemiology of fetal growth. *Paediatr Perinat Epidemiol* 2011;25(1):2–10. doi:10.1111/j.1365-3016.2010.01166.x.

6. Unterscheider J, Daly S, Geary MP, Kennelly MM, McAuliffe FM, O'Donoghue K, Hunter A, Morrison JJ, Burke G, Dicker P, Tully EC, Malone FD. Optimizing the definition of intrauterine growth restriction: The multicenter prospective PORTO study. *Am J Obstet Gynecol* 2013;208(4):290.e1-.e6. doi:10.1016/j.ajog.2013.02.007.

7. Yaron Y, Heifetz S, Ochshorn Y, Lehavi O, Orr-Urtreger A. Decreased first trimester PAPP-A is a predictor of adverse pregnancy outcome. *Prenat Diagn* 2002;22(9):778–82. doi:10.1002/pd.407.

8. Goetzl L, Krantz D, Group NBS. Low first-trimester PAPP-a identifies pregnancies requiring IUGR screening. *Am J Obstet Gynecol* December 2003;189(6): Supplement, Page S215

9. Krantz D, Goetz L, Simpson JL. Association of extreme first-trimester free human chorionic gonadotropin-beta, pregnancy-associated plasma protein A, and nuchal translucency with intrauterine growth restriction and other adverse pregnancy outcomes. *Am J Obstet Gynecol* 2004 Oct;191(4):1452–8.

10. Albaiges G. One-stage screening for pregnancy complications by color Doppler assessment of the uterine arteries at 23 weeks' gestation. *Obstet Gynecol* 2000;96(4):559–64.

11. Campbell S, Black RS, Lees CC, Armstrong V, Peacock JL. Doppler ultrasound of the maternal uterine arteries: Disappearance of abnormal waveforms and relation to birthweight and pregnancy outcome. http://dxdoiorg/101080/j1600-04122000079008631x. 2009;79(8):631–4. doi:10.1080/j.1600-0412.2000.079008631.x

12. Kingdom JCP, Burrell SJ, Kaufmann P. Pathology and clinical implications of abnormal umbilical artery Doppler waveforms. *Ultrasound Obstet Gynecol* 1997;9(4):271–86. doi:10.1046/j.1469-0705.1997.09040271.x.

13. Ott WJ. Diagnosis of intrauterine growth restriction: Comparison of ultrasound parameters. *Am J Perinatol* 2002;19(3):133–7. doi:10.1055/s-2002-25313.

14. Rowlands DJ, Vyas SK. Longitudinal study of fetal middle cerebral artery flow velocity waveforms preceding fetal death. *BJOG* 1995;102(11):888–90. doi:10.1111/j.1471-0528.1995.tb10876.x.

15. Baschat AA, Hecher K. Fetal growth restriction due to placental disease. *Semin Perinatol* 2004;28(1):67–80.

16. Lees CC, Marlow N, Van Wassenaer-Leemhuis A, Arabin B, Bilardo CM, Brezinka C, Calvert S, Derks JB, Diemert A, Duvekot JJ, Ferrazzi E, Frusca T, Ganzevoort W, Hecher K, Martinelli P, Ostermayer E, Papageorghiou AT, Schlembach D, Schneider KTM, Thilaganathan B, Todros T, Valcamonico A, Visser GHA, Wolf H. 2 year neurodevelopmental and intermediate perinatal outcomes in infants with very preterm fetal growth restriction (TRUFFLE): A randomised trial. *Lancet* March 2015. doi:10.1016/S0140-6736(14)62049-3.

17. Ferrazzi E, Bozzo M, Rigano S, Bellotti M, Morabito A, Pardi G, Battaglia FC, Galan HL. Temporal sequence of abnormal Doppler changes in the peripheral and central circulatory systems of the severely growth-restricted fetus. *Ultrasound Obstet Gynecol* 2002;19(2):140–6. doi:10.1046/j.0960-7692.2002.00627.x.

18. Hecher K, Campbell S, Doyle P, Harrington K, Nicolaides K. Assessment of fetal compromise by Doppler ultrasound investigation of the fetal circulation. Arterial, intracardiac, and venous blood flow velocity studies. *Circulation* 1995;91(1):129–38. doi:10.1161/01.CIR.91.1.129.

19. Vergani P, Roncaglia N, Locatelli A, Andreotti C, Crippa I, Pezzullo JC, Ghidini A. Antenatal predictors of neonatal outcome in fetal growth restriction with absent end-diastolic flow in the umbilical artery. *Am J Obstet Gynecol* 2005;193(3 Pt 2):1213–18. doi:10.1016/j.ajog.2005.07.032.

20. Khoury MJ, Erickson JD, Cordero JF, McCarthy BJ. Congenital malformations and intrauterine growth retardation: A population study. *Pediatrics* 1988;82(1):83–90.

21. Rosenthal GL, Wilson PD, Permutt T, Boughman JA, Ferencz C. Birth weight and cardiovascular malformations: A population-based study. The Baltimore-Washington Infant Study. *Am J Epidemiol* 1991;133(12):1273–81.

22. Rosenthal GL. Patterns of prenatal growth among infants with cardiovascular malformations: possible fetal hemodynamic effects. *Am J Epidemiol* 1996;143(5):505–13.

23. Spiers PS. Does growth retardation predispose the fetus to congenital malformation? *Lancet* 1982;1(8267):312–14.

24. Capper A. The fate and development of the immature and of the premature child: A clinical study. Review of the Literature and Study of Cerebral Hemorrhage in the New-Born Infant. *Am J Dis Child* 1928;35(2):262–88. doi:10.1001/archpedi.1928.01920200094012.

25. Kumar S. *Handbook of Fetal Medicine*. Cambridge University Press, 2010.

26. Hussain U, Daemen A, Missfelder-Lobos H, De Moor B, Timmerman D, Bourne T, Lees C. Umbilical artery pulsatility index and fetal abdominal circumference in isolated gastroschisis. *Ultrasound Obstet Gynecol* 2011;38(5):538–42. doi:10.1002/uog.8947.

27. Carroll SG, Kuo PY, Kyle PM, Soothill PW. Fetal protein loss in gastroschisis as an explanation of associated morbidity. *Am J Obstet Gynecol* 2001;184(6):1297–301. doi:10.1067/mob.2001.114031.

28. Norman SM, Odibo AO, Longman RE, Roehl KA, Macones GA, Cahill AG. Neural tube defects and associated low birth weight. *Am J Perinatol* 2012;29(6):473–6. doi:10.1055/s-0032-1304830.

29. Scott KE, Usher R. Fetal malnutrition: Its incidence, causes, and effects. *Am J Obstet Gynecol* 1966;94(7):951–63.

30. Snijders RJ, Sherrod C, Gosden CM, Nicolaides KH. Fetal growth retardation: Associated malformations and chromosomal abnormalities. *Am J Obstet Gynecol* 1993;168(2):547–55.

31. Wilkins-Haug L, Roberts DJ, Morton CC. Confined placental mosaicism and intrauterine growth retardation: A case-control analysis of placentas at delivery. *Am J Obstet Gynecol* 1995;172(1):44–50. doi:10.1016/0002-9378(95)90082–9.

32. Boghassian NS et al. Anthropometric charts for infants with trisomies 21, 18, or 13 born between 22 weeks gestation and term: The VON charts. *Am J Med Genet A* 2012 Feb;158A(2):322–32. doi: 10.1002/ajmg.a.34423. Epub 2012 Jan 13.

33. Morris JK, Cole TJ, Springett AL, Dennis J. Down syndrome birth weight in England and Wales: Implications for clinical practice. *Am J Med Genet A* 2015;167A(12):3070–5. doi:10.1002/ajmg.a.37366.

34. Yeo L, Guzman ER, Day-Salvatore D, Walters C, Chavez D, Vintzileos AM. Prenatal detection of fetal trisomy 18 through abnormal sonographic features. *J Ultrasound Med* 2003;22(6):581–90–quiz591–2.

35. Snijders RJ, Sebire NJ, Nayar R, Souka A, Nicolaides KH. Increased nuchal translucency in trisomy 13 fetuses at 10–14 weeks of gestation. *Am J Med Genet* 1999;86(3):205–7.

36. Kroes I, Janssens S, Defoort P. Ultrasound features in trisomy 13 (Patau syndrome) and trisomy 18 (Edwards syndrome) in a consecutive series of 47 cases. *Facts Views Vis Obgyn* 2014;6(4):245–9.

37. Abu-Amero S, Wakeling EL, Preece M, Whittaker J, Stanier P, Moore GE. Epigenetic signatures of Silver-Russell syndrome. *J Med Genet* 2010;47(3):150–4. doi:10.1136/jmg.2009.071316.

38. Prickett AR, Ishida M, Böhm S, Frost JM, Puszyk W, Abu-Amero S, Stanier P, Schulz R, Moore GE, Oakey RJ. Genome-wide methylation analysis in Silver-Russell syndrome patients. *Hum Genet* 2015;134(3):317–32. doi:10.1007/s00439-014-1526-1.

39. Price SM, Stanhope R, Garrett C, Preece MA, Trembath RC. The spectrum of Silver-Russell syndrome: A clinical and molecular genetic study and new diagnostic criteria. *J Med Genet* 1999;36(11):837–42.

40. Wakeling EL, Amero SA, Alders M, Bliek J, Forsythe E, Kumar S, Lim DH, MacDonald F, Mackay DJ, Maher ER, Moore GE, Poole RL, Price SM, Tangeraas T, Turner CLS, Van Haelst MM, Willoughby C, Temple IK, Cobben JM. Epigenotype–phenotype correlations in Silver-Russell syndrome. *J Med Genet* 2010;47(11):jmg.2010.079111-jmg.2010.079768. doi:10.1136/jmg.2010.079111.

41. Paladini D, Volpe P. *Ultrasound of Congenital Fetal Anomalies: Differential Diagnosis and Prognostic Indicators.* 2014.

42. Chen M, Hwu W-L, Kuo S-J, Chen C-P, Yin P-L, Chang S-P, Lee D-J, Chen T-H, Wang B-T, Lin CC. Subtelomeric rearrangements and 22q11.2 deletion syndrome in anomalous growth-restricted fetuses with normal or balanced G-banded karyotype. *Ultrasound Obstet Gynecol* 2006;28(7):939–43. doi:10.1002/uog.3884.

43. Volpe P, Marasini M, Caruso G, Marzullo A, Buonadonna AL, Arciprete P, Di Paolo S, Volpe G, Gentile M. 22q11 deletions in fetuses with malformations of the outflow tracts or interruption of the aortic arch: Impact of additional ultrasound signs. *Prenat Diagn* 2003;23(9):752–7. doi:10.1002/pd.682.

44. Tavormina PL, Shiang R, Thompson LM, Zhu YZ, Wilkin DJ, Lachman RS, Wilcox WR, Rimoin DL, Cohn DH, Wasmuth JJ. Thanatophoric dysplasia (types I and II) caused by distinct mutations in fibroblast growth factor receptor 3. *Nat Genet* 1995;9(3):321–8. doi:10.1038/ng0395-321.

45. Vanhoenacker FM, Van der Aa N, Blaumeiser B. The French telephone receiver sign in thanatophoric dysplasia. *JBR-BTR* 2009;92(1):63.

46. Langer LO, Yang SS, Hall JG, Sommer A, Kottamasu SR, Golabi M, Krassikoff N. Thanatophoric dysplasia and cloverleaf skull. *Am J Med Genet Suppl* 1987;3:167–79.

47. Picone O, Simon I, Benachi A, Brunelle F, Sonigo P. Comparison between ultrasound and magnetic resonance imaging in assessment of fetal cytomegalovirus infection. *Prenat Diagn* 2008;28(8):753–8. doi:10.1002/pd.2037.

48. Lazzarotto T, Guerra B, Lanari M, Gabrielli L, Landini MP. New advances in the diagnosis of congenital cytomegalovirus infection. *J Clin Virol* 2008;41(3):192–7. doi:10.1016/j.jcv.2007.10.015.

49. Feldman B, Yinon Y, Tepperberg Oikawa M, Yoeli R, Schiff E, Lipitz S. Pregestational, periconceptional, and gestational primary maternal cytomegalovirus infection: Prenatal diagnosis in 508 pregnancies. *Am J Obstet Gynecol* 2011;205(4):342.e1–342.e6. doi:10.1016/j.ajog.2011.05.030.

50. Ruellan Eugene G, Barjot P, Campet M, Vabret A, Herlicoviez M, Muller G, Levy G, Guillois B,

Freymuth F, Freymuth F. Evaluation of virological procedures to detect fetal human cytomegalovirus infection: Avidity of IgG antibodies, virus detection in amniotic fluid and maternal serum. *J Med Virol* 1996;50(1):9–15. doi:10.1002/(SICI)1096–9071(199609)50:1<9::AID-JMV3>3.0.CO;2–5.

51. Guerra B, Lazzarotto T, Quarta S, Lanari M, Bovicelli L, Nicolosi A, Landini MP. Prenatal diagnosis of symptomatic congenital cytomegalovirus infection. *Am J Obstet Gynecol* 2000;183(2):476–82. doi:10.1067/mob.2000.106347.

52. Gouarin S, Gault E, Vabret A, Cointe D, Rozenberg F, Grangeot-Keros L, Barjot P, Garbarg-Chenon A, Lebon P, Freymuth F. Real-time PCR quantification of human cytomegalovirus DNA in amniotic fluid samples from mothers with primary infection. *J Clin Microbiol* 2002;40(5):1767–72. doi:10.1128/JCM.40.5.1767-1772.2002.

53. Picone O, Costa J-M, Leruez-Ville M, Ernault P. Cytomegalovirus (CMV) glycoprotein B genotype and CMV DNA load in the amniotic fluid of infected fetuses. *Prenat Diagn* 2004.

54. Nedelec O, Bellagra N, Devisme L, Hober D, Wattré P, Dewilde A. [Congenital human cytomegalovirus infection: Value of human cytomegalovirus DNA quantification in amniotic fluid]. *Ann Biol Clin (Paris)* 2002;60(2):201–7.

55. Revello MG, Lazzarotto T, Guerra B, Spinillo A, Ferrazzi E, Kustermann A, Guaschino S, Vergani P, Todros T, Frusca T, Arossa A, Furione M, Rognoni V, Rizzo N, Gabrielli L, Klersy C, Gerna G, CHIP Study Group. A randomized trial of hyperimmune globulin to prevent congenital cytomegalovirus. *N Engl J Med* 2014;370(14):1316–26. doi:10.1056/NEJMoa1310214.

56. Jacquemard F, Yamamoto M, Costa J-M, Romand S, Jaqz-Aigrain E, Dejean A, Daffos F, Ville Y. Maternal administration of valaciclovir in symptomatic intrauterine cytomegalovirus infection. *BJOG* 2007;114(9):1113–21. doi:10.1111/j.1471-0528.2007.01308.x.

57. Kimberlin DW, Jester PM, Sánchez PJ. Valganciclovir for symptomatic congenital cytomegalovirus disease. *N Engl J Med* 2015;372(10):933–43. doi:10.1056/NEJMoa1404599.

58. Lipitz S, Yinon Y, Malinger G, Yagel S, Levit L, Hoffman C, Rantzer R, Weisz B. Risk of cytomegalovirus-associated sequelae in relation to time of infection and findings on prenatal imaging. *Ultrasound Obstet Gynecol* 2013;41(5):508–14. doi:10.1002/uog.12377.

59. Farkas N, Hoffmann C, Ben-Sira L, Lev D, Schweiger A, Kidron D, Lerman-Sagie T, Malinger G. Does normal fetal brain ultrasound predict normal neurodevelopmental outcome in congenital cytomegalovirus infection? *Prenat Diagn* 2011;31(4):360–6. doi:10.1002/pd.2694.

60. Malinger G, Lev D, Lerman-Sagie T. Imaging of fetal cytomegalovirus infection. *Fetal Diagn Ther* 2011;29(2):117–26. doi:10.1159/000321346.

61. Yinon Y, Farine D, Yudin MH. Screening, diagnosis, and management of cytomegalovirus infection in pregnancy. *Obstet Gynecol Surv* 2010;65(11):736–43. doi:10.1097/OGX.0b013e31821102b4.

62. Dunn D, Wallon M, Peyron F, Petersen E, Peckham C, Gilbert R. Mother-to-child transmission of toxoplasmosis: risk estimates for clinical counselling. *Lancet* 1999;353(9167):1829–33. doi:10.1016/S0140-6736(98)08220-8.

63. Romand et al. Usefulness of quantitative polymerase chain reaction in amniotic fluid as early prognostic marker of fetal infection with *Toxoplasma gondii*. *Am J Obstet Gynecol* March 2004;190(3):797–802.

64. Malinger G, Werner H, Rodriguez Leonel JC, Rebolledo M, Duque M, Mizyrycki S, Lerman Sagie T, Herrera M. Prenatal brain imaging in congenital toxoplasmosis. *Prenat Diagn* 2011;31(9):881–6. doi:10.1002/pd.2795.

65. Berrébi A, Assouline C, Bessières M-H, Lathière M, Cassaing S, Minville V, Ayoubi J-M. Long-term outcome of children with congenital toxoplasmosis. *Am J Obstet Gynecol* 2010;203(6):552.e1-e6. doi:10.1016/j.ajog.2010.06.002.

66. Tookey PA. Review of antenatal rubella susceptibility screening and the standard criteria for screening. *Institute of Child Health* May 2012:1–11.

67. Hardelid P, Cortina-Borja M, Williams D, Tookey PA, Peckham CS, Cubitt WD, Dezateux C. Rubella seroprevalence in pregnant women in North Thames: Estimates based on newborn screening samples. *J Med Screen* 2009;16(1):1–6. doi:10.1258/jms.2009.008080.

68. Robertson SE, Featherstone DA, Gacic-Dobo M, Hersh BS. Rubella and congenital rubella syndrome: Global update. *Rev Panam Salud Publica* 2003;14(5):306–15.

Fetal Growth Restriction and Hypertensive Diseases of Pregnancy

Christopher W. G. Redman and Anne Cathrine Staff

Introduction

Hypertension can present in pregnancy in three ways: chronic hypertension, a medical issue that precedes and continues during pregnancy, gestational hypertension (GH), or preeclampsia. New-onset non-obstetric hypertension is exceptionally rare and not considered here. Chronic hypertension (CHT) affects about 1–5% of pregnancies [1]. Preeclampsia complicates about 2–5% of pregnancies [2,3] and gestational hypertension 2–17%, depending on parity and patient population [4,5]. These different categories of hypertension do not occur in isolation. Chronic hypertension is a major risk factor for preeclampsia (named superimposed preeclampsia). GH may be an early sign of preeclampsia in some women. All three forms of hypertension increase the risk of fetal growth retardation (FGR).

Preeclamptic hypertension is a form of secondary hypertension. The cause is the placenta. When it is delivered, the problem for the mother is resolved, but may impose the difficulties of preterm delivery on the baby, preeclampsia being one of the most common reasons for iatrogenic prematurity [6].

The placenta is, of course, the supply line for the fetus. When FGR is caused by failure to achieve optimal fetal growth, this is often secondary to placentally mediated problems. In this review, the term FGR, unless otherwise stated, is used to mean FGR mediated by placental dysfunction, usually secondary to abnormal uteroplacental perfusion.

Preeclampsia is defined as a syndrome comprising new-onset hypertension and proteinuria in the second half of pregnancy, which was not present before pregnancy and does not persist afterward. Syndromes are common in all branches of medicine. They assist clinical practice, but do not help, and often hinder, understanding of pathogenesis by promoting a focus on secondary features evident to the clinician. Recent revised definitions from ACOG [7] do not include FGR as a possible component of the syndrome, but allow non-proteinuric variants, whereas the Australasian definition includes both [8].

GH typically precedes proteinuria. But not all GH evolves into preeclampsia. It is more likely the earlier the onset. Before 30 weeks, nearly half of those who present with GH develop preeclampsia compared to around 5% of those at term [9]. GH without proteinuria is more common than preeclampsia and has fewer adverse outcomes, which is consistent with it being a form of incipient preeclampsia. As for preeclampsia, it involves more primiparae [10], more FGR [11], and a greater susceptibility to long-term cardiovascular disease [12], especially if it recurs in more than one pregnancy [13]. A recent review concludes that GH is a mixture of women with incipient preeclampsia and of those with undiagnosed chronic hypertension [14]. CHT is a major risk factor for so-called superimposed preeclampsia, especially preterm preeclampsia. Even in the absence of proteinuria, it predisposes to FGR, for example [15].

Two questions can be asked. First, does maternal hypertension directly cause placental dysfunction and thereby FGR? Second, does placental dysfunction of other causes lead to FGR on the one hand and maternal hypertension on the other? The two possibilities are not mutually exclusive.

Uteroplacental Hemodynamics

The placenta is the key to understanding the relation between maternal hypertension and FGR; the issue centers on uteroplacental hemodynamic function and how, when it is disordered, the ensuing placental dysfunction causes preeclampsia and placentally mediated FGR.

The placenta is extraordinarily complex, with two circulations – uteroplacental and fetoplacental – that coexist with a genetically disparate mother. Unlike all other fetal organs, it reaches maximal capacity and function before birth. Its development has to be fast. Given its short life span, deviations from normality have major effects on intrauterine fetal health. The placenta is characterized by its unique cell type – trophoblast. Villous trophoblast is a major part of the placenta, with proliferative unicellular villous cytotrophoblast maintaining and replenishing the overlying non-proliferative multinucleate syncytiotrophoblast. The placenta is attached to the uterine wall by anchoring villi that are more than anchors. The anchoring villi represent bridges where proliferative extravillous trophoblast migrates to invade the placental bed and plays a major part in ensuring an adequate uteroplacental blood flow. These cytotrophoblast are, in effect, ambassadors for fetal trade that negotiate adequate supplies from the mother. Such "negotiations" require that the placenta must evade maternal immune rejection yet divert a large proportion (20%) of maternal cardiac output to supply its needs [16], receive an adequate but not excessive supply of oxygen for oxidative metabolism, and take control of maternal metabolism to ensure good nutrition for the fetus. Placentation is the term used to describe early placental development, when its maternal blood supply is established, and involves both an initial phase of endocrine priming followed by a second phase that is dependent on the presence of extravillous trophoblast cells [17].

The Uterine, Arcuate and Radial Arteries during Pregnancy

Volume blood flow to the placenta is determined by the larger radial, arcuate, and uterine arteries, which dilate enormously in very early pregnancy, amplifying changes that have already started in the luteal phase of the menstrual cycle [16]. The underlying mechanisms are not well defined, but do not involve direct contact with extravillous cytotrophoblast. Possible explanations invoke shear stress, more nitric oxide synthesis and increased hCG (human chorionic gonadotropin), estrogen, progesterone, relaxin, and placental growth factor (PlGF) production [16]. For example, endothelial nitric oxide synthase activity increases eightfold in uterine arteries from pregnant compared to non-pregnant women [18].

While intervillous maternal blood flow is controlled upstream by the larger radial arteries [19], profound dilatation and remodeling at the tips of the much smaller spiral arteries (see later in this chapter)

slows blood flow velocities [19]. Other aspects of the circulation may be important such as maternal venous hemodynamics, which may have substantial effects on intervillous blood pressure. Maternal venous hypertension is transmitted retrogradely into the intervillous space, where if it is high it can compress the chorionic villous capillaries [20], perfused at very low pressures, so reducing their function. The clinical implications are not well documented or yet understood.

Large hemodynamic changes occur during pregnancy: systemically in the mother and locally in the uterus. Maternal arterial pressure is only one aspect of a larger and more complex process that ensures perfusion of the placenta in terms of blood flow volume, velocity, and perfusing pressure. Clinicians pay so much attention to blood pressure not because it is necessarily important in the pathogenesis of disorders like preeclampsia, but simply because it is what can be measured and monitored in pregnant women.

Placentation

The early development of the placenta has been summarized ([21] and Figure 4.1). Trophoblast differentiates early into villous and extravillous subsets: the former is associated with formation of the chorionic villous tree (branching morphogenesis) and the latter with invasion of the placental bed by extravillous cytotrophoblast, which stimulates spiral artery remodeling and development of adequate uteroplacental perfusion. Before 8 weeks, invasive endovascular plugs of trophoblast block the spiral arteries [22]. As a result, there is minimal hemochorial perfusion. The fetus is sustained by "histotrophic" nutrition [23], mediated by uterine glandular secretions, in a hypoxic environment. The uteroplacental circulation opens in a staged way, beginning at the placental pole furthest from the insertion of the umbilical cord and progressing centripetally from there [24]. As each artery unplugs, oxygenation of the relevant sectors of peripheral placental lobule increases relatively quickly. The ensuing oxidative stress atrophies the immature chorionic villi, leaving the chorionic layer of the decidua parietalis as a remnant of this process. Antioxidant defenses begin to strengthen after 8 weeks such that when the more central spiral arteries open, villous integrity is preserved as the definitive placenta begins to form, including a functional fetoplacental circulation. The intervillous

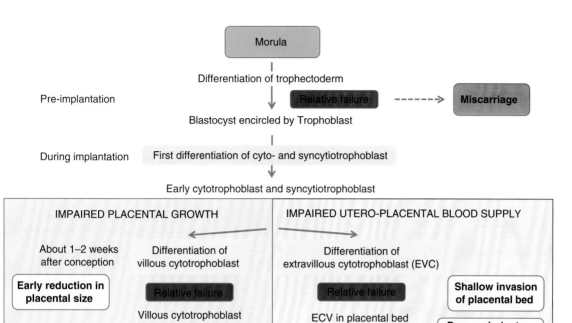

Figure 4.1 Trophoblast differentiation and early origins of preeclampsia and FGR.
This is a theoretical model to relate early placental development to preeclampsia (PE) and fetal growth restriction (FGR).
If the early differentiation of trophoblast into its villous and extravillous derivatives is suboptimal, this may result in a combination of PE and FGR. If only the villous pathway is affected, reduced placental growth and distal villous hypoplasia is likely to be more important (lower left, see text). If only the extravillous pathway is affected, preeclampsia is more likely (lower right).

circulation is fully established later, at the end of the first trimester [24].

Unplugging of the spiral arteries, which starts placental perfusion, is a key turning point in placental development. The remnants of the trophoblast plugs that remain adherent to the arterial wall form a transient pseudoendothelium. They also penetrate the underlying artery wall and either directly or, in concert with maternal cells, dramatically remodel the ends of the spiral arteries from small elastic arteries, encircled by smooth muscle cell layers, into structure-less funnels, widest at their distal tips, with non-contractile fibrinoid walls, devoid of internal and external elastic laminae, smooth muscle, or adventitia [25]. This remodeling has long been considered to be how uteroplacental blood flow is expanded.

However, the remodeled tips of spiral arteries do not *increase* blood flow into the intervillous space, but *reduce* its velocity, pressure, and pulsatility, which minimize hydrostatic and oxidative damage to the chorionic villi [18]. During pregnancy, uterine hemodynamics are adapted in two phases: first involving the large arteries that determine volume flow and later affecting the terminal spiral arteries that determine the flow velocity [16].

This restructuring is deficient in preeclampsia and placentally mediated FGR. The remodeling normally extends as far as the myometrial segments of the arteries but is shallower where there is FGR with or without preeclampsia (Figure 4.2). In this case the flow from the artery into the intervillous space is not so much reduced, but pulsatile and at an increased pressure. As explained later, this imposes stresses on the syncytiotrophoblast lining of the chorionic villi, leading to dysfunctional placental-maternal signaling.

33

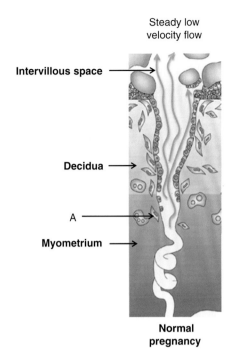
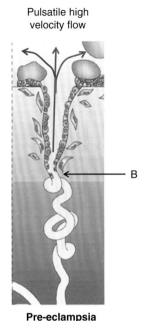

Steady low
velocity flow

Pulsatile high
velocity flow

Intervillous space

Decidua

A

Myometrium

B

Normal
pregnancy

Pre-eclampsia
FGR

Figure 4.2 Poor placentation in FGR (fetal growth retardation) with or without preeclampsia.
A. Spiral artery remodeling (from weeks 8–18) normally extends into the myometrial segments, associated with endovascular invasion of trophoblast, which before 8–10 weeks plugs the arteries prior to the hemochorial circulation opening. This promotes low-velocity, steady blood flow into the intervillous space.
B. In FGR, with or without preeclampsia, the remodeling is abnormally shallow and fails to reach the myometrium.
A collar of vascular smooth muscle (at point B) is retained that can contract and impede flow, which is at high velocity and pulsatile.
Adapted from Moffett-King A. *Nat Rev Immunol* 2002; 2: 656–63.

Maternal Hypertension and Fetal Growth Restriction: Mechanisms

The impact of antecedent maternal hypertension on placentation is not understood. Its association with FGR can be rationalized only by understanding the biological mechanisms. The fetus does not "sense" maternal hypertension. Nor does the placenta, in direct contact with the maternal circulation, appear to have baroceptors. However, it is crucial that the blood pressure in the intervillous space is kept low (below 20 mm Hg [25], so that it does not compress the capillaries of the chorionic villi, which are fragile structures filled at very low blood pressure, which can be easily collapsed and thereby lose effective function.

Placental Dysfunction as a Cause of Secondary Maternal Hypertension

By the year 2000, it was understood that preeclampsia was associated with dysfunctional uteroplacental perfusion that caused hypoxia with or without oxidative stress (not the same thing – see later in this chapter) and release of one or more, as yet unknown, placental factors into the maternal circulation that stimulate hypertension and other features of the syndrome. This was summarized in our two-stage model of preeclampsia [27]. In line with this model, we consider first what is happening in the placenta and second the downstream consequences in maternal systems. The unifying process in the placenta is biological stress [28].

Biological Stress, Pregnancy and Placentally Mediated Disease

Biological stress arises when a cell, tissue, or body system deviates from its set point of homeostasis. Such deviations are intrinsic to every moment of life and are managed by stress responses, which quickly restore equilibrium. It is self-evident that they encompass a huge range of responses that ensure survival. At the cellular level, there are four outcomes to stress: normality is restored; the cell gives up, is disassembled and cleared away (apoptosis); the cell disintegrates and spills its contents into its surrounds (necrosis); or the cell survives, but homeostasis is not restored and is replaced by chronic stress. The last is the basis of many if not all chronic illnesses. One aspect of the stress response is autophagy. While intracellular components are normally degraded and reused for cell maintenance, in stressed cells, this process is increased. Another aspect of cell stress is release of membrane microvesicles (summarized in [28]).

It is important to recognize that normal pregnancy itself is a major biological stress for the mother, imposed by the placenta. Most mothers adapt and cope, using stress responses that we artlessly call normal pregnancy physiology, for example, the early increases in the maternal pulse rate and leucocyte count already evident in the first trimester. If the placenta becomes stressed, it imposes an extra burden for the mother to be added to the already considerable load of her normal pregnancy. A common and important placental stress arises from dysfunctional maternal-placental perfusion. Because the placenta is the fetal lifeline, this can lead to FGR and chronic fetal hypoxemia. But placental signaling to the mother also becomes deranged, for example, causing maternal cardiovascular dysfunction – which is what we call preeclampsia.

Stress Responses and Syncytiotrophoblast (STB)

A wide range of stresses are resolved by a relatively small number of integrated responses that restore equilibrium. A classical stress response is inflammation, which is activated by external or internal triggers, not just infection (external danger), but also by accumulation of dangerous waste products, or biochemical damage to basic cellular molecules (internal danger). Stress may be generated by deficient or excess supplies to meet metabolic needs: oxygen, glucose,

protein, water, and so on. Hypoxia and hyperoxia are both dangerous, as are both hypoglycemia and hyperglycemia, for example.

The placental syncytiotrophoblast is a microvillus epithelium and the functional interface between mother and baby, sustaining fetal respiration, nutrition, and waste disposal. Because it lines the intervillous space, perfused by maternal blood, it serves as a virtual maternal endothelium. Dysfunctional maternal perfusion usually causes intervillous hypoxia. During hypoxia, cellular protein synthesis slows [28]. If severe, what is called the unfolded protein response is activated in the protein factory of the cell, the endoplasmic reticulum, which then prioritizes synthesis of proteins that promote recovery at the expense of other proteins. There are negative aspects (shut down of some functions) and positive aspects (increased production of rescue factors, such as antioxidants). This is called endoplasmic reticulum stress (ER stress). Under these conditions, the recovering cell may be vulnerable to sudden restoration of normoxia, which causes oxidative damage, otherwise known as oxidative stress (Figure 4.3). Normally the cell can quench leakages of reactive oxygen species (ROS). Unquenched ROS indiscriminately oxidize all cellular constituents and impair or change their functions. Intermittent fluctuations in oxygenation may result from uterine contractions (such as during labor) or changes in maternal posture or perfusion; the ensuing oxidative damage is termed ischemia-reperfusion injury [30].

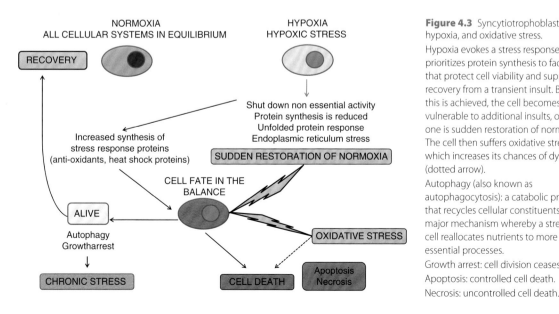

Figure 4.3 Syncytiotrophoblast, hypoxia, and oxidative stress.
Hypoxia evokes a stress response that prioritizes protein synthesis to factors that protect cell viability and support recovery from a transient insult. Before this is achieved, the cell becomes vulnerable to additional insults, of which one is sudden restoration of normoxia. The cell then suffers oxidative stress, which increases its chances of dying (dotted arrow).
Autophagy (also known as autophagocytosis): a catabolic process that recycles cellular constituents. It is a major mechanism whereby a stressed cell reallocates nutrients to more essential processes.
Growth arrest: cell division ceases.
Apoptosis: controlled cell death.
Necrosis: uncontrolled cell death.

35

The target tissue in preeclampsia is the maternal endothelium [31]. Its dysfunction can explain many if not all features of the maternal syndrome [32]. Generalized endothelial activation affects arterial function, but also underlies the much more widespread pathology of vascular inflammation [33], which includes altered metabolism, the complex liver dependent acute phase response, and increased insulin resistance [32]. Diverse inflammatory stimuli reduce nitric oxide bioavailability in the endothelium, thereby impairing flow-mediated vasodilation and increasing arterial pressure [34]. Chronic vascular inflammation underlies chronic hypertension and arterial disease, specifically the artery disease associated with obesity and the metabolic syndrome [35]. The same mechanisms underlie the hypertension of preeclampsia [33].

STB Stress, Hypertension, and FGR

In more severe preeclampsia, there is clear histopathological evidence of STB stress: increased necrosis, apoptosis, and autophagy. The placental release of STB microvesicles, another stress response, is also increased [28]. The maternal vascular inflammatory response is what would be predicted because maternal stress systems respond to the damaged syncytial surface of the placenta as if it were maternal tissue. Vascular inflammation explains more features of preeclampsia than any other biological mechanism [33], but cannot account directly for maternal hypertension, the key feature of the disorder.

This difficulty was largely resolved by the discovery of how angiogenic and antiangiogenic factors of placental origin contribute to the preeclampsia syndrome [36]. Vascular endothelial growth factor (VEGF) is the best known of several angiogenic factors. It is not produced by syncytiotrophoblast, whereas its close cousin, placental growth factor (PlGF), is. Note that PlGF is not placental specific. PlGF is normally produced in non-pregnant individuals from the heart and other tissues at low levels [37]. Antiangiogenic factors dysregulated in preeclampsia include soluble VEGF receptor-1 (sVEGFR-1, also known as sFLT1) and soluble endoglin (sENG). The typical but by no means consistent pattern of preeclampsia is an excess of circulating anti-angiogenic sVEGFR-1 and sENG, and a deficit of pro-angiogenic PlGF, also preceding the clinical onset of the syndrome.

The availability of circulating free VEGF and PlGF is reduced in preeclampsia. Both VEGF and PlGF help maintain the integrity of maternal endothelium. The consequences of VEGF deficiency have been well documented by the use of synthetic inhibitors of VEGF to treat cancer in non-pregnant patients. Proteinuria as well as hypertension, sometimes severe, are side effects. The evidence is that maternal hypertension is not mediated directly by a deficiency of vascular nitric oxide, which is the expected consequence of VEGF deprivation [38]. Instead it seems to arise from vascular oxidative stress, which is a by-product of disordered nitric oxide synthesis (Figure 4.4). Endothelin is a powerful endothelium derived vasoconstrictor that promotes vascular inflammation and oxidative stress, as observed in preeclampsia [39].

FGR and ER Stress

The relation between STB stress and FGR is intuitively easy to envisage. Apart from loss of maternal-placental transport functions, the presence of ER stress distinguishes a preeclampsia placenta with FGR from a preeclampsia placenta without FGR. This is clearly seen by electron microscopy in the syncytium. Measurements specific to the syncytium are not yet available, but analysis of whole placental villous tissue confirms that ER stress is strongly linked to FGR [40]. This makes sense because the endoplasmic reticulum is the major producer of proteins within cells.

Biomarkers of STB Stress

In preeclampsia and FGR mediated by placental vascular dysfunction, both sFlt-1 and soluble endoglin production by syncytiotrophoblast increase despite ER stress, which would be expected to lead to less protein production. There are several other markers that increase similarly, for example, leptin, activin-A, inhibin-A, and corticotrophin-releasing hormone, all of which are potential biomarkers for preeclampsia. There are likely to be many more since the stress response is wide ranging. They will all reflect the problem in the placental syncytium. How they might modify the maternal syndrome is not fully clarified, but it is to be expected that they will, in concert, by their peripheral actions add to the complexity and heterogeneity of the maternal syndrome, while signaling the placental problem that affect fetal growth. Increased production from a tissue suffering ER stress is typical of what might be termed a positive stress response. These circulating proteins are therefore STB stress response markers and not preeclampsia biomarkers, as is often considered. The reduction in circulating

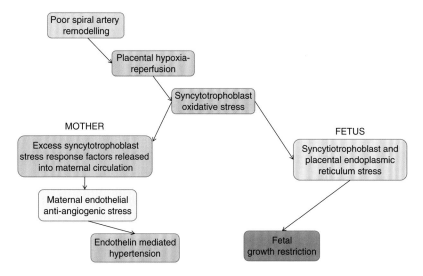

Figure 4.4 The association of FGR and hypertension with poor placentation. Poor spiral artery remodeling leads to syncytiotrophoblast oxidative stress, which has two downstream consequences. The mother's circulation is destabilized by excess STB-derived sFlt-1 (and other factors), which deprive her vascular endothelium of VEGF and stimulate overproduction of endothelin and maternal hypertension (see Figure 4.7a). The placenta suffers impairment of protein synthesis (endoplasmic reticulum stress), which is strongly associated with FGR.

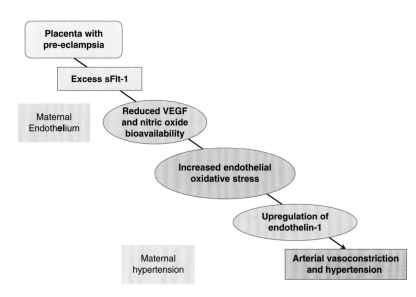

Figure 4.5 How does circulating sFlt-1 cause hypertension? Passing the stresses from placenta to mother.
sFlt-1, a product of syncytiotrophoblast stress, in turn acts on maternal endothelium and causes a downstream stress response, which provokes upregulation of endothelin, which is the most potent cause of arterial constriction. The exact signaling mechanisms are unclear. The evidence suggests a more direct role for excess endothelin than nitric oxide deficiency [38].

PlGF in these contexts is typical of a negative stress response. The cause of this placental stress is dysfunctional uteroplacental perfusion, which may lead to hypoxia, ischemia or ischemia reperfusion, and oxidative stress. This is a plausible model of maternal hypertension as a secondary consequence of STB stress caused by uteroplacental mal-perfusion secondary to poor placentation (Figure 4.5).

Fetal Growth Restriction in Relation to Early- and Late-Onset Preeclampsia

Fetal growth restriction is not a major feature of preeclampsia at term [41], the most common variant of the syndrome. The high preponderance of SGA in early-onset preeclampsia (presenting before 34 weeks) was noted more than 30 years ago [42]. Of a large cohort of pregnancies selected before 32 weeks by a diagnosis of FGR, 60% were associated with some form of gestational hypertension and a further 11% with chronic hypertension [43]. In contrast, preeclampsia at and beyond term involves more often large-for-gestational-age babies than normal [41,44]. A well-grown or even larger-than-average baby would seem to be incompatible with poor placentation, so what is happening in late-onset preeclampsia disease?

37

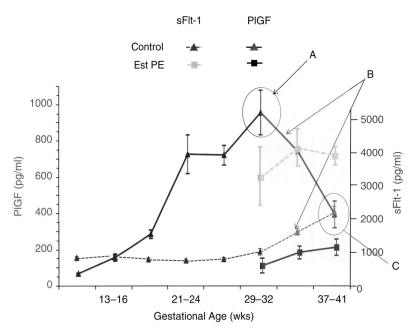

Figure 4.6 Markers of syncytiotrophoblast stress – positive and negative – in normal pregnancy. In normal pregnancy PlGF (▲) rises steadily to 29–32 weeks (**A**) and falls thereafter until delivery (**B**). On the same time course, sFlt-1 (▲) increases (B). By term, the normal values of both biomarkers are close to those of established preeclampsia (**C**, ■,■). Observations on preeclampsia began at the end of the second trimester in this study. But note that preeclampsia can occur at any time after 20 weeks.
Adapted from Levine RJ et al. *N Engl J Med* 2004;350:672e83.

Two Causes of Uteroplacental Malperfusion Underlying Preeclampsia

Circulating biomarkers of STB stress display interesting features at term (Figure 4.6). After 30–34 weeks of any uncomplicated and normotensive pregnancy, there is evidence of increasing STB stress, in terms of a (on average) rising maternal circulating sFlt-1 and falling PlGF. Why is this? We propose that it is most likely due to placental hypoxia or oxidative stress. Available evidence (summarized in [28]) suggests that oxygen tension in intervillous blood progressively falls with advancing gestational age. This may be due either to declining uteroplacental perfusion or to increased uptake of oxygen by the maturing placenta, or both. Reduced oxygen tension is consistent with the slowing of placental growth toward and beyond full term, which is most evident for the higher placental weight centiles and least evident for the smallest placentas [45].

Post-term pregnancies are associated with increased rates of adverse outcomes: unexplained stillbirth, neonatal dysmaturity, and mortality (reviewed in [46]). They are also more often complicated by preeclampsia and eclampsia [47]. There is also more STB necrosis [48]. Indeed, STB histopathology of post-term pregnancies is strikingly similar to that of preeclampsia of any gestational age [48]. That circulating biomarkers of syncytial stress are altered (for example, low PlGF) with gestational age toward or into a zone that

is characteristic of preeclampsia is consistent with, but does not prove that, placental malperfusion toward term is not secondary to poor placentation, but to physical limits on placental growth or age or both, which are evident in placental growth charts [45].

We propose there are at least two placental causes of preeclampsia (Figure 4.7). The first is extrinsic to the placenta, namely incomplete spiral artery remodeling, affecting uteroplacental circulation by causing pulsatile high-velocity intervillous flow (Figure 4.2). The second is intrinsic to the growing placenta, which sooner or later triggers processes that restrict intervillous perfusion. Combinations of these two pathologies are likely. For example, very mildly impaired placentation might precipitate preeclampsia owing to advancing placental maturity at 37–40 weeks in a pregnancy, which with unimpaired placentation could have continued safely until 41–42 weeks. This concept predicts that more women with larger-than-average placentas should develop preeclampsia at term, which is what is observed [49], as we saw for women with multiple pregnancies who have an increased risk for preeclampsia.

Mixed Origins of Late-Onset Preeclampsia Associated with LGA and SGA Infants

Late-onset preeclampsia is associated with a bilaterally skewed distribution of birth weight with small

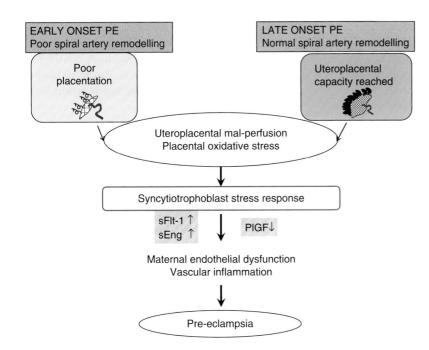

EARLY ONSET PE
Poor spiral artery remodelling

Poor
placentation

LATE ONSET PE
Normal spiral artery remodelling

Uteroplacental
capacity reached

Uteroplacental mal-perfusion
Placental oxidative stress

Syncytiotrophoblast stress response

sFlt-1 ↑
sEng ↑   PlGF↓

Maternal endothelial dysfunction
Vascular inflammation

Pre-eclampsia

Figure 4.7 Early- and late-onset preeclampsia (PE) arise from different causes of dysfunctional uteroplacental perfusion.

We suggest that these lead to the same downstream problems of STB stress, maternal endothelial dysfunction with vascular inflammation, and hypertension secondary, in part, to endothelin over-secretion and other features of the preeclampsia syndrome [39].

excesses of both LGA (large for gestational age) and SGA (small for gestational age) infants, relative to normal [44,50]. The excess of LGA in late preeclampsia appears to depend entirely on maternal obesity [50]. Doppler ultrasound analyses of fetal cerebral and placental blood flows in mildly underweight fetuses (birth weights mainly 10th–50th centiles) demonstrate that while they are technically well grown, more of these fetuses show evidence of brain-sparing redistribution [51], which is a feature of hypoxia. In terms of the concepts we present in this chapter, these are the babies whose placentas have reached the limits of what their relatively adequate uteroplacental circulation can provide. Every fetus has such limits, but most will be delivered before they reach them.

Does Maternal Cardiovascular Dysfunction Cause Placental Pathology?

That chronic hypertension predisposes to preeclampsia is well established [52], particularly of the early-onset type [53]. Many have considered the association to be causal (reviewed in [52]), that the hypertension itself causes the problem, which is potentially preventable by appropriate anti-hypertensive treatment, for which there is little evidence at the moment. By its association with early-onset preeclampsia, it must be assumed

that a dysfunctional placentation and consequent FGR are involved. Current theories of placentation emphasize the importance of immunological maternal-fetal disparity in relation to placentation problems [54], but this or other mechanisms that might inhibit or promote placentation are not well delineated.

Long-term hypertension, in non-pregnant individuals, is closely linked to endothelial dysfunction, associated with vascular inflammation and invariably with some degree of vascular oxidative stress. Several studies attest to the vulnerability of the invasive extracellular trophoblast to inflammatory, oxidative, and other stresses. In general, experimental and human observations are consistent in that inflammatory stimuli in their broadest sense, which can also include hypoxia and classical bacterial endotoxin-induced responses, inhibit trophoblast invasion, for example, in pregnant rats [55]. Analysis of early pregnancy termination samples from pregnancies with abnormal uterine artery Doppler velocity waveforms (increased risk of early-onset preeclampsia) demonstrate trophoblast stress in terms of more apoptosis or increased sensitivity to apoptosis [56]. If this is correct, then hypertension does not directly cause placental damage, but is one aspect of a broader systemic inflammatory process that in its local manifestation in the first trimester decidua has adverse effects on placentation and in its systemic aspect causes arterial hypertension.

It is a recent concept that gestational myocardial dysfunction may similarly increase the risk of preeclampsia [57]. Women who develop early- rather than late-onset preeclampsia have multiple indices of symptomless, myocardial dysfunction, including impaired relaxation and both diastolic and ventricular dysfunction. This is at 20–23 weeks, prior to signs of preeclampsia. On average, there is also a higher mean arterial pressure and reduced cardiac output. Early pregnancy is a time of major maternal cardiovascular adaptation (reduced peripheral resistance, expanded plasma volume, and increased cardiac output) stimulated directly or indirectly by placental function. Since early-onset preeclampsia is a disorder that begins with poor placentation in the first trimester, it is likely that these cardiovascular changes are not fully achieved. Preexisting chronic hypertension may contribute to this cardiovascular profile. To what extent these changes amplify fetal growth restriction caused by poor placentation is unknown.

Does Placental Pathology in Hypertensive Diseases of Pregnancy Suggest Hypertensive Damage?

The placental lesions of dysfunctional maternal perfusion are shown in Table 4.1. Most are not specific to preeclampsia, but are also associated with normotensive FGR [58], which is consistent with the concept that hypertension is an epiphenomenon to a more profound placental problem. The most relevant lesion to FGR is distal villous hypoplasia, which results from failure of the villous tree to branch and grow adequately. It is the lesion most associated with impaired umbilical arterial Doppler blood flow velocity waveforms [59]. Acute atherosis, once considered pathognomonic of preeclampsia, can also occur in normal and FGR pregnancies without hypertension [60].

Summary and Conclusion

Hypertension is a major, but not inevitable maternal sign of placental problems, associated with impaired uteroplacental perfusion. It is primarily correlated with maternal arterial endothelial dysfunction, which is part of a larger problem of generalized vascular inflammation. It is caused by release of multiple factors from the placental syncytiotrophoblast surface, which is stressed by hypoxia or ischemia or both. sFLt-1 is an example of a factor increased by stress. PlGF is an example of the second type of response, which is diminished by stress. Both are considered potential biomarkers for preeclampsia. In many women, the markers combine to perturb maternal endothelial function and hence provoke hypertension, typical of preeclampsia. In other women, they indicate placental dysfunction that may occur with FGR only.

Two main causes of placental under-perfusion can be recognized. Very early failure of placentation results in abnormal spiral arteries, which perturbs placental growth and function from early in pregnancy and is associated with early-onset preeclampsia and FGR. Second, around term, the placenta begins to outgrow uterine capacity and becomes relatively under-perfused. This particularly happens with placental overgrowth associated with maternal obesity

Table 4.1 Placental lesions associated with preeclampsia, FGR, or both

Location of Lesion	Specific Lesion
Chorionic villi	Mal-development of the villous tree, distal villous hypoplasia Chronic villitis of unknown etiology
Spiral arteries	Deficient remodeling of spiral arteries Acute atherosis Spiral artery thrombosis
Placental lobule or part of lobule	Placental infarction
Syncytiotrophoblast	Excess syncytial knots Syncytiotrophoblast necrosis
Intervillous space	Perivillous fibrin deposition Placental floor infarction

and large placentas and correlates with late-onset preeclampsia, which typically is not associated with FGR. However more precise analysis reveals that at term, preeclampsia is associated with a small excess of LGA and SGA fetuses. The latter probably represent women affected by minor degrees of poor placentation.

At term, the circulating angiogenic biomarkers demonstrate that all pregnant women are beginning to develop a degree of STB stress. Hence the background of "normality" at this stage more closely resembles that of preeclampsia, which makes a preeclampsia diagnosis based on circulating biomarkers more difficult in late gestational ages.

Although CHT, GH, and preeclampsia all correlate with FGR, the placental dysfunction is probably not due to the hypertension itself, but to the underlying vascular inflammation.

Key Points

- The placenta is the cause of exacerbations of blood pressure associated with pregnancy.
- Abnormalities of uteroplacental blood supply can perturb placental function.
- The placental dysfunction can lead to FGR.
- The placental dysfunction stimulates release of several factors into the maternal circulation that disrupt endothelial function (of which hypertension is one sign).
- Hypertension and FGR tend to be correlated, but normotensive FGR also arises with the same placental pathology.
- Hypertension is not the direct cause, but the result of these problems.
- The placental pathology in FGR and preeclampsia is consistent with this view.
- Poor placentation leads to early problems and early-onset clinical disease.
- Placental "overgrowth" is a late event in pregnancy that causes relative under-perfusion of the placenta and late-onset preeclampsia disease.
- Late-onset preeclampsia is not associated with FGR, but there is a small excess of LGA babies and evidence for a minor degree of fetal hypoxemia in some smaller fetuses that are probably mildly undergrown.

References

1. Bramham K, Parnell B, Nelson-Piercy C, et al. Chronic hypertension and pregnancy outcomes: Systematic review and meta-analysis. *BMJ* 2014;348:g2301.

2. Dahlstrom BL, Engh ME, Bukholm G, et al. Changes in the prevalence of pre-eclampsia in Akershus County and the rest of Norway during the past 35 years. *Acta Obstet Gynecol Scand* 2006;85:916–21.

3. Klungsøyr K, Morken NH, Irgens L, Vollset SE, Skjaerven R. Secular trends in the epidemiology of pre-eclampsia throughout 40 years in Norway: Prevalence, risk factors and perinatal survival. *Paediatr Perinat Epidemiol* 2012;26:190–8.

4. Sibai BM. Diagnosis and management of gestational hypertension and reeclampsia. *Obstet Gynecol* 2003;102:181–92.

5. Saftlas AF, Olson DR, Franks AL, et al. Epidemiology of preeclampsia and eclampsia in the United States, 1979–1986. *Am J Obstet Gynecol* 1990;163:460–5.

6. Ananth CV, Vintzileos AM. Maternal-fetal conditions necessitating a medical intervention resulting in preterm birth. *Am J Obstet Gynecol* 2006;195:1557–63.

7. American College of Obstetricians and Gynecologists. Report of the American College of Obstetricians and Gynecologists' Task Force on Hypertension in Pregnancy. *Obstet Gynecol* 2013;122:1122–31.

8. Lowe SA, Brown MA, Dekker GA, et al. Guidelines for the management of hypertensive disorders of pregnancy 2008. *Aust N Z J Obstet Gynaecol* 2009;49:242–6.

9. Saudan P, Brown MA, Buddle ML et al. Does gestational hypertension become pre-eclampsia? *BJOG* 1998;105:1177–84.

10. Roberts CL, Algert CS, Morris JM, et al. Hypertensive disorders in pregnancy: A population-based study. *Med J Australia* 2005;182:332–5.

11. Macdonald-Wallis C, Tilling K, Fraser A, et al. Associations of blood pressure change in pregnancy with fetal growth and gestational age at delivery: Findings from a prospective cohort. *Hypertension* 2014;64:36–44.

12. Marin R, Gorostidi M, Portal CG, et al. Long-term prognosis of hypertension in pregnancy. *Hypertens Pregnancy* 2000;19:199–209.

13. Magnussen EB, Vatten LJ, Smith GD, Hypertensive disorders in pregnancy and subsequently measured cardiovascular risk factors. *Obstet Gynecol* 2009; 114:961–70.

14. Melamed N, Ray JG, Hladunewich M, et al. Gestational hypertension and preeclampsia: Are they the same disease? *J Obstet Gynaecol Can* 2014 Jul; 36(7):642–7.

15. Zetterström K, Lindeberg SN, Haglund B, et al. Chronic hypertension as a risk factor for offspring to be born small for gestational age. *Acta Obstet Gynecol Scand* 2006;85(9):1046–50.

16. Osol G, Moore LG. Maternal uterine vascular remodeling during pregnancy. *Microcirculation* 2014;21:38–47.

17. Burton GJ, Fowden A. The placenta: A multifaceted, transient organ. *Phil Trans R Soc* 2015;370(1663):20140066.

18. Nelson SH, Steinsland OS, Wang Y, et al. Increased nitric oxide synthase activity and expression in the human uterine artery during pregnancy. *Circ Res* 2000;87:406–11.

19. Burton GJ, Woods AW, Jauniaux E, et al. Rheological and physiological consequences of conversion of the maternal spiral arteries for uteroplacental blood flow during human pregnancy. *Placenta* 2009;30:473–82.

20. Gyselaers W, Mullens W, Tomsin K, et al. Role of dysfunctional maternal venous hemodynamics in the pathophysiology of pre-eclampsia: A review. *Ultrasound Obstet Gynecol* 2011;38:123–9.

21. Huppertz B. Placental origins of preeclampsia: Challenging the current hypothesis. *Hypertension* 2008;5:970–5.

22. Jauniaux E, Watson AL, Hempstock J, et al. Onset of maternal arterial blood flow and placental oxidative stress. A possible factor in human early pregnancy failure. *Am J Pathol* 2000;157:2111–22.

23. Burton GJ, Watson AL, Hempstock J, et al. Uterine glands provide histiotrophic nutrition for the human fetus during the first trimester of pregnancy. *J Clin Endocrinol Metab* 2002;87:2954–9.

24. Burton GJ, Jauniaux E, Charnock-Jones DS. The influence of the intrauterine environment on human placental development. *Int J Dev Biol* 2010;54:303–12.

25. Redman CW, Sargent IL. Latest advances in understanding preeclampsia. *Science* 2005;308:1592–4.

26. Moll W. Structure adaptation and blood flow control in the uterine arterial system after hemochorial placentation. *Eur J Obstet Gynecol Reprod Biol* 2003;110 Suppl 1:S19–27.

27. Redman CW. Current topic: Pre-eclampsia and the placenta. *Placenta* 1991;12:301–8.

28. Redman CW, Sargent IL, Staff AC. IFPA Senior Award Lecture: Making sense of pre-eclampsia – Two placental causes of preeclampsia? *Placenta* 2014;35 Suppl:S20–5.

29. Senft D, Ronai ZA. UPR, autophagy, and mitochondria crosstalk underlies the ER stress response. *Trends Biochem Sci* 2015 Feb 2. pii:S0968-0004(15)00003-1.

30. Burton GJ, Jauniaux E. Placental oxidative stress: From miscarriage to preeclampsia. *J Soc Gynecol Investig* 2004;11:342e52.

31. Roberts JM, Taylor RN, Musci TJ et al. Preeclampsia: An endothelial cell disorder. *Am J Obstet Gynecol* 1989;161:1200–4.

32. Redman CW, Sargent IL. Placental stress and pre-eclampsia: A revised view. *Placenta* 2009;30 Suppl A:S38–42.

33. Redman CW, Sargent IL. Pre-eclampsia, the placenta and the maternal systemic inflammatory response – a review. *Placenta* 2003;Suppl A:S21–7.

34. Sitia S, Tomasoni L, Atzeni F, et al. From endothelial dysfunction to atherosclerosis. *Autoimmun Rev* 2010;9:830–4.

35. Prieto D, Contreras C, Sánchez A. Endothelial dysfunction, obesity and insulin resistance. *Curr Vasc Pharmacol* 2014;12:412–26.

36. Maynard SE, Min JY, Merchan J, et al. Excess placental soluble fms-like tyrosine kinase 1 (sFlt1) may contribute to endothelial dysfunction, hypertension, and proteinuria in preeclampsia. *J Clin Invest* 2003;111:649e58.

37. De Falco S. The discovery of placenta growth factor and its biological activity. *Exp Mol Med* 2012;44:1–9.

38. Lankhorst S, Saleh L, Danser AJ, et al. Etiology of angiogenesis inhibition-related hypertension. *Curr Opin Pharmacol* 2014;21C:7–13.

39. LaMarca BD, Alexander BT, Gilbert JS, et al. Pathophysiology of hypertension in response to placental ischemia during pregnancy: A central role for endothelin? *Gend Med* 2008;5 Suppl A:S133–8.

40. Yung HW, Hemberger M, Watson ED, et al. Endoplasmic reticulum stress disrupts placental morphogenesis: Implications for human intrauterine growth restriction. *J Pathol* 2012;228:554–64.

41. Xiong X, Demianczuk NN, Saunders LD, et al. Impact of preeclampsia and gestational hypertension on birth weight by gestational age. *Am J Epidemiol* 2002;155:203–9.

42. Moore MP, Redman CW. Case-control study of severe pre-eclampsia of early onset. *Br Med J Clin Res Ed* 1983;287:580–3.

43. Lees C, Marlow N, Arabin B, et al. Perinatal morbidity and mortality in early-onset fetal growth restriction: Cohort outcomes of the

trial of randomized umbilical and fetal flow in Europe (TRUFFLE). *Ultrasound Obstet Gynecol* 2013;42:400–8.

44. Verlohren S1, Melchiorre K, Khalil A, et al. Uterine artery Doppler, birth weight and timing of onset of pre-eclampsia: Providing insights into the dual etiology of late-onset pre-eclampsia. *Ultrasound Obstet Gynecol* 2014;44:293–8.

45. Almog B, Shehata F, Aljabri S, et al. Placenta weight percentile curves for singleton and twins deliveries. *Placenta* 2011;32:58e62.

46. Norwitz ER, Snegovskikh VV, Caughey AB. Prolonged pregnancy: When should we intervene? *Clin Obstet Gynecol* 2007;50:547e57.

47. Caughey AB, Stotland NE, Escobar GJ. What is the best measure of maternal complications of term pregnancy: Ongoing pregnancies or pregnancies delivered? *Am J Obstet Gynecol* 2003;189:1047e52.

48. Jones CJ, Fox H. Ultrastructure of the placenta in prolonged pregnancy. *J Pathol* 1978;126:173e9.

49. Dahlstrøm B, Romundstad P, Øian P et al. Placenta weight in pre-eclampsia. *Acta Obstet Gynecol Scand* 2008;87:608e11.

50. Rasmussen S, Irgens LM, Espinoza J. Maternal obesity and excess of fetal growth in pre-eclampsia. *BJOG* 2014;121:1351–7.

51. Morales-Roselló J, Khalil A, Morlando M, et al. Changes in fetal Doppler indices as a marker of failure to reach growth potential at term. *Ultrasound Obstet Gynecol* 2014;43:303–10.

52. Redman CW, Jacobson S-L, Russell R. Hypertension in pregnancy. In Powrie RO, Greene ME, Camann W, eds. *Medical Disorders in Obstetric Practice*. Wiley-Blackwell, Chichester. 2010:153–81.

53. Lisonkova S, Joseph KS. Incidence of preeclampsia: Risk factors and outcomes associated with early- versus late-onset disease. *Am J Obstet Gynecol* 2013;209:544.e1–544.e12.

54. Redman CW, Sargent IL. Immunology of pre-eclampsia. *Am J Reprod Immunol* 2010;63:534–43.

55. Cotechini T, Komisarenko M, Sperou A, et al. Inflammation in rat pregnancy inhibits spiral artery remodeling leading to fetal growth restriction and features of preeclampsia. *J Exp Med* 2014;211:165–79.

56. Whitley GS, Dash PR, Ayling LJ, Prefumo F, Thilaganathan B, Cartwright JE. Increased apoptosis in first trimester extravillous trophoblasts from pregnancies at higher risk of developing preeclampsia. *Am J Pathol* 2007;170:1903–9.

57. Melchiorre K, Sutherland G, Sharma R, Nanni M, Thilaganathan B. Mid-gestational maternal cardiovascular profile in preterm and term pre-eclampsia: A prospective study. *BJOG* 2013;120:496–504.

58. Parks WT. Placental hypoxia: The lesions of maternal malperfusion. *Semin Perinatol* 2015;39:9–19.

59. Fitzgerald B, Levytska K, Kingdom J, et al. Villous trophoblast abnormalities in extremely preterm deliveries with elevated second trimester maternal serum hCG or inhibin-A. *Placenta* 2011;32:339–45.

60. Staff AC, Dechend R, Pijnenborg R. Learning from the placenta: Acute atherosis and vascular remodeling in preeclampsia-novel aspects for atherosclerosis and future cardiovascular health. *Hypertension* 2010;56:1026–34.

Chapter 5

Assisted Reproduction Techniques (ART) and Fetal Growth

Christoph Brezinka and Shirin Khanjani

Infertility is extremely prevalent, with one in seven couples experiencing difficulty in conceiving. Assisted reproduction techniques (ART) have therefore become increasingly popular. In 2011, 2% of all babies born in the UK were conceived through in vitro fertilization (IVF). In 2013, in the UK, 49,636 women had a total of 64,600 cycles of IVF or intra-cytoplasmic sperm injection (ICSI). The live birth rate after IVF has increased from 14% per cycle in 1991 to 25% in 2011 [1,2].

In a normal, unaided cycle, one follicle matures – and in "natural-cycle" IVF, this single follicle is then retrieved in the hope of obtaining a viable oocyte on which to perform IVF or ICSI. However, to improve success rates, most ART procedures are performed using protocols to induce multi-follicular growth, mostly with the use of gonadotropins (i.e., FSH, hMG).

Studies have suggested a higher prevalence of pregnancy complications in women with subfertility irrespective of the infertility treatment received (i.e., IVF, ICSI, IUI, and ovulation induction) [3–6]. Many studies have shown a significant association between receiving fertility treatment and having preterm neonates and/or babies born small for gestational age (SGA) [7]. Probable causes have been discussed in the literature, including higher incident of multiple pregnancies, maternal factors such as placental insufficiency, and genetic predisposition [8]. A study from Denmark showed that singletons born after intrauterine insemination (IUI) had higher risk of adverse perinatal outcomes compared with spontaneous conception. Stimulation with clomiphene citrate was associated with a higher risk of SGA compared with natural-cycle IUI. Interestingly, follicle-stimulating hormone (FSH) treatment did not seem to be associated with adverse outcomes [9]. Alarming, a prospective study of 20,166 singleton pregnancies published in 2010 showed that women who conceived through ART had an increased risk of stillbirth compared to

women who conceived naturally. This correlation was not explained by confounding factors, suggesting that the increased risk of stillbirth can be a result of the fertility treatment or unknown factors relating to couples who undergo ART [10].

There is an increased incidence of multiple pregnancies with ART, and this explains most of the pregnancy complications. A recent study showed no increase in maternal or fetal complications in dizygotic twins conceived through ART compared to dizygotic twins conceived naturally [11]. The introduction of elective single embryo transfer has significantly reduced the rate of pregnancy complications [12].

Singleton IVF pregnancies in nulliparous women over 35 years of age have been associated with higher rates of caesarean section, preterm births, and infants of lower average birth weight, but the risk is similar between the women who conceived spontaneously compared to women undergoing ART [13]. Interesting, a recent study showed that although singleton conceptions after ART result in higher maternal and neonatal complications, the impact of maternal age is more pronounced with spontaneous conception [14].

Ovarian hyperstimulation syndrome (OHSS) is a condition that presents with significantly enlarged ovaries and third-space fluid accumulation and that affects 1% of all stimulated cycles. A study published in 2010 showed that singleton pregnancies affected by OHSS exhibited an increased risk of low birth weight by 40% [15]. In the absence of clinical OHSS, ART pregnancies conceived with elevated estradiol levels (E2 >3950 pg/l) on the day of hCG administration had higher rates of preeclampsia and SGA by nine and four fold, respectively, compared to women undergoing ART with E2 levels <3950 pg/l. The authors of this chapter argue that estradiol-induced changes in trophoblast maturation can lead to changes in placental function [16]. The possible association between

OHSS and/or markedly elevated estradiol levels at the time of ET and adverse perinatal outcome was studied in a large registry-based study of more than 30,000 singletons born after ART. Low birth weight in newborns (but not preterm delivery) was more likely when fresh embryos were transferred and less likely when frozen embryos were used. The more physiological milieu in the uterus at the time of implantation of cryopreserved as opposed to freshly retrieved blastocysts was discussed as a possible cause [17]. Data associating OHSS and the hormonal environment at the time of embryo transfer with pregnancy outcome are blurred by the fact that OHSS is more frequent and more severe in twin pregnancies, which by themselves contribute greatly to the overall morbidity of ART pregnancies.

Embryo quality based on morphokinetic analysis has been the subject of heated debate among fertility specialists. It's been generally accepted that transferring "good-quality embryos" increases chances of pregnancy and reduces the risk of miscarriage. However, a recent study showed that embryo quality is not significantly associated with pregnancy complications [18]. Embryo vitrification and frozen embryo transfer cycles have become increasingly popular. A population-based cohort study showed that singleton babies born after transfer of vitrified blastocysts compared with singletons born after transfer of fresh blastocysts were at 33% and 40% less risk of low birth weight and SGA, respectively [19]. Another study from Japan showed that vitrification of embryos did not increase the incidence of adverse neonatal outcomes or birth defects following single embryo transfer [20].

Gene expression and histology of the placenta in ART pregnancies has been extensively studied. In a study from Norway, more than half a million spontaneously conceived pregnancies were compared with 8,529 singleton pregnancies arising from ART: mean birth weight of the newborns was lower in the ART group, but these babies had bigger and heavier placentae than those from spontaneous conceptions. The authors argue since the endometrium in subfertile women provides a suboptimal environment for implantation and development of the blastocyst, this might necessitate a compensatory growth of the placenta, once implantation is successful [21]. In a Dutch-French study, genome-wide mRNA expression analysis was performed in placentae from ART pregnancies and from naturally conceived pregnancies.

Up-regulation of several biological pathways, among them two growth-inhibitory genes, was a significant feature of altered gene expression in the ART placentae [22]. However, the authors found no difference in birth weight between the ART babies and the spontaneously conceived cohort. Comparing intrauterine growth in several species, it was found that a period of fetal growth restriction up until mid-pregnancy is followed by accelerated fetal growth and increased placental size toward the end of gestation [23]. A clearly biphasic growth pattern was observed in calf fetuses conceived by ART that had smaller size on ultrasound biometry in early pregnancy but higher birth weights at the end of their 285-day gestation than spontaneously conceived controls. The placentomes of ART calf fetuses showed increased thickness and diameter [24]. Ultra-structural analysis of human placentae from ART pregnancies showed terminal villi with degenerative alterations, a decrease in apical microvilli, and more vacuoles than in placentae from spontaneously conceived pregnancies. This could reflect disturbances during the establishment of the placental blood barrier, leading to intrauterine growth restriction [25].

In the largest study to date, a significant correlation between an increase in congenital malformations and a decreased paternal sperm count was observed [26]. Subfertility is associated with a higher risk of imprinting disorder in offspring, and, in the next generation, subfertility is one of the consequences of imprinting disorders, irrespective of mode of conception [27]. Rare imprinting disorders, particularly Beckwith-Widemann syndrome (an overgrowth syndrome) and Angelman syndrome, appear more frequently after ART conceptions [28]. Imprinting disorders like Russel-Silver (which leads to severe FGR) and Prader-Willi do not show an association with ART; however, more epidemiological studies are needed [29]. In a large Danish study, Zhu and colleagues found that couples who had taken more than 12 months to conceive had the same, slightly elevated rate of congenital malformations in their offspring, as those with ART pregnancies, leading to the conclusion that "the underlying disease is more important than the treatment" [30].

Conclusions

Advanced maternal age, a long history of infertility, and medical conditions causing infertility among

Table 5.1 Key references studying assisted reproduction and fetal growth restriction

Study	Population	Findings
Perinatal outcome of singleton pregnancies following in vitro fertilization	634 pregnancies	Singletons from IVF/ICSI pregnancies have poorer perinatal outcome [3]
Obstetric outcome of singleton pregnancies after IVF: a matched control study in four Dutch university hospitals	307 IVF compared with 307 control pregnancies	The proportion of SGA was significantly higher in the IVF group [4]
Differential effect of mode of conception and infertility treatment on fetal growth and prematurity	200 fertile and 748 infertile	Higher prevalence of pregnancy complications in infertile women irrespective of receiving infertility treatment [7]
Perinatal outcomes in 6,338 singletons born after intrauterine insemination in Denmark, 2007 to 2012: the influence of ovarian stimulation	6,338 singletons	Singletons born after IUI had higher risk of adverse perinatal outcomes compared with natural conception children [9]
Dizygotic twin pregnancies after medically assisted reproduction and after natural conception: maternal and perinatal outcomes	6,694 Dizygotic twin pregnancies	Maternal and perinatal risks are similar for twin pregnancies conceived after ART and after natural conception [11]
Neonatal outcome of IVF singletons versus naturally conceived in women aged 35 years and over	283 IVF, 283 matched natural conception	No difference in neonatal outcomes between IVF and natural conception groups [13]
Ovarian stimulation and low birth weight in newborns conceived through in vitro fertilization	56,792	The ovarian stimulation-induced maternal environment can represent an independent mediator contributing to the risk of low birth weight [17]

other impairments, as well as a high rate of multiple and higher multiple pregnancies, all lead to ART pregnancies having higher-risk pregnancies by all criteria from premature deliveries and underweight newborns to birth defects (Table 5.1). It is difficult to tease out the effect of ART from the other clinical factors pertaining to the pregnancy. Patterns observed in ART in animal models may provide helpful insights and analogies; however, primate and particularly human pregnancy preclude easy comparisons with animals with different uteri, placentae and fertility [31]. One must always keep in mind that without ART – with rare exceptions – these pregnancies would not have come into being at all.

Key Points

- Pregnancies conceived from ART are at higher risk of pregnancy complications, particularly multiple pregnancies. These are at much higher risk of fetal growth restriction.
- There is no clear evidence as to whether ART per se is associated with a higher incidence of SGA or FGR.

- Imprinting disorders may lead to excessive or reduced fetal growth: these may be more common in ART-conceived pregnancies.

References

1. (HFEA), H.F.a.E.A. *Fertility Treatment in 2013: Facts and Figures.*

2. O'Flynn N. Assessment and treatment for people with fertility problems: NICE guideline. *Br J Gen Pract* 2014;64(618):50–1.

3. Stojnic J, et al. Perinatal outcome of singleton pregnancies following in vitro fertilization. *Clin Exp Obstet Gynecol* 2013;40(2):277–83.

4. Koudstaal J, et al. Obstetric outcome of singleton pregnancies after IVF: a matched control study in four Dutch university hospitals. *Hum Reprod* 2000;15(8):1819–25.

5. Wang JX et al. The obstetric outcome of singleton pregnancies following in-vitro fertilization/gamete intra-fallopian transfer. *Hum Reprod* 1994;9(1):141–6.

6. Doyle P, Beral V, Maconochie N. Preterm delivery, low birthweight and small-for-gestational-age in liveborn singleton babies resulting from in-vitro fertilization. *Hum Reprod* 1992;7(3):425–8.

7. Valenzuela-Alcaraz B, et al. Differential effect of mode of conception and infertility treatment on fetal growth and prematurity. *J Matern Fetal Neonatal Med* 2016:1–6.

8. Kondapalli LA, Perales-Puchalt A. Low birth weight: Is it related to assisted reproductive technology or underlying infertility? *Fertil Steril* 2013. 99(2):303–10.

9. Malchau SS, et al. Perinatal outcomes in 6,338 singletons born after intrauterine insemination in Denmark, 2007 to 2012: The influence of ovarian stimulation. *Fertil Steril* 2014;102(4):1110–16 e2.

10. Wisborg K, Ingerslev HJ, Henriksen TB. IVF and stillbirth: A prospective follow-up study. *Hum Reprod* 2010;25(5):1312–16.

11. Bensdorp AJ, et al. Dizygotic twin pregnancies after medically assisted reproduction and after natural conception: Maternal and perinatal outcomes. *Fertil Steril* 2016.

12. Takeshima K, et al. Impact of single embryo transfer policy on perinatal outcomes in fresh and frozen cycles-analysis of the Japanese Assisted Reproduction Technology registry between 2007 and 2012. *Fertil Steril* 2016;105(2):337–46 e3.

13. Tomic V, Tomic J. Neonatal outcome of IVF singletons versus naturally conceived in women aged 35 years and over. *Arch Gynecol Obstet* 2011;284(6)1411–16.

14. Wennberg AL, et al. Effect of maternal age on maternal and neonatal outcomes after assisted reproductive technology. *Fertil Steril* 2016.

15. Luke B, et al. Factors associated with ovarian hyperstimulation syndrome (OHSS) and its effect on assisted reproductive technology (ART) treatment and outcome. *Fertil Steril* 2010;94(4):1399–404.

16. Imudia AN, et al. Peak serum estradiol level during controlled ovarian hyperstimulation is associated with increased risk of small for gestational age and preeclampsia in singleton pregnancies after in vitro fertilization. *Fertil Steril* 2012;97(6):1374–9.

17. Kalra SK, et al. Ovarian stimulation and low birth weight in newborns conceived through in vitro fertilization. *Obstet Gynecol* 2011;118(4):863–71.

18. Zhu J, et al. Does IVF cleavage stage embryo quality affect pregnancy complications and neonatal outcomes in singleton gestations after double embryo transfers? *J Assist Reprod Genet* 2014;31(12):1635–41.

19. Li Z, et al. Clinical outcomes following cryopreservation of blastocysts by vitrification or slow freezing: A population-based cohort study. *Hum Reprod* 2014;29(12):2794–801.

20. Kato O, et al. Neonatal outcome and birth defects in 6623 singletons born following minimal ovarian stimulation and vitrified versus fresh single embryo transfer. *Eur J Obstet Gynecol Reprod Biol* 2012;161(1):46–50.

21. Haavaldsen C, Tanbo T, Eskild A. Placental weight in singleton pregnancies with and without assisted reproductive technology: a population study of 536,567 pregnancies. *Hum Reprod* 2012;27(2):576–82.

22. Nelissen EC, et al. Altered gene expression in human placentas after IVF/ICSI. *Hum Reprod* 2014;29(12):2821–31.

23. Bloise E, Feuer SK, Rinaudo PF. Comparative intrauterine development and placental function of ART concepti: Implications for human reproductive medicine and animal breeding. *Hum Reprod Update* 2014;20(6):822–39.

24. Bertolini M, et al. Morphology and morphometry of in vivo- and in vitro-produced bovine concepti from early pregnancy to term and association with high birth weights. *Theriogenology* 2002;58(5):973–94.

25. Zhang Y, et al. Ultrastructural study on human placentae from women subjected to assisted reproductive technology treatments. *Biol Reprod* 2011;85(3):635–42.

26. Bonduelle M, et al. Prenatal testing in ICSI pregnancies: Incidence of chromosomal anomalies in 1586 karyotypes and relation to sperm parameters. *Hum Reprod* 2002;17(10):2600–14.

27. Whitelaw N, et al. Epigenetic status in the offspring of spontaneous and assisted conception. *Hum Reprod* 2014;29(7):1452–8.

28. Allen C, Reardon W. Assisted reproduction technology and defects of genomic imprinting. *BJOG* 2005;112(12):1589–94.

29. Dupont C, Sifer C. A review of outcome data concerning children born following assisted reproductive technologies. *ISRN Obstet Gynecol* 2012:405382.

30. Zhu JL, et al. Infertility, infertility treatment, and congenital malformations: Danish national birth cohort. *BMJ* 2006;333(7570):679.

31. Sanchez-Calabuig MJ, et al. Potential health risks associated to ICSI: Insights from animal models and strategies for a safe procedure. *Front Public Health* 2014;2:241.

6 Fetal Growth Restriction Study Design and Outcomes

Hans Wolf and J. W. Ganzevoort

Introduction

Fetal growth restriction (FGR) is a frequent complication of pregnancy with considerable impact on mothers and their infants. Notwithstanding this, knowledge regarding the cause, prevention, the timely detection, or treatment is limited and the number of studies addressing these topics is small. In the Current Controlled Trials Register, only four ongoing or planned trials concerning FGR are detected (three for treatment for FGR with Low Molecular Weight Heparin, sildenafil or allopurinol, and one for smoking cessation among pregnant women with nicotine replacement therapy). Apparently, current research concerning FGR is inadequate.

Cause

Research to explore the underlying cause (ischemic placental disease) touches genetics, immunology, and molecular changes as possible mechanisms. Although associations have been detected, the underlying mechanisms have not been discovered. A major difficulty in basic research is the lack of a proper animal model for growth restriction as human placentation differs widely from placentation in other species.

Prevention

Prevention of FGR from ischemic placental disease is unavailable. Possible preventive treatments such as low-dose aspirin, calcium supplementation, or specific nutritional supplementation have not proven effective for general use. This is in contrast with other causes for fetuses to be small for gestational age (SGA). The most common cause for SGA is smoking, and the well-known measure is smoking cessation [1]. Furthermore, women are advised on proper nutrition and to take measures to reduce the risk for toxoplasmosis and cytomegalovirus infection during pregnancy.

Timely Detection

Studies on prediction of FGR during the first trimester have targeted hormonal assays used for prenatal assessment for the risk of chromosomal abnormalities, uterine artery Doppler measurement, and maternal cardiovascular parameters (blood pressure or cardiac output) [2]. However, in multiparous women, previous obstetric history is an even stronger predictor [3]. As effective prevention is not available, there is no use for predictive tests in this respect, although, given the difficulty we have in timely diagnosing FGR, it might be useful to define a high-risk group for more extensive antenatal surveillance than standard care.

Diagnosis of FGR in the second or third trimester is hampered by the lack of precision of the available methods (palpation and sonographic biometry) and by the fact that FGR is a dynamic process that cannot be diagnosed by one observation of a fetal size smaller than average. Not all small-for-size fetuses are growth restricted, and only those with ischemic placental disease are at risk for hypoxia, acidosis, and death and need surveillance and possibly early delivery. Fetal Doppler has proven helpful to discriminate those fetuses at risk, but does not help selection in an unselected population [4,5].

Interventions

The decision for early delivery of a FGR fetus is usually based on cardiotocography and fetal Doppler. The cut-off limits for these measurements have been determined by "experience" from cohort studies. Only three studies explored if early delivery was useful and at which cut-off long-term infant outcome could be best (Digitat, GRIT, TRUFFLE) [6–8]. Outcomes of these studies suggest a more expectant approach with FGR in the late preterm to early term period and to a management combining the use of strict computerized cardiotocography criteria with ductus venosus Doppler measurement in the early preterm period.

Study Design – General Considerations

Ask the Right Question

Each study starts with a clinical question. In daily practice, we may be so overwhelmed by the magnitude of our clinical work that we do not realize that the underlying foundation of many things that we do is flimsy. It takes an open mind to realize this uncertainty instead of going with the flow of a daily routine. Subsequently, it is a challenge to ask the proper questions and form a hypothesis to be studied. This hypothesis needs clear and unambiguous formulation.

Define What Is Already Known

Before engaging in a new study, a search for relevant publications should be done to see if others have not already solved the question. If there are more studies available, it may be appropriate to combine results in a meta-analysis. Meta-analysis can be very challenging if entry criteria, interventions, or endpoints are not completely similar. Furthermore, publication bias may be significant, as some studies may not be registered in PubMed or not be published at all. Especially small studies may be published only when results were positive while negative results may remain unpublished, thereby exaggerating the effects [9]. A good example of this bias can be seen in the many meta-analyses of low-dose aspirin for the prevention of preeclampsia. A plot of number of study participants on the Y-axis to the odds ratio of the effect of the study on the X-axis (Forrest plot) shows a highly skewed pattern where all the small trials are to the far left, showing a far higher effect than the large trials, while there is only one small trial without effect [10].

Obtaining all the study databases in a meta-analysis of individual patient data (IPD) may allow better analysis because now adjustment for relevant clinical parameters can be done. Often high-quality studies will include their data, while low-quality studies do not. If a thorough literature search cannot answer the question, and the clinical relevance is strong enough, a new study is appropriate.

Use Internationally Agreed Definitions

It is of paramount importance to have an international agreement on the definitions of the population to be studied (see also Chapter 2). It allows for adequate comparison of studies and their outcomes. Currently, there is some agreement to which cut-offs of parameters of fetal growth should be used, but this predominantly defines small for gestational age (SGA), rather than strict FGR. All research in FGR is hampered by the difficulty to discriminate between fetuses that are small for their gestational age without any pathology and growth-restricted fetuses that are at risk for malnutrition, hypoxia, acidosis, and death due to placental ischemic disease. To discriminate between SGA and FGR, additional parameters should be used like longitudinal growth pattern and Doppler flow measurement of uterine and fetal blood vessels. Cut-off values for these parameters are available from internationally accepted population studies providing a percentile distribution.

Use Internationally Agreed Outcomes

Not only should the study population be defined according to internationally agreed standards, the same holds true for the choice of outcomes. It is important to determine which outcomes are most meaningful and which are adequate surrogates. This can be done under the umbrella of the CROWN-initiative [11]. In this light, the relevance of long-term follow-up cannot be stressed enough. Fetal growth restriction and malnutrition may have long-term effects on health and disease [12]. Advantages or disadvantages in the short term may be different in the long term.

Engage in (Inter)national Collaboration

The time has gone where single centers can successfully perform relevant studies, specifically in the field of clinical studies. The required sample sizes are too big, and the expertise of a single center to meet all demands of clinical trials is too limited. Small, underpowered studies should not be performed. They contribute to publication bias, as negative results of small studies will often not be published.

If the ambition is to perform adequately sized trials on meaningful outcomes that have good internal and external validity, it is highly recommended to perform these in collaboration. Trials performed in collaborative networks can be performed at lower costs, in a shorter time, and have more meaningful outcome results and make successful implementation more likely [13].

There are more arguments for collaboration that include cross-pollination, the improvement of academic thinking, and enjoyment. This is even more so if studies are performed in international networks, although these constructs do have more challenges. In those circumstances, it may also be an option to perform separate trials on a national level with identical criteria and outcomes, with a specific intent to perform individual participant data meta-analysis, a prospective IPD.

Combining efforts in such a manner is strongly advised. It should become far more honorable to be a member of a large study group than to be the first author of an underpowered study.

Study Design – Specific Considerations

Use Appropriate Study Designs

Specifically in FGR it is not only important to evaluate the proposed interventions, but more so to evaluate the combinations of screening or diagnostic tools with interventions. Both screening and diagnosis are uncertain in the absence of a gold standard for FGR. Any study that aims to determine the efficacy of a diagnostic method, treatment, or management should be designed as a randomized study. Case control or cohort studies may be used for the development of a hypothesis or an intervention limit, but further proof should come from randomized designs.

Choose Relevant Targets

Possible useful studies could aim at improved diagnosis during pregnancy (e.g., routine three-weekly biometry combined with fetal Doppler versus standard care), and at improving fetal monitoring during pregnancy as condition is more important than growth. Studies for prevention or treatment may focus on medication that affects vascular tone (like sildenafil or NO donors) to improve placenta circulation. Preventive medication should be harmless as many women with FGR cannot be recognized by screening and thus universal treatment might be more effective than treatment targeting risk indicators. Continuation of research early in pregnancy for parameters associated with the development of FGR may combine maternal cardiovascular parameters (blood pressure, cardiac output), uterine Doppler measurement, 3D sonographic volume measurement, and hormonal assays as these parameters could independently be attributed to FGR risk.

Choose the Relevant Population

Inclusion criteria should be so specific that after completion of the trial the study results can be applied properly and time-independent to the right group of patients. A criterion like "suspicion of growth restriction" is insufficient as suspicions or beliefs change with time and may be different by the time the study is completed. Thus, if one wants to include women with a pregnancy complicated by FGR, one should use fetal biometry and Doppler criteria.

For a prediction or treatment study, inclusion should be random and not influenced because cases are recruited from a university outpatient clinic or an antenatal diagnosis clinic that will have a selected population.

Informed consent is a standard part of study recruitment. Information should be in writing and explained orally. It is very useful to appoint a person specifically to help clinicians in study recruitment, to ensure that no eligible cases are missed, that the study is performed properly, and that the necessary data are entered. A research nurse is ideal for this.

All cases who refuse participation should be registered with at least the parameters necessary for inclusion to determine afterward if participating cases are similar to nonparticipating cases and preclude selection bias.

Design Adequate Randomization

Randomization should be "anonymous" by computer. It is easiest to generate random number lists with trial allocation before a study starts as random number generators in computers are not completely random in starting the process. Stratification might be useful to prevent randomization inequality for parameters that are thought to be very important for study outcome, like gestational age. For power issues, the stratification instrument should not be used lightly and is not necessary in larger studies as the randomization process should then result in equal groups. Randomization methods that are sensitive to manipulation, like sealed envelopes, throwing of coins, or alternate dates should not be used.

Use a Well-Described Intervention

The intervention or the criteria on which to perform an intervention should be described explicitly and exactly in a way that others can act identically as the partakers in the study. For instance, it is better to specify a cut-off for fetal heart rate short-term variation or for fetal Doppler than to decide on an intervention for a clinical suspicion of fetal distress. Suspicions and beliefs change and could be different by the time the study is completed.

Although deviations from study protocol should be absent, in reality, clinicians always find reasons to diverge from a protocol. Possible deviations from protocol should be described in advance and criteria to allow this should be specified. The randomization groups should be managed identically except for the intervention to be studied, and this intervention should consist of a single action and not of a complex strategy.

Data Entry

The database should be located on a secure website, both for entry of the data necessary for randomization and the study data. The program should control for "unlikely" data entries, and randomization may be allowed only after all criteria are met. Frequent warnings should be sent for absent or incomplete data. Records should be locked after completion and mutations allowed only through the database supervisor. Many clinical studies are not blinded, and it is useful to enter the follow-up data in a separate database to prevent the person performing follow-up being influenced by observing trial data.

If data can be obtained from primary databases (e.g., for laboratory or ultrasound data), then it may prevent transcription errors by using the primary data. The study website should then enable data upload. It takes careful consideration to decide which data have to be collected. Ideally, one would like to know "everything," but the time needed for extensive data entry may preclude this.

Outcome

The outcome of a study should be the clinically most relevant observation that can be obtained, and it should be possible to measure this unbiased. Intermediate measurement data like Doppler results or biochemical test results are far less relevant as a study outcome. Generally, one primary and a number of secondary endpoints are defined.

As in modern obstetrics long-term maternal sequelae are unlikely, most obstetric intervention studies will target neonatal outcome. Perinatal mortality is a clear outcome, but usually the frequency of this is insufficient for significant statistical calculation. Because severe morbidity and mortality are associated, they are often combined as a composite outcome, although the impact is quite different. If both point in the same direction, this use of a composite endpoint is defensible, but if they do not, interpretation becomes difficult.

For a rare outcome like mortality, specification might be useful to determine if death is specifically associated with conditions in the intervention arm where it occurred or if it could have happened just as well in the other study arm.

Although there is some association between severe neonatal morbidity and later development, this association is not strong. Using neonatal morbidity as a primary outcome may over- or underestimate effects. A good example is the ORACLE trial, where antibiotic treatment after preterm pre-labor rupture of membranes reduced neonatal morbidity, while at the age of 2 years no differences were observed between groups [14]. The opposite was found in the TRUFFLE trial, where severe neonatal morbidity was similar between groups, but less impaired neurodevelopment was observed in surviving infants at the age of 2 years [7]. Generally, a developmental score after 2 or more years can be considered more relevant than short-term outcome as it is associated better with long-term health and the ability to become self-supporting when an adult. Intervention studies should always plan long-term follow-up, notwithstanding the fact that this is time-consuming and increases the costs of a study.

Study Performance

Study performance should be monitored closely. It may be advisable to visit the participating centers at regular intervals to check protocol adherence and data compliance and to hold regular meetings of all persons involved in the execution of the trial. Appointing a research nurse for the study locally will make it more likely to recruit all eligible cases and perform the study appropriately.

Safety

All studies should have medical ethics approval and should be registered in a trials register. Adverse events should be registered, and at regular intervals, study data should be overlooked by a safety committee.

Follow-Up

As specified earlier, long-term follow-up data should be used for intervention studies. Care should be taken not to lose participants. After 2 years, many will have moved, and finding them could be difficult or impossible. It is useful to ask consent at inclusion for later request of medical information, because an attending pediatrician or gynecologist may have the new address of the participant. A mailing with some information regarding study progress or a birthday card may make the participant remember the study and may induce the sending of a new address card.

Statistics – Exclusion

Study results should remain unknown until the end of the study, except to the monitoring committee, who should mainly focus on safety. All statistical analyses should have been decided before the data become available, and preferably all tables are designed beforehand. It is advisable to assign a person who does not participate in the study performance to supervise statistical analysis as this person will have less preference for either randomization allocation.

Primary analysis should be based on intention to treat – once a participant is included he/she can never leave the trial, even if he/she refuses further participation after randomization. Only after primary analysis may certain cases with incomplete management or incomplete data be excluded.

Cases lost to follow-up should be compared for entry criteria to the complete cases to exclude selection bias. Imputation could be used to complete missing data.

Publication

It is an obligation to publish any randomized trial with sufficient power, irrespective of outcome. Nonpublication of negative results is unethical because it may prolong the use of harmful or inane treatments.

Key Points

- Though the definition of fetal growth restriction varies between different countries, recent large studies have converged towards one based on biometry and Doppler.

- Use of a well defined intervention with a realistic estimate of an effect size is crucial.

- Designing a study around a common outcome datasets will allow easier comparison, facilitating meta analysis and individual patient data analysis.

- International collaborations and recruitment improve the generalizability of results.

Conclusion

Clinical research is time-consuming and demands a large effort from all participants. For effective research, multicenter cooperation is necessary to ensure that study size is large enough for conclusive results. The reward of participating in a large multicenter trial will usually not be worldwide fame, but the fun of regular contact with likeminded colleagues should be sufficient compensation.

References

1. Magee BD, Hattis D, Kivel NM. Role of smoking in low birth weight. *J Reprod Med* 2004;49(1):23–7.

2. Akolekar R, Syngelaki A, Poon L, Wright D, Nicolaides KH. Competing risks model in early screening for preeclampsia by biophysical and biochemical markers. *Fetal Diagn Ther* 2013;33(1):8–15.

3. Ananth CV, Peltier MR, Chavez MR, Kirby RS, Getahun D, Vintzileos AM. Recurrence of ischemic placental disease. *Obstet Gynecol* 2007;110(1):128–33.

4. Alfirevic Z, Stampalija T, Gyte GM. Fetal and umbilical Doppler ultrasound in normal pregnancy. *Cochrane Database Syst Rev* 2010;(8):CD001450.

5. Alfirevic Z, Milan SJ, Livio S. Caesarean section versus vaginal delivery for preterm birth in singletons. *Cochrane Database Syst Rev* 2013;9:CD000078.

6. Boers KE, Vijgen SM, Bijlenga D, van der Post JA, Bekedam DJ, Kwee A, et al. Induction versus expectant monitoring for intrauterine growth restriction at term: Randomised equivalence trial (DIGITAT). *BMJ* 2010;341:c7087.

7. Lees C, Marlow N, Van Wassenaer A, et al. The Trial of Randomized Umbilical and Fetal Flow in Europe (TRUFFLE) study: Two year neurodevelopmental and intermediate perinatal outcomes. *Lancet* 2015;385:2162–72.

8. Thornton JG, Hornbuckle J, Vail A, Spiegelhalter DJ, Levene M. Infant wellbeing at 2 years of age in the Growth Restriction Intervention Trial

(GRIT): Multicentred randomised controlled trial. *Lancet* 2004;364(9433):513–20.

9. Egger M, Juni P, Bartlett C, Holenstein F, Sterne J. How important are comprehensive literature searches and the assessment of trial quality in systematic reviews? Empirical study. *Health Technol Assess* 2003;7(1):1–76.

10. Friedman AM, Cleary KL. Prediction and prevention of ischemic placental disease. *Semin Perinatol* 2014;38(3):177–82.

11. Khan K. The CROWN initiative: Journal editors invite researchers to develop core outcomes in women's health. *Obstet Gynecol* 2014;124(3):487–8.

12. Wadhwa PD, Buss C, Entringer S, Swanson JM. Developmental origins of health and disease: Brief history of the approach and current focus on epigenetic mechanisms. *Semin Reprod Med* 2009;27(5):358–68.

13. Moss AJ, Francis CW, Ryan D. Collaborative clinical trials. *N Engl J Med* 2011;364(9):789–91.

14. Kenyon S, Pike K, Jones DR, Brocklehurst P, Marlow N, Salt A, et al. Childhood outcomes after prescription of antibiotics to pregnant women with preterm rupture of the membranes: 7-year follow-up of the ORACLE I trial. *Lancet* 2008;372(9646):1310–18.

Analysis of National and International Guidelines on Placental–Fetal Growth Restriction

Gemma Malin, Lesley McCowan, K. E. Boers, and Jim G. Thornton

Introduction

Neither diagnosis nor management of fetal growth restriction is straightforward. Serial symphysio-fundal height measurement is commonly used as a screening tool in the general obstetric population. Observational studies have reported that plotting serial measurements of fundal height on customized growth charts doubles the detection of small-for-gestational age fetuses with detection rates of approximately 50% [1,2]. Ultrasound measurement of fetal biometry is moderately accurate in predicting fetal weight [3–5]. but to date routine third trimester scanning has not been associated with reduced perinatal morbidity or mortality [6]. Umbilical artery and ductus venosus Doppler, along with reduced short-term fetal heart rate variability on computerized CTG, has been correlated with fetal hypoxemia [7–9]. However, few of the screening or diagnostic tests for the fetal effects of growth restriction have been evaluated for prediction of substantive adverse outcomes, death, or brain damage. With the notable exception of umbilical artery Doppler waveforms [10], most reported test-accuracy studies have been susceptible to treatment paradox.

Timed delivery is the only current intervention likely to have a significant effect on rates of perinatal death and brain damage. Although it may prevent stillbirth, it also has the potential to do harm by adding the effects of premature birth to the existing problems of growth restriction. The optimum timing of delivery depends on both the severity of fetal growth restriction (FGR) and the degree of prematurity.

Fortunately, there have been some trials of timed delivery [11–15]. However, the GRIT study has been difficult to interpret for two reasons. First, the entry criterion of clinician uncertainty, while ethically mandated, may have restricted participation to women who could not benefit from either immediate or deferred delivery. Second, no clear guidelines for delivery were mandated for participants in the control arm. This latter problem was avoided in the TRUFFLE trial [16], where criteria for delivery were defined in all three arms, albeit not always followed.

The DIGITAT trial of timed delivery for growth restriction at term was easier to interpret because policies for both groups were defined. However, it was too small to show the effect of either policy on substantive adverse fetal outcomes; there were no fetal or neonatal deaths in either arm [14].

In the absence of clear trial evidence, clinicians are forced to follow expert opinion from textbooks, review articles, and guidelines. However, the content of national guidelines regarding the management of FGR has inconsistencies. The aim of this chapter was to review and compare existing guidance.

Methods

We searched PubMed and Google for national guidelines on the diagnosis and management of fetal growth restriction. Guidelines were included if they had the backing of a national obstetric and gynecological society, and had been developed by consultation with a committee or similar structure of experts. Guidelines prepared by single authors or by small groups of self-selected authors, even if acting for a national specialist organization, were not included.

Each guideline was read by the first author (GM), who prepared summary tables of screening policy, diagnosis policy, monitoring of pregnancies where the diagnosis had been made, and finally delivery timing policy. The fourth author (JGT) checked the tables against the original guideline documents. The tables prepared from the NVOG guideline were checked against the original Dutch-language guideline by a native Dutch speaker (KEB).

Results

Six guidelines were identified. These were produced by the American College of Obstetricians and Gynecologists (ACOG), the Royal College of Obstetricians and Gynaecologists (RCOG) (UK), the New Zealand Maternal and Fetal Medicine Network (NZMFMN), the Health Service Executive (HSE) (Ireland), and the Nederlandse Vereniging voor Obstetrie & Gynaecologie (NVOG) (Netherlands) [17–22]. The only guideline more than 2 years old [21] is currently under revision; however, at the time of writing, the update had not been released. The Dutch guideline is therefore not based on the most recent evidence for the diagnosis and management of fetal growth restriction, which was considered in the remaining five guidelines.

Note: All the guidelines reviewed preceded the publication of fetal growth standards by the Intergrowth-21 project and by WHO [23–25]. Readers should be aware that guideline recommendations about need for customization and choice of particular charts might change in response to these new charts.

The countries of origin, sponsoring national bodies, and dates of preparation or latest revision are shown in Table 7.1.

The recommendations for fetal growth restriction prevention and screening are shown in Table 7.2. Screening measures considered include clinical risk factors, uterine artery Doppler, serum tests, clinical palpation, fundal height measurement, or routine third trimester growth scans.

The recommendations for diagnosis of growth restriction among women identified as at increased risk are shown in Table 7.3, for monitoring fetuses who have been identified as growth restricted in Table 7.4, and for timing of delivery in Table 7.5.

Areas of Differing Practice

Aspirin

Low-dose aspirin is recommended by national and international societies for women at increased risk of preeclampsia [26–28]. However, recommendations for its use to prevent growth restriction vary. NZMFMN, SOGC, and HSE Ireland explicitly recommend low-dose aspirin for this indication. The justification is presumably that although the evidence

for benefit from low-dose aspirin is largely related to women at increased risk of preeclampsia, there is considerable overlap between the conditions, and the trials show not only a reduction in preeclampsia, but also a reduction in growth restriction [29].

Screening Using PAPP-A or other Serum Markers

None of the guidelines recommends using PAPP-A or any other serum test as a screening test for fetal growth restriction, but two, RCOG and NZMFMN, recommend that if PAPP-A is measured for another reason, namely aneuploidy screening, and found to be below 0.4 multiples of the median (MoM), then it should be regarded as a major risk factor for growth restriction. The Canadian guideline recommends that abnormality of two or more serum parameters of the aneuploidy screening test be regarded as an increased risk. This recommendation is based on a multicenter cohort study evaluating outcomes after quadruple testing [30,31].

Interpretation of Risk

None of the guidelines explicitly states that tests should be interpreted in the light of the patient's prior risk. A specific test result or combination of results is much more likely to predict an adverse outcome in a woman with a clinical risk factor for growth restriction, such as bleeding, previous FGR-related fetal death, or preeclampsia, than in a woman who was tested for screening or maternal anxiety. Failure of clinicians to consider prior risk properly may partly explain the apparent inconsistency between the benefit of measuring fetal Doppler waveforms in high-risk pregnancy [32] and the lack of benefit in low-risk pregnancies [6]. The problem would be minimized by the recommendation that all women were risk assessed at booking and the information used when interpreting the results of subsequent ultrasound scans. All guidelines recommend that any women in whom growth restriction is suspected clinically undergo ultrasound regardless of their prior risk.

Fundal Height Measurement

Five guidelines recommend the use of symphysial-fundal height measurement of which two, SOGC and ACOG, recommend charting on a conventional chart, one, RCOG, states that either a conventional or customised chart may be used, and NZMFMN, and HSE Ireland, recommend a customized chart.

Table 7.1 The guidelines

Title	The Investigation and Management of the Small-for-Gestational-Age Fetus	Guideline for the Management of Suspected Small-for-Gestational-Age Singleton Pregnancies and Infants after 34 Weeks' Gestation	Intrauterine Growth Restriction: Screening, Diagnosis and Management	Fetal Growth Restriction-Recognition, Diagnosis and Management	Practice bulletin no. 134: "Fetal Growth Restriction"	Foetale Groeibeperking
Sponsoring organization	Royal College of Obstetricians and Gynaecologists (RCOG)	New Zealand Maternal and Fetal Medicine Network (NZMFMN)	Society of Obstetricians and Gynecologists of Canada (SOGC)	Institute of Obstetricians and Gynaecologists, Royal College of Physicians of Ireland and Health Service Executive (HSE)	American College of Obstetricians and Gynecologists (ACOG)	Nederlandse Vereniging voor Obstetrie & Gynaecologie (NVOG)
Year	2014	2014	2013	2014	2013	2008
Country	United Kingdom	New Zealand	Canada	Ireland	United States	Netherlands
Guideline development process	Developed by guideline leads after reviewing evidence. Peer reviewed.	Written by experts in the field after reviewing the evidence. Peer reviewed. Feedback obtained from members of professional body.	Prepared by the Maternal Fetal Medicine Committee after reviewing the literature. Approved by the Executive and Council of SOGC.	Written by three experts, peer reviewed by a further five then reviewed and endorsed by the program's advisory board.	Developed by the ACOG Committee on Practice Bulletins after reviewing published evidence.	Developed by the NVOG Committee on Guidelines, under responsibility of the board of NVOG.

Table 7.2 Definition, prevention, and screening for the small-for-gestational-age fetus

Country	United Kingdom	New Zealand	Canada	Ireland	United States	Netherlands
Definition of small for gestational age	Estimated fetal weight <10th centile or AC <10th centile	Estimated fetal weight <10th centile or abdominal circumference ≤5th centile	Estimated fetal weight <10th centile	Estimated fetal weight <10th centile	Estimated fetal weight <10th centile	Estimated fetal weight <10th centile
Risk assessment at booking?	Yes	Yes	Yes	Yes	Yes	Yes
Biomarkers part of risk assessment?	If Pregnancy Associated Plasma Protein-A <0.4 MoM consider major risk. Use of PAPP-A for population screening not recommended	If Pregnancy Associated Plasma Protein-A <0.4 MoM consider major risk. Use of PAPP-A for population screening not recommended	If two or more serum parameters of aneuploidy screen abnormal (threshold unspecified) fetus at increased risk	Not discussed	No evidence for improved outcome	No
Uterine artery Doppler for high risk women?	At 20 weeks for those with ≥3 minor risk factors	At 20–24 weeks in high risk women	At 19–23 weeks, in women with risk factors	Not discussed	No evidence for improved outcome	At 18–24 weeks in high-risk women
Screening for low risk women	Serial symphysio-fundal height from 24 weeks, plotted on conventional or customized chart. Ultrasound biometry if <10th centile or slow or static growth	Serial symphysio-fundal height plotted on customized chart. Ultrasound biometry if reducing velocity or <10th centile	Serial symphysio-fundal height. If height in centimeters is less than gestational age (in weeks) by > 3 centimeters, arrange ultrasound scan	Symphysio-fundal height at every visit, plotted on customized chart if available	Symphysio-fundal height. Ultrasound biometry if >3 centimeters discrepancy with gestational age	Serial abdominal palpation. No evidence that symphysio-fundal height measurement is superior
Prevention	Aspirin 75mg daily, prior to 16 weeks in women with risk factors for preeclampsia	Women at high risk of growth restriction, consider aspirin 100mg daily	Low-dose aspirin for prior history of preeclampsia, growth restriction, or ≥ risk factors	Low-dose aspirin in presence of significant risk factors. Consider low molecular weight heparin in individual cases.	Insufficient evidence to recommend	Aspirin not recommended to prevent fetal growth restriction
Other preventative measures	Smoking cessation. No evidence for dietary measures	Smoking cessation in early pregnancy	Smoking cessation	Smoking cessation	No evidence for bed rest or dietary measures	Smoking cessation. Bed rest not indicated

Table 7.3 Ultrasound surveillance of high-risk women

Country	United Kingdom	New Zealand	Canada	Ireland	United States	Netherlands
Criteria for serial scanning	Uterine artery Doppler increased resistance, ≥1 major risk factor, or unsuitable for symphysio-fundal height monitoring. Biometry & umbilical artery Doppler from 26–28 weeks	Major risk factors or unsuitable for symphysio-fundal height monitoring. Gestation to start depends on risk factors. If previous small-for-gestational-age infant < 32 weeks start at 24 weeks	Major risk factors, or increased resistance on uterine artery Doppler. Commence serial ultrasound from 26 weeks	Women with risk factors from 26 weeks	Women with prior small-for-gestational-age newborn or other risk factors or unsuitable for symphysio-fundal height monitoring.	Women with risk factors, between 26 and 34 weeks, possibly after uterine artery Doppler
Recommended biometry	Estimated fetal weight and abdominal circumference on conventional or customized chart	Estimated fetal weight on customized chart, and abdominal circumference on population chart	Estimated fetal weight or abdominal circumference on population chart	Estimated fetal weight and abdominal circumference on customized chart	Estimated fetal weight on population chart	Estimated fetal weight on population or customized chart
Umbilical artery Doppler?	Yes	Only if fetus small on biometry, or reduced growth velocity	Only if fetus small on biometry	Yes	Yes	Yes
Biochemical tests	Not recommended	Not recommended	Not recommended	Not recommended	Not recommended	Not recommended
Interval	Minimum 3 weeks	2–3 weeks	2 weeks	2–4 weeks	3–4 weeks	3 weeks

Two guidelines recommend diagnosing fetal growth restriction when the fundal height measurement is more than 3 cm below the gestational age in weeks. Neither provides a reference to support this recommendation. If fundal height in centimeters is considered to approximate gestational age in weeks, this corresponds to the 50th–75th centiles on published population growth charts [33,34]. However, given the rise in maternal obesity since these charts were produced, this may not apply to the current population. The 2008 Netherlands guideline states that clinical palpation is superior to fundal height measurement, but does not provide a reference for this statement. A single randomized trial identified within a Cochrane review to address this question did not show any difference between palpation and symphysial-fundal height measurement with a tape measure [35].

Use of Customized Ultrasound Growth Charts for Diagnosis

These are recommended by the, New Zealand, and Ireland guidelines. The New Zealand guidelines recommend the use of the GROW chart [2], while the Irish guidelines recommend an alternative chart developed using pregnancy data from their national population [36]. The Netherlands guidelines advise that population or RCOG and customized charts may be used, and the U.S. and Canadian ones both recommend only population charts within their guidelines. However, a recent Canadian publication has suggested that adjusting growth charts for ethnicity alone would reduce over-diagnosis of small for gestational age by 36–45% [37].

Table 7.4 Surveillance once growth restriction has been identified

Country	United Kingdom	New Zealand	Canada	Ireland	United States	Netherlands
U.S. biometry	Estimated fetal weight on conventional or customized chart every 2 weeks	Estimated fetal weight on customized chart every 2 weeks	Estimated fetal weight on population chart every 2 weeks	Estimated fetal weight on customized chart every 2 weeks	Estimated fetal weight on population chart every 3–4 weeks	Estimated fetal weight on customized or population chart every 2–4 weeks
Liquor volume measurement	Deepest vertical pocket. Not as the only surveillance tool	Deepest vertical pocket. Assess if Doppler abnormal, 1–2 times weekly	Amniotic fluid index	Amniotic fluid index in all cases	Amniotic fluid volume with serial measurements, timing unspecified	Assess to decide need for karyotype, but not for delivery timing
Umbilical artery Doppler	Every 2 weeks	Every 2 weeks, more frequently if abnormal	Every 2 weeks	Every 2 weeks	From gestational age where delivery considered for fetal benefit. Frequency unspecified	1–2 times per week
Other Doppler	Middle cerebral artery and ductus venosus if umbilical artery Doppler abnormal. Ductus venosus if absent or reversed end diastolic UA flow	If SGA ≥34 weeks, middle cerebral artery Doppler, and cerebral placental ratio every 2–3 weeks	Middle cerebral artery and ductus venosus studies	Middle cerebral artery or ductus venosus should not be used to indicate delivery	Insufficient evidence to support the use of middle cerebral artery or ductus venosus Doppler in clinical practice	Insufficient evidence to recommend other methods of surveillance
Cardiotocograph surveillance	Do not use alone Daily computerized cardiotocograph for absent or reversed end diastolic UA flow if ductus venosus Doppler unavailable	Do not use as the only surveillance tool	Only if biophysical profile abnormal	Daily if absent or reversed end diastolic flow on umbilical artery Doppler	Only initiate if gestational age reached where delivery would be considered for perinatal benefit. Frequency unspecified	In the first instance Doppler may be used, in the second instance cardiotocography. Frequency not specified.
Biophysical profile	Do not use	Do not use as the only surveillance tool	Consider weekly	Adding to Doppler may improve detection of the acidotic fetus	Not discussed	No evidence of superiority to cardiotocography alone
Other	Offer detailed fetal survey, karyotype and cytomegalovirus, and toxoplasmosis screen for severely small for gestational age fetuses at 18–20 weeks scan. Consider syphilis and malaria screen.	Consider further investigations into underlying cause, depending on the presentation and presence of other explanatory factors. Tests to consider include placental histology, karyotype of the fetus or neonate, screening for rare infections	Offer invasive testing to rule out aneuploidy where fetal abnormalities suspected, soft markers seen, or no supportive evidence for underlying placental insufficiency. Maternal screening for infectious etiology may be considered.	Amniocentesis if additional findings, such as poly- or an-hydramnios, soft markers or structural abnormalities present. Cytomegalovirus and toxoplasmosis testing may be indicated.	Consider prenatal karyotype if fetal structural defect in the presence of growth restriction, or mid-trimester onset	Karyotype only if normal or increased amniotic fluid and normal Doppler in the presence of fetal growth restriction Toxoplasmosis and cytomegalovirus testing only if other abnormalities suggestive

Table 7.5 Timing and mode of delivery

Country	United Kingdom	New Zealand	Canada	Ireland	United States	Netherlands
Doppler criteria for delivery	Viable (≥24 weeks and EFW>500g) with absent or reversed end diastolic flow on umbilical artery Doppler, or ductus venosus absent or reversed "A" wave, or umbilical vein pulsations deliver by 32 weeks Middle cerebral artery Doppler pulsatility index <5th centile, deliver by 37 weeks	Deliver the fetus with suspected SGA by 38 weeks if middle cerebral artery Doppler <5th centile, Cerebral placental Ratio<5th centile, UtAD >95th centile at time of diagnosis of SGA.	Deliver if middle cerebral Artery or ductus venosus Doppler is abnormal or umbilical artery Doppler deteriorates	If absent EDF, delivery should be considered no later than 34 weeks If reversed EDF, delivery should be considered no later than 30 weeks' gestation	If small for gestational age with additional factors (oligohydramnios, maternal comorbidity, raised pulsatility index) deliver at 34+0 to 37+6 weeks Small for gestation age with no other abnormal parameters, deliver at 38+0 to 39+6 weeks.	If <32 weeks, use CTG to time delivery, if UAD abnormal. >34 weeks, consider delivery if umbilical artery Doppler abnormal
Cardiotocograph criteria for delivery	Short-term variability ≤ 3ms	Not specified	"abnormal" (criteria not specified)	Delivery indicated in a viable fetus by reduced short term variability	Not specified	If < 32 weeks, deliver based on "abnormal" (criteria not specified) short term variability <4ms can be used
Timing of delivery if Dopplers normal	If >34 weeks deliver if static growth over 3 weeks If estimated fetal weight <10th centile offer delivery at 37 weeks	If estimated fetal weight <3rd centile deliver by 38 weeks If estimated fetal weight >3rd centile <10th centile deliver at 40 weeks unless other clinical concern Deliver at 38 weeks if uterine artery and middle cerebral artery Dopplers not available	Discuss delivery or ongoing monitoring after 37 weeks. If amniotic fluid volume < 5 cm or deepest vertical pocket <2 cm or biophysical profile abnormal, consider delivery.	Isolated growth restriction (EFW <10th centile and normal umbilical artery Doppler), delay delivery until at least 37 weeks, and even until 38–39.	Not specified. Advise participation in DIGITAT study	
Preparation for delivery	Corticosteroids prior to delivery 24+0 to 35+6 weeks.	Corticosteroids if delivery <34 weeks	Corticosteroids if delivery <34 weeks	Corticosteroids prior to delivery between 24+0 and 34+0 weeks. Consider up to 38+0 for elective Caesarean section Magnesium sulphate <32 weeks	Corticosteroids ≤34 weeks Magnesium sulphate ≤ 32 weeks	Corticosteroids if delivery <34 weeks
Mode of delivery	If ARED deliver by caesarean section If EDF present, induction of labor with continuous CTG.	If middle cerebral artery Doppler abnormal consider Caesarean rather than induction	Not specified	Caesarean section is likely when ARED flow on umbilical artery Doppler, or <34 weeks	Depends on gestation and etiology.	If concerns regarding fetal condition, deliver by Caesarean. Fetal size only concern, offer induction. Avoid vaginal breech at term if EFW <2800 grams

Gestation at Which Fetal Monitoring Is Recommended to Start

The New Zealand guideline recommends that ultrasound examinations begin at 24 weeks for pregnancies at high risk. The RCOG, SOGC, HSE Ireland, and the NVOG recommend starting growth scans at 26 weeks. The American practice bulletin states that serial ultrasonography in women with a prior growth-restricted fetus may be reasonable, but that the optimum surveillance regimen has not been determined.

Use of Biophysical Profile Scoring

This is recommended by SOGC and HSE Ireland, but not by the RCOG, NZMFMN, or the NVOG. The ACOG guideline highlights that the optimal surveillance regime is unknown, and recommends not commencing antepartum testing (including non-stress and biophysical profile) before a gestation when delivery would be considered for perinatal benefit.

Use of Umbilical Artery Doppler

All countries recommend the use of umbilical artery Doppler for surveillance. This recommendation is evidence-based in that this is the only test shown to predict fetal death in studies that avoided the treatment paradox [10] and because randomized trials of its use, at least in high-risk pregnancy, have shown that its use can reduce perinatal death [31], presumably via timely delivery of at risk babies with abnormal Doppler studies.

Use of CTG, Conventional or Computerized

The RCOG, NZMFMN, and NVOG guidelines recommend that cardiotocograph (CTG) should not be used alone for surveillance. Instead it should be combined with regular umbilical artery Doppler. In the presence of absent or reversed end diastolic flow velocities, the UK (RCOG) recommends daily computerized CTG and Ireland (HSE) daily conventional CTG. The U.S. (ACOG) guideline recommends conventional CTG for surveillance.

Recommendations for Preterm Delivery

Almost all guidelines suggest that terminal or near-terminal fetal heart rate patterns are an indication for delivery at any gestation. For example, the UK guidelines give short-term variability (STV)

$< = 3$ milliseconds (msec), Ireland reduced STV, the Netherlands <4msec, and Canada abnormal CTG (threshold unspecified) as indications for delivery at any gestation.

The RCOG guidelines recommend delivery by 32 weeks in the presence of absent or reversed end diastolic velocity in umbilical artery Doppler waveform, or earlier if the venous Doppler becomes abnormal. This recommendation is based on the guideline authors' interpretation of the Growth Restriction Intervention trial (GRIT) trial [11,12] and other observational evidence.

After 34 weeks, the RCOG guideline recommends delivery if growth has been static for more than 3 weeks. In the flow diagram, this recommendation applies to fetuses in whom umbilical artery Doppler is also abnormal, albeit to a lesser degree than absent or reversed end diastolic flow velocities. ACOG recommends delivery between 34+0 and 37+6 weeks in growth-restricted fetuses with additional risk factors for adverse outcome, including oligo-hydramnios or abnormal umbilical artery Doppler.

At or near term, the recommendations are stronger. For example, the RCOG guideline recommends offering delivery at 37 weeks if the EFW is less than the 10th centile. However, this guidance was published before follow-up of infants in the DIGITAT trial, which suggested that neonatal morbidity was lowest overall in infants delivered beyond 38 weeks' gestation [14]. There was no difference in long-term neurodevelopmental outcomes between induction of labor or expectant management in the term small-for-gestational-age infant [38]. The recommendation of the NZMFMN guideline is in keeping with this finding, with delivery recommended at 38 weeks if the EFW is below the 3rd centile and delivery at term if it is between the 3rd and 10th centiles and all Doppler indices are normal. This guideline also recommends delivery at 38–39 weeks, if uterine and middle cerebral artery Doppler are not available to stratify risk, in pregnancies with normal umbilical artery Doppler findings.

Conclusion

Unsurprisingly, given the paucity of evidence, guidelines for management of fetal growth restriction vary widely. There is general agreement that some sort of screening should be undertaken, but the details vary. All guidelines recommend that pregnancies judged to be at high risk of fetal growth restriction should be monitored with ultrasound biometry and umbilical artery Doppler waveforms; the basis for the latter are the trials summarized in the Cochrane review [32]. Guidelines for other Doppler waveforms and fetal heart rate monitoring vary.

When it comes to the timing of delivery, the guidelines do not emphasize the interpretation of test results in the light of prior risk. The only definitive criteria for delivery before 34 weeks, recommended by multiple guidelines, are reduced short-term fetal heart rate variability in the cardiotocograph (CTG) or a pre-terminal pattern. Recommendations for delivery for growth restriction nearer to term also vary widely, highlighting the fact that the current tools are still a long way from being able to accurately predict which babies truly need early delivery to avoid death or morbidity as a result of growth restriction. Interpretation of the existing evidence and its translation into clinical guidelines, despite being performed in a robust and similar fashion by all of the publishing bodies, is therefore ultimately subjective.

Key Points

- Though symphysis fundal height features in most guidelines as a method of screening for fetal growth restriction, this modality is based on very little evidence.

- The use of customization of both symphysis fundal height and/or fetal ultrasound measurements is inconsistently recommended by national guidelines.

- Once fetal growth restriction is recognized, follow up with ultrasound and umbilical artery Doppler is recommended, usually combined with CTG.

- Recommendations for delivery are based on abnormal umbilical Doppler, abnormal venous Doppler or computerised CTG short term variability depending on the guideline and the fetal gestation.

References

1. Roex A, Nikpoor P, Van Eerd, Hodyl N, Dekker G. Serial plotting on customised fundal height charts results in doubling of the antenatal detection of small for gestational age fetuses in nulliparous women. *Aust NZ J Obstet Gynecol* 2012;52:78–82.

2. Gardosi J, Francis A. Controlled trial of fundal height measurement plotted on customised antenatal growth charts. *BJOG* 1999;106:309–17.

3. Chang TC, Robson SC, Boys RJ, Spencer JA. Prediction of the small for gestational age infant: Which ultrasonic measurement is best? *Obstet Gynecol* 1992;80:1030–8.

4. Coomarasamy A, Connock M, Thornton JG, Khan KS. Accuracy of ultrasound biometry in the prediction of macrosomia: A systematic quantitative review. *BJOG* 2005;112(11):1461–6.

5. Chauhan SP, Magann EF. Screening for fetal growth restriction. *Clin Obstet Gynecol* 2006;49:284–94.

6. Alfirevic Z, Stampalija T, Medley N. Fetal and umbilical Doppler ultrasound in normal pregnancy. *Cochrane Database Syst Rev* 2015, Issue 4. Art. No.: CD001450. DOI: 10.1002/14651858.CD001450.pub4.

7. Morris RK, Malin G, Robson SC, Kleijnen J, Zamora J, Khan KS. Fetal umbilical artery Doppler to predict compromise of fetal/neonatal wellbeing in high-risk populations: systematic review and bivariate meta-analysis. *Ultrasound Obstet Gynecol* 2011;37:135–42.

8. Serra V, Moulden M, Bellver J, Redman CW. The value of the short-term fetal heart rate variation for timing the delivery of the growth-retarded fetuses. *BJOG* 2008;115:1101–7.

9. Yagel S, Kivilevitch Z, Cohen SM, Valsky DV, Messing B, Shen O, et al. The fetal venous system, Part II: Ultrasound evaluation of the fetus with congenital venous system malformation or developing circulatory compromise. *Ultrasound Obstet Gynecol* 2010;36:93–111.

10. Thornton JG, Lilford RJ. Do we need randomised trials of antenatal tests of fetal wellbeing? *BJOG* 1993; 100:197–200.

11. The GRIT Study Group. A randomised trial of timed delivery for the compromised preterm fetus: Short term outcomes and Bayesian interpretation. *BJOG* 2003;110:27–32.

12. The GRIT Study Group. Infant wellbeing at 2 years of age in the Growth Restriction Intervention trial (GRIT): A multicentred randomised controlled trial. *Lancet* 2004;364:513–19.

13. Walker D-M, Marlow N, Upstone, L, Gross, H. Hornbuckle J, Vail A, Wolke D, Thornton JG on behalf of the GRIT Study Group. The Growth Restriction Intervention Trial (GRIT): Long-term outcomes in a randomised trial of timing of delivery in fetal growth restriction. *Am J Obstet Gynecol* 2011;204(1):341–9.

14. Boers K, Bijlenga D, Vijgen S, Van der Post J, Bekedam D, Kwee A, Van der Salm P, Van Pampus M, Spaanderman M, De Boer K, Bremer H, Duvekot

J, Hasaart T, Delemarre F, Bloemenkamp K, Van Meir C, Willekes C, Wijnen E, Rijken M, le Cessie S, Roumen F, Thornton JG, Van Lith J, Mol BW, Scherjon S (2011) Induction versus expectant monitoring for intrauterine growth restriction at term (the DIGITAT trial). *BMJ* 2011;342:35.

15. Boers KE, Van Wyk L, Van der Post JAM, et al. Neonatal morbidity after induction vs expectant monitoring in intrauterine growth restriction at term: A subanalysis of the DIGITAT RCT. *Am J Obstet Gynecol* 2012;206:344.e1–7.

16. Lees CC, Marlow, N, Van Wassenaer-Leemhuis, A, et al. for the TRUFFLE study group. Two year neurodevelopmental and intermediate perinatal outcomes in infants with very preterm fetal growth restriction (TRUFFLE): A randomised trial. *Lancet* 2015;385:2162–72.

17. American College of Obstetricians and Gynecologists. ACOG Practice Bulletin no 134: Fetal growth restriction. *Obstet Gynecol* 2013;121(5):1122–33.

18. Royal College of Obstetricians and Gynecologists (RCOG) Guideline Committee. The investigation and management of the small for gestational age fetus. Green top guideline No. 31. Jan 2014 www.rcog.org.uk/en/guidelines-research-services/guidelines/gtg31/.

19. New Zealand Maternal and Fetal Medicine Network (NZMFMN) Guideline for the management of suspected small for gestational age singleton pregnancies and infants after 34 weeks gestation. 2014 www.asum.com.au/newsite/Files/Documents/Resources/NZMFM%20SGA%20Guideline_September%202013.pdf.

20. Health Service Executive (Ireland). Fetal growth restriction – recognition, diagnosis and management. 2014 www.hse.ie/eng/about/Who/clinical/natclinprog/obsandgynaeprogramme/29-_Fetal_Growth_Restriction-IUGR_CPG_final_.pdf.

21. Nederlandse Vereniging voor Obstetrie & Gynaecologie (NVOG). Foetale Groeibeperking 2008. http://nvog-documenten.nl/index.php?pagina=/richtlijn/item/pagina.php&richtlijn_id=828.

22. Society of Obstetricians and Gynecologists Canada (SOGC) Intrauterine growth restriction: screening, diagnosis and management. 2013 http://sogc.org/guidelines/intrauterine-growth-restriction-screening-diagnosis-management/.

23. Papageorghiou AT, Ohuma EO, Altman DG, Todros T, Cheikh Ismail L, Lambert A, Jaffer YA, Bertino E, Gravett MG, Purwar M, Noble JA, Pang R, Victora CG, Barros FC, Carvalho M, Salomon LJ, Bhutta ZA, Kennedy SH, Villar J; International Fetal and Newborn Growth Consortium for the 21st Century (INTERGROWTH-21st). International standards for fetal growth based on serial ultrasound measurements: the Fetal Growth Longitudinal Study of the INTERGROWTH-21st Project. *Lancet* 2014 Sep 6;384(9946):869–79.

24. Papageorghiou AT, Ohuma EO, Gravett MG, Hirst J, da Silveira MF, Lambert A, Carvalho M, Jaffer YA, Altman DG, Noble JA, Bertino E, Purwar M, Pang R, Cheikh Ismail L, Victora C, Bhutta ZA, Kennedy SH, Villar J; International Fetal and Newborn Growth Consortium for the 21st Century (INTERGROWTH-21st). International standards for symphysis-fundal height based on serial measurements from the Fetal Growth Longitudinal Study of the INTERGROWTH-21st Project: prospective cohort study in eight countries. *BMJ* 2016 Nov 7;355:i5662.

25. Kiserud T, Piaggio G, Carroli G, Widmer M, Carvalho J, Neerup Jensen L, Giordano D, Cecatti JG, Abdel Aleem H, Talegawkar SA, Benachi A, Diemert A, Tshefu Kitoto A, Thinkhamrop J, Lumbiganon P, Tabor A, Kriplani A, Gonzalez Perez R, Hecher K, Hanson MA, Gülmezoglu AM, Platt LD. The World Health Organization fetal growth charts: A multinational longitudinal study of ultrasound biometric measurements and estimated fetal weight. *PLoS Med* 2017 Jan 24;14(1):e1002220.

26. National Institute for Health and Care Excellence (NICE). Hypertension in pregnancy: The management of hypertensive disorders during pregnancy. 2010 www.nice.org.uk/guidance/cg107.

27. Magee LA, Pels A, Helewa M, Rey E, Von Dadelszen P, Hypertension Guideline Committee. Prediction and prevention. In: Diagnosis, evaluation, and management of the hypertensive disorders of pregnancy: Executive summary. *J Obstet Gynaecol Can.* 2014 May;36(5):425–6.

28. World Health Organization (WHO). WHO recommendations for the prevention and treatment of pre-eclampsia and eclampsia. 2011. http://whqlibdoc.who.int/publications/2011/9789241548335_eng.pdf.

29. Askie LM, Duley L Henderson-Smart DJ, Stewart LA, on behalf of the PARIS Collaborative Group. (2007) Antiplatelet agents for prevention of pre-eclampsia: A meta-analysis of individual patient data. *Lancet* 2007;369:1791–8.

30. Dugoff L, Hobbins JC, Malone FD, Vidaver J, Sullivan L, Canick JA, et al. Quad screen as a predictor of adverse pregnancy outcome. *Obstet Gynecol* 2005;106(2):260–7.

31. Dugoff L. First- and second-trimester maternal serum markers for aneuploidy and adverse obstetric outcomes. *Obstet Gynecol* 2010;115:1052–61.

32. Alfirevic Z, Stampalija T, Gyte GML. Fetal and umbilical Doppler ultrasound in high-risk pregnancies. *Cochrane Database Syst Rev* 2013, Issue 11. Art. No.: CD007529. DOI: 10.1002/14651858. CD007529.pub3.

33. Calvert JP, Crean EE, Newcombe RG, Pearson JF. Antenatal screening by measurement of symphysis-fundus height. *BMJ* 1982;285:846.

34. Quaranta P, Currell R, Redman CW, Robinson JS. Prediction of small-for-dates infants by measurement of symphysial-fundal-height. *BJOG* 1981;88(2):115–19.

35. Robert PJ, Ho JJ, Valliapan J, Sivasangari S. Symphysial fundal height (SFH) measurement in pregnancy for detecting abnormal fetal growth. *Cochrane Database Syst Rev* 2012, Issue 7. Art.

No.: CD008136. DOI: 10.1002/14651858.CD008136. pub2.

36. Unterscheider J, Geary MP, Daly S, McAuliffe FM, Kennelly MM, Dornan J, et al. The customised fetal growth potential: A standard for Ireland. *Eur J Obstet Gynecol Reprod Biol* 2013 Jan;166(1):14–17.

37. Melamed N, Ray JG, Shah PS, Berger H, Kingdom JC. Should we use customized fetal growth percentiles in urban Canada? *J Obstet Gynaecol Canada* 2014;36(2):164–70.

38. Van Wyk L, Boers KE, Van der Post JAM, et al. Effects on (neuro)developmental and behavioral outcome at 2 years of age of induced labor compared with expectant management in intrauterine growth-restricted infants: Long-term outcomes of the DIGITAT trial. *Am J Obstet Gynecol* 2012;206:406.e1–7.

Chapter

8

Maternal Cardiovascular Function and Fetal Growth Restriction

Rosemary Townsend and Asma Khalil

Introduction

Women undergo a variety of physiological cardio-vascular adaptations in normal pregnancy. Marked changes from the non-pregnant state can be seen from as early as 6 weeks' gestation [1]. In normal pregnancy, cardiac output (CO) rapidly increases and there is generalized peripheral vasodilatation, resulting in a fall in total peripheral resistance (TPR) [2]. These cardiovascular changes are different in pregnancies affected by preeclampsia or fetal growth restriction (FGR) [3,4]. Women who present with preeclampsia form a heterogeneous group, with some features particularly discordant between the group of women with early-onset preeclampsia (necessitating delivery prior to 34 weeks' gestation) or preeclampsia associated with FGR compared to late-onset preeclampsia with appropriate-for-gestational age (AGA) fetuses [3,4].

Since both preeclampsia and FGR are linked to failure of early placentation, it would be anticipated that impaired placentation may also be detectable prior to clinical presentation through a failure to achieve the physiological cardiovascular changes normally seen in early pregnancy. Indeed, on investigating women in the first trimester, measurable differences in cardiac and vascular parameters have been identified. Interestingly, there are significant differences between those women who go on to develop FGR alone and those who develop preeclampsia [5].

Cardiac Changes in Uncomplicated Pregnancies

CO has been extensively studied in uncomplicated and complicated pregnancies both at term and throughout pregnancy. In this chapter, we will refer to CO rather than cardiac index (CI) (CO related to body surface area), as the use of CI in pregnancy is controversial [6]. Traditionally, CO is measured by echocardiography, but as this is a highly skilled and time-consuming test,

other modalities have been employed. For example, the finger arterial pressure wave can be used to extrapolate the aortic pressure, stroke volume, and heart rate, and to calculate the CO [7]. Alternatively, an ultrasound CO monitor (USCOM®), which uses ultrasound to assess aortic or pulmonary valve flow, is a simple device for assessing cardiac function (Figure 8.1). Devices such as these may facilitate large-scale studies of maternal cardiovascular changes in pregnancy, which are necessary to build on the current knowledge base and to arrive at potential screening and management tools. The currently available modalities for assessment of CO are summarized in Table 8.1.

CO is defined as the product of stroke volume and heart rate. CO is increased by 5 weeks after the last menstrual period and continues to increase up to 45% above the non-pregnant level until 24 weeks' gestation. Both heart rate and stroke volume contribute to this increase. The increase in heart rate is already seen by 5 weeks of gestation and continues to increase until 32 weeks. Stroke volume increases a little later by 8 weeks' gestation and reaches its maximum at about 20 weeks. Approximately 70% of the increase in CO occurs by the 16th week of gestation, which is well before the marked increase in uterine blood flow (Figure 8.2). During multiple gestations, there is a further increment of about 15% in CO [8]. The increase in CO is linked to a rise in preload, a decrease in afterload, an increased compliance of conduit vessels, ventricular remodeling, and activation of the renin-angiotensin-aldosterone system. The rise in CO is further influenced by enhanced myocardial performance. The ejection fraction of the left ventricle remains constant throughout gestation [8] (Figure 8.3).

Preload

Left atrial dimensions increase gradually from early pregnancy, reaching a plateau at 30–34 weeks' gestation. Left atrial enlargement appears to result from

65

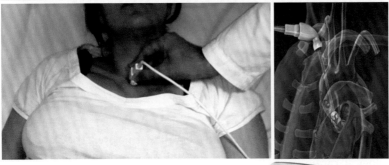

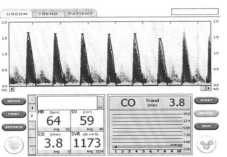

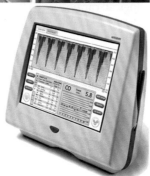

Figure 8.1 Cardiac output assessment using the ultrasound cardiac output monitor (USCOM®).
Source: Karamermer Y, Roos-Hesselink JW. Coronary heart disease and pregnancy. *Future Cardiol* 2007.

an increase in preload and circulating blood volume. Valensise described an enlargement of both the left atrium and ventricle, suggesting that left atrial enlargement might be an expression of preload increase [9]. The increases in stroke volume and CO during pregnancy are linked to the increase of the left atrial diameter, suggesting a relationship between these preload parameters [8].

Afterload

Cardiac afterload represents the mechanical resistance to the movement of blood driven out of the left ventricle and can be divided into:

- a steady component (total or systemic or peripheral vascular resistance, TPR); and
- a pulsatile component.

TPR is determined primarily by the cross-sectional diameter of the resistance vasculature. The marked increase in CO coupled with a decline in MAP indicates a marked reduction of systemic vascular resistance. The steady component of the afterload decreases during pregnancy, leveling off after the second trimester [8].

During uncomplicated pregnancy, a significant reduction of TPR occurs concomitantly with an increased CO and a decreased mean arterial pressure (MAP) [9,10]. A strong correlation exists between the uterine Resistance Index (RI) and TPR. This correlation suggests that a decrease of the uterine RI by a factor 1 causes a decrease of the TPR by a factor 0.26 (correlation coefficient 0.26) [9]. This supports a reduction of the TPR with as much as 20% by the placental bed [11].

The pulsatile component is defined by the load faced by the heart due to the response of the arterial tree to oscillations in pressure and flow.

The reduced TPR (steady component) represents an important adaptive response that maintains MAP within the normal range at the time of the greatly increased CO. Therefore, concomitant changes in arterial pulsatile load during normal pregnancy, including arterial compliance, counterbalance the potentially deleterious effects of this TPR reduction alone [12].

Cardiac Dimensions

Hypertrophic cardiac changes are observed in normal pregnancy [13]. This effect may be due in part to the continuous state of volume overload and increased heart rate (HR) that is characteristic of pregnancy and

Table 8.1 Measurement of cardiac output

Modality of measurement	Validated in pregnancy	Continuous or intermittent monitoring	Invasive or non-invasive	Advantages	Disadvantages
Thermodilution (via Pulmonary Artery Catheter)	Yes	Continuous (but with slight delay)	Invasive with risk of significant harm	Historical gold standard with high accuracy. Allows assessment of additional hemodynamic parameters (SVO2 or pulmonary artery pressures)	Risk of significant harm due to its invasive nature. Expensive. Available only in intensive care setting
Echocardiography (transoesophageal or transthoracic)	Yes	Non-continuous	Non-invasive	Allows additional assessment of cardiac structure and function. Accurate	Requires skilled operator with ability to correlate findings with changes in normal pregnancy. Transesophageal echo is superior, but requires sedation or anesthesia and is less acceptable to patients
Doppler ultrasound (esophageal or suprasternal) (e.g., USCOM® for suprasternal Doppler)	No	Intermittent	Non-invasive (if suprasternal technique used)	Acceptable accuracy and intra-observer variability compared to thermodilution	Operator dependent – relatively high inter-observer variability. Depends on an algorithm/ model of fixed aortic diameter that may not be applicable in pregnant or unstable patients
Pulse waveform analysis (e.g., LIDCO®)	Yes	Continuous	Invasive (peripheral rather than central line)	If properly calibrated accuracy is thought to be high. Uncalibrated systems (eg Flotrac-Vigileo) have limited accuracy in validation studies.	Requires arterial line insertion. Requires regular calibration (sometimes via central venous line). Vulnerable to movement and arrhythmia. Less accurate during rapid hemodynamic changes
Bioreactance (e.g., NICOM®)	No	Continuous	Non-invasive	More accurate than bioimpedance techniques. Simple to use and sensors can be located anywhere on the thorax	Subject to movement artefact. Expensive consumables
Bioimpedance (e.g., BioZ® ICG)	Inconsistent validation data	Continuous	Non-invasive	Simple. Low cost	Affected by changes in peripheral vascular resistance or pulmonary edema which may occur in the unwell pregnant woman
Carbon dioxide rebreathing	No	Continuous	Non-invasive	Commonly used in intensive care settings	Only possible in ventilated patients
Finger pulse wave analysis (e.g., Modelflow®)	No	Continuous	Non-invasive	Easy to use	Limited accuracy compared to thermodilution and ultrasound techniques. Depends on mathematical assumptions that may introduce bias

Svo2: percentage of oxygen saturation in the pulmonary arterial blood

is analogous to exercise-induced cardiac hypertrophy [14]. Additionally, there is evidence that the hormonal changes associated with pregnancy promote cardiac remodeling. Progesterone induces myocyte hypertrophy, and exogenous administration of progesterone in animal models mimics the increase of CO in pregnancy [15]. Cardiac hypertrophy, increased plasma volume in pregnancy, and increased HR all contribute to an increase in CO [16].

Cardiac Changes in Fetal Growth Restriction

Cardiac Output

In contrast to the physiological rise in CO in normal pregnancy, in normotensive FGR pregnancies, we see a blunted rise in the CO in the first trimester [17].

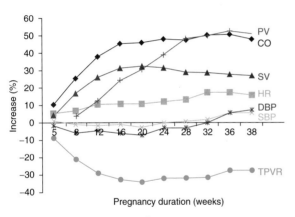

Figure 8.2 Blood pressure waveform.
Source: Karamermer Y, Roos-Hesselink JW. Coronary heart disease and pregnancy. *Future Cardiol* 2007; 3:559–67.

Furthermore, in pregnancies that ultimately develop preeclampsia, the CO is initially abnormally high in the first trimester, reflecting a hyperdynamic circulation [18]. Women can therefore be classified into three distinct groups in the first trimester – normal rise in CO, suboptimal rise in CO, and an abnormal hyperdynamic rise in CO. So in the first trimester, CO is elevated in pregnancies destined to develop preeclampsia, but reduced in pregnancies destined to develop FGR. Although there is a clear difference in CO in the first trimester in women destined to develop preeclampsia, CO falls toward the end of pregnancy, so that by term, both FGR and preeclampsia pregnancies have a low CO [18]. This points to several pathways of pathophysiology that may lead to the same clinical (change in CO) endpoint.

Stroke Volume

A comparison of echocardiographic findings in the third trimester in women with pregnancies complicated by FGR with and without preeclampsia found a number of differences in the factors mediating the low CO found in both groups [19]. In both groups, CO was similar but SV was lower in the normotensive group, as was MAP. This suggests that, while systolic function is affected in both processes, in preeclampsia, women are also affected by reduced left ventricle (LV) contractility and impaired diastolic function (which is relatively preserved in normotensive women with FGR), whereas in FGR, the reduced CO is mainly related to reduced SV. This correlates with another prospective study evaluating first trimester echocardiography findings for the prediction of preeclampsia. In this cohort, the group of small for gestational age (SGA) without PE had the lowest stroke volume of all groups evaluated,

Figure 8.3 Augmentation index.

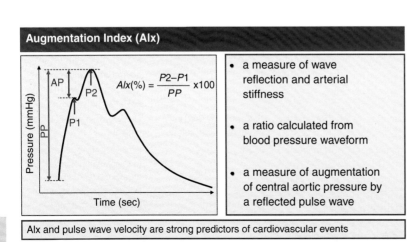

including preeclampsia with and without SGA fetuses and uncomplicated pregnancies [18].

Vascular Changes in Fetal Growth Restriction

Total Peripheral Resistance

The vasodilation of normal pregnancy is detectable even from the luteal phase of the menstrual cycle, mediated in part by relaxin released from the corpus luteum and a number of other factors [20]. Impaired placentation in the first half of pregnancy correlates with lower angiogenic and vasodilatory circulating factors and consequently higher peripheral vascular tone. In the first trimester, in women who later develop preeclampsia without FGR, the CO is increased (as described earlier), but TPR is not. This suggests that the higher blood pressure seen in the first trimester in these women is due to the increased CO rather than increased TPR. In contrast, in the first trimester, TPR is raised in women destined to develop FGR (with or without preeclampsia) [7]. Later in pregnancy, lack of vasodilation and an abnormally high TPR are associated with both preeclampsia and FGR, but seem to be particularly related to growth restriction.

This distinction that is apparent in early pregnancy is important, and it may not be apparent in the second half of pregnancy [21]. It suggests that preeclampsia with FGR and preeclampsia without FGR are clinically similar presentations of distinct pathological processes; in preeclampsia with FGR, the clinically detectable rise in blood pressure is associated with an early increase in TPR, whereas in preeclampsia with AGA fetuses, the blood pressure rise may be mediated by other factors. FGR without preeclampsia is more similar to the first than the second presentation. There is some evidence to suggest that pre-pregnancy vascular health affects the form of disease that presents in pregnancy [22]. If the prime cause of preeclampsia is impaired placentation, it is necessary to understand how some women with clear placental insufficiency show no maternal signs of preeclampsia.

Blood Pressure

In general, pregnancies with FGR alone have a low-to-normal MAP throughout pregnancy compared to women with preeclampsia, with or without FGR [7]. Chronic hypertension is a risk factor for the development of preeclampsia, but those women with chronic hypertension who do not develop preeclampsia may still be at increased risk of developing FGR in pregnancy [23]. This is consistent with the understanding that chronic hypertension is associated with atherosclerosis and endothelial damage that can also affect the placental bed [24]. In fact, chronic hypertension may cause a reduction in uteroplacental flow that compromises fetal growth while an otherwise normal pregnancy progresses without evidence of preeclampsia.

Key studies reporting on changes in CO, SV, and TPR in pregnancies complicated by FGR or SGA, where the data could be extracted, are shown in Table 8.2.

Arterial Stiffness

Increased arterial stiffness may represent a marker for preexisting generalized endothelial dysfunction and low-grade chronic inflammation, features also associated with the syndrome of preeclampsia [29–32]. The augmentation index (AIx) is a measure of arterial stiffness known to be a marker for a range of cardiovascular conditions in the non-pregnant population, such as diabetes, hypertension, and stroke [29–32]. Arterial stiffness can be assessed by arteriography on an outpatient basis and is associated with the risk of preeclampsia [33,34].

One study compared women with SGA fetuses with and without preeclampsia, using data prospectively gathered in the first trimester [35]. It was found that while in the first trimester high uterine artery pulsatility index (UAPI) and low serum PAPP-A are present in both groups, the AIx is normal in women with normotensive SGA pregnancies but elevated in women who later present with preeclampsia and SGA fetuses [35]. However, this study found no difference between the two groups in pulse wave velocity (PWV), another marker of arterial stiffness measured with arteriography, and which has been previously linked with preeclampsia [36]. Although this study did not discriminate between SGA and FGR fetuses, the difference begs the question whether the combination of impaired placentation (as demonstrated by the high UAPI and low PAPP-A) and maternal vascular health (as demonstrated by the high AIx) is what determines the phenotype of presentation in later pregnancy. In women with abnormal placentation, those with normal AIx may have sufficient cardiovascular reserve to

Table 8.2 Changes in maternal cardiac output, stroke volume, and vascular resistance in pregnancies complicated by fetal growth restriction (FGR) or small for gestational age (SGA)

Author	Year	Definition SGA/FGR	Gestation at assessment (week)	Marker	Level in FGR/SGA	Level in controls	P value
Cardiac output (CO)/cardiac index (CI)							
Rosso [25]	1993	BW <10th centile	36–38	CO	5483 (186)*	6191 (132)	<0.01
Rosso [25]	1993	BW <10th centile	36–38	CI	3357 (114)*	3788 (106)	<0.02
Bamfo [19]	2008	EFW <3rd centile, asymmetry, cerebral redistribution and oligohydramnios	24–35	CO	4.79 (0.52)	5.52 (1.21)†	0.02
Bamfo [19]	2008	EFW <3rd centile, asymmetry, cerebral redistribution and oligohydramnios	24–35	CI	3.12 (0.71)	2.94 (0.30)†	0.32
Melchiorre [26]	2012	AC <10th centile, UAPI >95th centile and need for delivery <37 weeks	at diagnosis	CI	2.73 (2.55–3.26)	3.48 (3.09–3.9)	<0.001
Lopes van Balen [27]	2013	BW <10th centile	18+/-2	CO	5.6 (5.3–5.9)	5.9 (2.6–6.3)	0.143
Oben [28]	2014	BW <5th centile	12	CO	6.4 (5.4–7.3)	7.1 (6.2–8.2)	0.025
Stroke volume (SV)/Stroke volume index (SVI)							
Bamfo [18]	2008	EFW <3rd centile, asymmetry, cerebral redistribution and oligohydramnios	24–35	SV	75.1 (15.88)	61.06 (8.8)†	<0.01
Melchiorre [26]	2012	AC <10th centile, UAPI >95th centile and need for delivery <37 weeks	at diagnosis	SVI	42 (35–48)	40 (38–46)	0.6
Oben [28]	2014	BW <5th centile	12	SV	65 (58–75)	75 (66–86)	0.033
Total peripheral vascular resistance (TPVR/TVR/their indices (TPVRI/TVRI))							
Rosso [25]	1993	BW <10th centile	36–38	TPVR	1306 (62)*	1031 (33)	<0.001
Bamfo [18]	2008	EFW <3rd centile, asymmetry, cerebral redistribution and oligohydramnios	24–35	TVR	1573.51 (268.87)	1434.05 (255.93)†	0.12
Melchiorre [26]	2012	AC <10th centile, UAPI >95th centile and need for delivery <37 weeks	at diagnosis	TVRI	2456 (2197–2894)	1857 (1553–2005)	<0.001
Lopes van Balen [27]	2013	BW <10th centile	18+/-2	PVR	1227 (1167–1288)	1138 (1064–1212)	0.065

values are reported as mean (standard deviation) or median (interquartile range)
* value are reported as mean (standard error of the mean); † controls were pregnancies complicated by hypertension and FGR
BW, Birth Weight; EFW, Estimated Fetal Weight; AC, Abdominal Circumference

avoid preeclampsia, but women with raised AIx (indicating preexisting endothelial dysfunction) are more likely to present with both preeclampsia and FGR.

This model has previously been proposed and a number of maternal factors have been identified that could cause endothelial dysfunction and interact with impaired placentation to produce preeclampsia [37]. These include insulin resistance, hyperlipidemia and disorders of coagulation [37,38]. It is also valid to propose that preexisting maternal endothelial dysfunction causes impaired placentation, which then later presents with preeclampsia, whereas impaired placentation in otherwise healthy women produces only fetal effects.

Arterial stiffness can also be measured by flow-mediated dilatation (FMD) responsiveness. A study in postnatal women using this technique demonstrated a persistent difference between women with pregnancies affected by FGR and those with AGA fetuses, whether hypertensive or not [39]. This difference is not seen when comparing glyceryl trinitrate (GTN) responsiveness between the study groups, which supports the view that endothelial dysfunction (rather than vascular smooth muscle dysfunction) is the primary pathology. It is not possible to ascertain from this study whether the vascular dysfunction predated pregnancy in only the preeclamptic patients. Neither does it tell us how long these changes will persist in normotensive women affected by FGR, but the findings of Khalil and colleagues would suggest that this similarity in vascular resistance does not exist in the first trimester until the endothelial damage associated with FGR is triggered [35].

Conclusions

Women with pregnancies complicated by FGR have reduced CO and increased TPR throughout pregnancy. Although CO in the third trimester is similar to that in pregnancies affected by preeclampsia, they have lower SV, better-preserved diastolic function, and low-to-normal MAP. In the first trimester, pregnancies complicated by SGA have less evidence of endothelial dysfunction than those that will develop preeclampsia, but do have evidence of endothelial dysfunction that persists past pregnancy.

These findings identify FGR as a unique pathophysiological process and help clarify the difference in pathogenesis of early-onset and late-onset preeclampsia. First trimester cardiovascular measurements may offer benefit if incorporated into screening tools for FGR and preeclampsia.

Key Points

- Women undergo a variety of physiological cardiovascular adaptations in normal pregnancy, in order to support the development of the fetoplacental unit.
- Marked changes from the non-pregnant state can be seen from as early as 6 weeks' gestation.
- Women with pregnancies complicated by fetal growth restriction (FGR) have reduced cardiac output and increased total peripheral resistance throughout pregnancy.
- Although cardiac output in the third trimester is similar to that in pregnancies affected by preeclampsia, they have lower stroke volume, better-preserved diastolic function, and low-to-normal mean arterial pressure.
- In the first trimester, pregnancies complicated by small for gestational age have less evidence of endothelial dysfunction than those that will develop preeclampsia, but do have evidence of endothelial dysfunction that persists past pregnancy.

References

1. Mahendru AA, Everett TR, Wilkinson IB, Lees CC, McEniery CM. Maternal cardiovascular changes from pre-pregnancy to very early pregnancy. *J Hypertens* 2012;30:2168–72.

2. Duvekot JJ, Cheriex EC, Pieters FA, Menheere PP, Peeters LH. Early pregnancy changes in hemodynamics and volume homeostasis are consecutive adjustments triggered by a primary fall in systemic vascular tone. *Am J Obstet Gynecol* 1993;169:1382–92.

3. Valensise H, Vasapollo B, Gagliardi G, Novelli GP. Early and late preeclampsia: Two different maternal hemodynamic states in the latent phase of the disease. *Hypertension* 2008;52:873–80.

4. Khalil A, Jauniaux E, Harrington K. Antihypertensive therapy and central hemodynamics in women with hypertensive disorders in pregnancy. *Obstet Gynecol* 2009;113:646–54.

5. Khaw A, Kametas NA, Turan OM, Bamfo JEAK, Nicolaides KH. Maternal cardiac function and uterine

artery Doppler at 11–14 weeks in the prediction of pre-eclampsia in nulliparous women. *BJOG* 2008;115:369–76.

6. Van Oppen AC, Van der Tweel I, Duvekot JJ, Bruinse HW. Use of cardiac index in pregnancy: Is it justified? *Am J Obstet Gynecol* 1995;173(3 Pt 1):923–8.

7. Rang S, Van Montfrans GA, Wolf H. Serial hemodynamic measurement in normal pregnancy, preeclampsia, and intrauterine growth restriction. *Am J Obstet Gynecol* 2008;198:519.e1–9.

8. Valensise H, Vasapollo B, Novelli GP. Maternal cardiovascular hemodynamics in normal and complicated pregnancies. *Fetal Matern Med Rev* 2003;14:355–85.

9. Valensise H, Novelli GP, Vasapollo B, Borzi M, Arduini D, Galante A, Romanini C. Maternal cardiac systolic and diastolic function: Relationship with uteroplacental resistances. A Doppler and echocardiographic longitudinal study. *Ultrasound Obstet Gynecol* 2000;15:487–97.

10. Tkachenko O, Shchekochikhin D, Schrier RW. Hormones and hemodynamics in pregnancy. *Int J Endocrinol Metab* 2014;12:e14098.

11. Curran-Everett D, Morris KG Jr, Moore LG. Regional circulatory contributions to increased systemic vascular conductance in pregnancy. *Am J Physiol* 1991;261:H1842–7.

12. Poppas A, Shroff SG, Korcarz CE, Hibbard JU, Berger DS, Lindheimer MD, Lang RM. Serial assessment of the cardiovascular system in normal pregnancy. Role of arterial compliance and pulsatile arterial load. *Circulation* 1997;95:2407–15.

13. Savu O, Jurcuţ R, Giuşcă S, Van Mieghem T, Gussi I, Popescu BA, Ginghină C, Rademakers F, Deprest J, Voigt JU. Morphological and functional adaptation of the maternal heart during pregnancy. *Circ Cardiovasc Imaging* 2012;5:289–97.

14. Chung E, Leinwand LA. Pregnancy as a cardiac stress model. *Cardiovasc Res* 2014;101:561–70.

15. Chung E, Yeung F, Leinwand LA. Calcineurin activity is required for cardiac remodelling in pregnancy. *Cardiovasc Res* 2013;100:402–10.

16. Karamermer Y, Roos-Hesselink JW. Coronary heart disease and pregnancy. *Future Cardiol* 2007;3:559–67.

17. Bosio PM, McKenna PJ, Conroy R, O'Herlihy C. Maternal central hemodynamics in hypertensive disorders of pregnancy. *Obstet Gynecol* 1999;94:978–84.

18. Bamfo JEAK, Kametas NA, Chambers JB, Nicolaides KH. Maternal cardiac function in normotensive and pre-eclamptic intrauterine growth restriction. *Ultrasound Obstet Gynecol* 2008;32:682–6.

19. Bamfo JEAK, Kametas NA, Chambers JB, Nicolaides KH. Maternal cardiac function in fetal growth-restricted and non-growth-restricted small-for-gestational age pregnancies. *Ultrasound Obstet Gynecol* 2007;29:51–7.

20. Conrad KP. Maternal vasodilation in pregnancy: The emerging role of relaxin. *Am J Physiol Regul Integr Comp Physiol* 2011;301:R267–75.

21. Visser W, Wallenburg HC. Central hemodynamic observations in untreated preeclamptic patients. *Hypertension* 1991;17:1072–7.

22. Spaanderman MEA, Willekes C, Hoeks APG, Ekhart THA, Aardenburg R, Courtar DA, et al. Maternal nonpregnant vascular function correlates with subsequent fetal growth. *Am J Obstet Gynecol* 2005;192:504–12.

23. Haelterman E, Bréart G, Paris-Llado J, Dramaix M, Tchobroutsky C. Effect of uncomplicated chronic hypertension on the risk of small-for-gestational age birth. *Am J Epidemiol* 1997;145:689–95.

24. Robertson WB, Brosens I, Dixon HG. The pathological response of the vessels of the placental bed to hypertensive pregnancy. *J Pathol Bacteriol* 1967;93:581–92.

25. Rosso P, Donoso E, Braun S, Espinoza R. Maternal hemodynamic adjustments in idiopathic fetal growth retardation. *Gynecol Obstet Invest* 1993;35:162–5.

26. Melchiorre K, Sutherland GR, Liberati M, Thilaganathan B. Maternal cardiovascular impairment in pregnancies complicated by severe fetal growth restriction. *Hypertension* 2012;60:437–43.

27. Lopes van Balen VA, Spaan JJ, Ghossein C, Van Kuijk SM, Spaanderman ME, Peeters LL. Early pregnancy circulatory adaptation and recurrent hypertensive disease: an explorative study. *Reprod Sci* 2013;20:1069–74.

28. Oben J, Tomsin K, Mesens T, Staelens A, Molenberghs G, Gyselaers W. Maternal cardiovascular profiling in the first trimester of pregnancies complicated with gestation-induced hypertension or fetal growth retardation: A pilot study. *J Matern Fetal Neonatal Med* 2014;27:1646–51.

29. Roman MJ, Devereux RB, Kizer JR, Lee ET, Galloway JM, Ali T, Umans JG, Howard BV. Central pressure more strongly relates to vascular disease and outcome than does brachial pressure: The Strong Heart Study. *Hypertension* 2007;50:197–203.

30. Terai M, Ohishi M, Ito N, Takagi T, Tatara Y, Kaibe M, et al. Comparison of arterial functional evaluations as a predictor of cardiovascular events in hypertensive patients: The Non-invasive Atherosclerotic Evaluation in Hypertension (NOAH) study. *Hypertens Res* 2008;31:1135–45.

31. O'Rourke MF. Arterial pressure waveforms in hypertension. *Minerva Med* 2003;94:229–50.

32. Laurent S, Cockcroft J, Van Bortel L, Boutouyrie P, Giannattasio C, Hayoz D, Pannier B, Vlachopoulos C, Wilkinson I, Struijker-Boudier Hl; European Network for Non-invasive Investigation of Large Arteries. Expert consensus document on arterial stiffness: Methodological issues and clinical applications. *Eur Heart J* 2006;27:2588–605.

33. Horváth IG, Németh A, Lenkey Z, Alessandri N, Tufano F, Kis P, Gaszner B, Cziráki A. Invasive validation of a new oscillometric device (Arteriograph) for measuring augmentation index, central blood pressure and aortic pulse wave velocity. *Hypertens* 2010;28:2068–75.

34. Hausvater A, Giannone T, Sandoval YH, Doonan RJ, Antonopoulos CN, Matsoukis IL, Petridou ET, Daskalopoulou SS. The association between preeclampsia and arterial stiffness. *J Hypertens* 2012;30:17–33.

35. Khalil A, Sodre D, Syngelaki A, Akolekar R NK. Maternal hemodynamics at 11–13 weeks of gestation in pregnancies delivering small for gestational age neonates. *Fetal Diagn Ther* 2012;32:231–8.

36. Spasojevic M, Smith SA, Morris JM, Gallery EDM. Peripheral arterial pulse wave analysis in women with pre-eclampsia and gestational hypertension. *BJOG* 2005;112:1475–8.

37. Ness RB, Sibai BM. Shared and disparate components of the pathophysiologies of fetal growth restriction and preeclampsia. *Am J Obstet Gynecol* 2006;195:40–9.

38. Thadhani R, Ecker JL, Mutter WP, Wolf M, Smirnakis K V., Sukhatme VP, et al. Insulin resistance and alterations in angiogenesis: Additive insults that may lead to preeclampsia. *Hypertension* 2004;43:988–92.

39. Yinon Y, Kingdom JCP, Odutayo A, Moineddin R, Drewlo S, Lai V, et al. Vascular dysfunction in women with a history of preeclampsia and intrauterine growth restriction: Insights into future vascular risk. *Circulation* 2010;122:1846–53.

9 Placental Histopathology Findings in Fetal Growth Restriction

Neil Sebire and William Mifsud

Introduction

Pathological changes identified post-delivery in placentas from pregnancies associated with FGR are highly variable, ranging from characteristic abnormalities typical of uteroplacental vasculopathy to morphologically normal. This is likely because FGR is associated with a wide range of underlying mechanisms, and the placenta is a heterogeneous organ with geographical differences in pathological responses. Since only a small proportion of the placenta is typically examined histologically, there may be inadvertent sampling bias and lower detection rates for pathological changes, as well as variable sampling strategies between different studies. Furthermore, there are inter-observer differences in interpretation of many findings; some lesions are identified on the basis of arbitrary thresholds (for example, villitis of unknown etiology (VUE) is reportedly associated with FGR at highly variable rates). In addition, the terminology for placental morphological changes is not standardized, and different lesions and groupings may be reported in separate studies.

FGR may be secondary to systemic diseases and placental findings may reveal characteristic changes, for example, cytomegalic inclusions and villitis may suggest CMV infection and dysmorphic edematous villi may suggest a chromosomal anomaly. However, for the purposes of this chapter, the discussion will be confined to cases of FGR that are not associated with obvious other underlying conditions, hence representing the majority of clinical FGR cases.

FGR is a dynamic process, but in the majority of studies the population is defined based on fetal size below a particular centile at a single time point. With such groups, a significant proportion of cases therefore represents constitutionally small rather than pathologically FGR cases, emphasizing the need to distinguish FGR from smallness for gestational age (SGA) when interpreting studies.

With these caveats in mind, the majority of placentas associated with primary FGR have no identifiable gross pathological changes, and approximately a quarter are histologically normal on routine microscopic examination [1]. Improved correlations occur when study populations are tightly defined, especially by abnormal Doppler studies and serum markers, as well as with identification of high-risk subgroups. Specific morphological changes are reported with uteroplacental malperfusion, and additional morphological features reflect fetal compromise detected by abnormal umbilical artery Doppler studies.

The patterns of placental changes occurring in FGR cases with abnormal uterine artery (UtA) Doppler indices are similar to those occurring with preterm preeclampsia, and likely reflect a shared underlying defect of trophoblastic invasion of the maternal spiral arteries with secondary fetoplacental changes. (Broadly similar changes may also be detected in placentas from pregnancies complicated by genetic thrombophilic states, and conditions such as systemic lupus erythematosus and antiphospholipid syndrome.) Morphological changes of uteroplacental malperfusion include infarcts, decidual vascular atherosis, villous agglutination, and small straight, hypovascular terminal villi with increased syncytial knots. It is likely that with increasingly accurate methods of antenatal phenotyping of patients and detection of pathological FGR, understanding of specific pathological mechanisms and subtypes will improve.

Placental Macroscopic Features in Fetal Growth Restriction

Placental size is broadly related to fetal size, and is therefore proportionally reduced in FGR pregnancies [2–5]. The most frequent macroscopic lesion that occurs with increased frequency in FGR placentas compared to controls is patchy infarction [2,3]. The frequency varies, but in one series of 128 SGA placentas at term (birth weight less than 10th centile for gestational age), infarcts were present in 24% of SGA cases vs. 10% of non SGA controls. Only a minority (approximately 10%–15%) of placental infarcts are detected by antenatal ultrasound [6]. While the incidence of macroscopic infarction is increased in SGA compared to controls, infarcts affect only a minority of SGA cases. Furthermore, since non-SGA pregnancies are far more frequent than SGA pregnancies, the positive predictive value of such a finding in an unselected case is very low. Other macroscopic features that are variably reported with increased frequency in FGR/SGA placentas include placental abruption [1,3], hypercoiled cord [7], single umbilical artery, marginal cord insertion, velamentous cord insertion, and circumvallate placental morphology [2,4], although their clinical significance in this context in most cases remains uncertain.

Placental Histological Features Associated with Fetal Growth Restriction and Uteroplacental Malperfusion

The introduction of uterine artery (UtA) Doppler studies identified a subgroup of SGA fetuses with evidence of uteroplacental malperfusion, and placental bed biopsies in these cases showed a strong association with lesions of defective spiral artery remodeling by intermediate trophoblast: these include inadequate physiological change of the spiral arteries, fibrinoid necrosis, dense perivascular lymphocytic infiltrate, and the presence of mural foam cells (acute atherosis) [8–10]. These lesions may collectively be referred to as "decidual vasculopathy" (Figures X-Y), and while they are easy to detect on placental bed biopsies, they often cannot be adequately assessed in delivered placental samples, which typically include only a relatively small amount of superficial decidua, even with sampling regimes that increase the yield of decidual vessels [11].

Abnormal UtA Doppler indices have a strong positive predictive value (PPV; >90%) for defective trophoblast migration in placental bed biopsies, although a normal UtA Doppler profile has only a low negative predictive value (NPV) of less than 50% [10], indicating that there is a group of pregnancies with defective trophoblast migration in whom uteroplacental perfusion remains initially adequate based on Doppler findings.

In addition to decidual changes, uteroplacental malperfusion is associated with secondary morphological changes of the chorionic villi, including increased syncytiotrophoblast knotting, excess cytotrophoblast cells, thickened trophoblastic basement membrane, villous fibrosis, hypovascularity, and small, poorly branched villi. These features of "hypoxic villous damage," as well as non-peripheral infarcts involving more than 5% of placental parenchyma, and placental abruption, are associated with SGA cases with abnormal UtA velocimetry [12]. Furthermore, the majority of cases with such findings and abnormal UtA velocimetry are delivered before 37 weeks' gestation, with associated increased perinatal mortality. The presence or absence of pregnancy-induced hypertension per se does not appear to significantly affect these findings [12]. In contrast, most clinically identified SGA pregnancies with normal UtA velocimetry are usually delivered after 37 weeks' gestation, without markedly increased perinatal mortality. These findings identify a high-risk subgroup of SGA in which UtA velocimetry is a marker for defective remodeling of spiral arteries into uteroplacental vessels with consequent placental malperfusion, ischemia/reperfusion, impaired fetal growth, and greater perinatal mortality.

It remains uncertain why defective trophoblast migration only results in abnormal UtA Doppler velocimetry in a subset of cases: trophoblast migration occurs over a long period of gestation up to 24 weeks, and is likely not a homogenous process, and impairment of overall uteroplacental perfusion is likely to require a certain critical proportion of maternal vessels to remain untransformed.

Other studies, both with and without UtA Doppler correlation, have reported similar placental histological findings in SGA, and have also identified increased rates of other lesions, including increased/massive perivillous fibrin deposition, increase in nucleated fetal red blood cells, reduction in intervillous space and villous volume, and patchy villous inflammatory changes amounting to villitis of unknown etiology (VUE) [2,3,12–24]. However, no single histological change is present in more than 50% of cases, regardless of correlation with UtA Doppler velocimetry.

Abnormal UtA Doppler profiles are also reported in association with preterm preeclampsia, and correspond to a very similar pattern of microscopic lesions in the placental bed and placenta [9,25–30]. While it is difficult to exhaustively compare placental findings in SGA versus preeclampsia due to the limitations described previously, two studies [16,31] were carried out by the same group on the same study population (with delivery between 22 and 32 weeks' gestation), with tissue apparently sampled consistently, and the same pathologist assessing virtually identical sets of placental lesions across all cases. Of the 48 cases with "symmetrical" SGA (with both birth weight and fetal length below the 10th centile), 31 (65%) also had preeclampsia, a considerable overlap, especially since Doppler velocimetry was not a selection criteria. In a previous comparison of these and other studies [32], apart from some minor discrepancies in reporting lesions, preeclampsia cases are generally associated with greater proportions with certain findings compared to non-preeclampsia SGA, including "severe villous fibrosis" (80%, vs. 30%, respectively) and "severe villous hypovascularity" (70%, vs. 25%, respectively). These microscopic features (discussed further in the section on umbilical artery Doppler abnormalities) suggest that in that study population, preterm preeclampsia was associated with a higher rate of fetal compromise than preterm pure SGA, despite comparable rates of other placental microscopic changes. In addition, around 10% of the preterm SGA group had amnionitis, whereas none of the cases with preeclampsia had acute inflammation. All other features reported in both studies were detected at comparable frequencies [16,31,32]. The findings suggest that there is a common pathway of inadequate trophoblastic migration and conversion of maternal arteries, and when this is significant enough to impair overall uteroplacental perfusion, it may become clinically manifest as FGR and/or preeclampsia, presumably dependent on other, likely maternal factors.

The extent of impaired trophoblast invasion in the placental bed is broadly associated with the severity of the UtA Doppler abnormality [10,33–35], and the presence of acute atherosis and/or fibrinoid necrosis especially is associated with more severe FGR [36,37]. However, the clinical severities of FGR and preeclampsia are not closely related to the severity of "ischemic"-type changes in the placental parenchyma. In a study of preterm SGA placentas (<32 weeks' gestation), histological parameters that showed significant association with SGA were used as variables in a multiple regression analysis, in which FGR was the dependent variable. These placental variables could account for only around 30% of the variation in fetal growth, increasing only slightly if the presence of preeclampsia was added to the model. This indicates that histological measures of "severity" of placental lesions do not correlate well with the clinical severity of FGR, due either to methodological and sampling issues or genuine variation in pathology/phenotype relationship. When multiple regression was applied to only those cases with preeclampsia, the predictive value was only around 10%, and the individual contributions of the independent variables became much lower, indicating that placental parenchymal histological features correlate better with the presence of preeclampsia rather than with the severity of FGR in those with preeclampsia. Furthermore, the histological "severity" of placental parenchymal lesions is poorly correlated with the clinical severity of the preeclampsia. Thus, while disease associations are described and general pathological mechanisms can be implied, it is not possible to establish the severity of either preeclampsia or FGR from placental features.

In summary, uteroplacental malperfusion secondary to insufficient trophoblast migration and conversion of maternal spiral arteries is an underlying common mechanism leading to the largest group of FGR and/or preeclampsia. Its cause in any single case is often unclear, but there are considerable subsets of cases where there is a probable causative contribution from underlying conditions such as genetic thrombophilia or an autoimmune process typified by antiphospholipid antibodies; in both situations, the uteroplacental malperfusion is most likely not related to direct thrombotic events, but complex interactions with endothelium and trophoblast.

Genetic Thrombophilia and Uteroplacental Malperfusion

The background rate of genetic thrombophilias varies in different populations, but is generally relatively high at approximately 15–20%. There is a significantly greater frequency of genetic thrombophilias in women with severe preeclampsia [38,39], and FGR is more commonly found in those cases with severe preeclampsia who also have thrombophilia [38], while thrombophilic mutations, especially factor V Leiden, in cases with preeclampsia, are significantly more common in the subset with abnormal UtA Doppler indices [39]. These findings suggest that genetic thrombophilias increase the likelihood of impaired uteroplacental perfusion, possibly through a similar mechanism of impaired trophoblastic invasion and conversion of the maternal spiral arteries. To test this suggestion conclusively requires an analysis of the placental bed in these cases, but to date no such published studies are available. Morphological changes in the placenta, however, demonstrate a similar pattern of histological findings in placentas from complicated pregnancies with and without genetic thrombophilia (FGR, preeclampsia, placental abruption) leading to preterm birth [40–42], with one study finding significantly higher rates of infarction and fibrinoid necrosis of decidual vessels in thrombophilia-associated cases [41]; importantly, the data do not suggest a significant difference in the proportion of cases with maternal or fetal vessel thrombi or massive perivillous fibrin deposition. Thus, genetic thrombophilia is associated with an increased risk of preeclampsia and FGR, with placental morphology similar to cases with uteroplacental malperfusion due to idiopathic defective trophoblast migration.

Antiphospholipid Antibodies, Systemic Lupus Erythematosus and Uteroplacental Malperfusion

There are higher rates of SGA and of preeclampsia, as well as recurrent miscarriage and stillbirth, in women with antiphospholipid antibodies [43,44], and similarly in women with systemic lupus erythematosus (SLE) [45]. The presence of antiphospholipid antibodies is also associated with abnormal UtA Doppler waveforms [46], suggesting that antiphospholipid antibodies may impair trophoblast migration and conversion of maternal spiral arteries. Indeed, mothers with SLE have an increased incidence of decidual vasculopathy in placental samples [47]. In one study there was defective trophoblast migration in almost 90% of decidual material from "products of conception" in recurrent miscarriages with primary antiphospholipid syndrome (PAPS) compared to around 40% in PAPS-negative cases, in which the proportion was comparable to that found in social terminations of pregnancy without a history of recurrent pregnancy loss [48]. Another study of histological findings in placental bed biopsies in PAPS reported an increased incidence of decidual chronic inflammatory cell infiltrates (which were found in most cases), especially macrophages, but, surprisingly, no significant difference in spiral artery remodeling when compared to a control group of placental bed biopsies from women without PAPS [49]. However, in this study, only 3 of the 10 placental bed biopsies in the PAPS group had FGR and none had preeclampsia, and, apart from another case with uterine rupture in labor, the remaining cases had no antenatal complications. The comparison was thus between PAPS cases that were uncomplicated and a control group without PAPS, and therefore may not be representative of PAPS pathologies. The overall findings suggest that women with PAPS have an increased likelihood of defective trophoblast migration, which may occur on a background of increased decidual recruitment of macrophages and other chronic inflammatory cells. Indeed, in a culture model, first-trimester trophoblast cells showed reduced migration when antiphospholipid antibodies bound trophoblast-expressed β2-glycoprotein I, with concomitant reduction in STAT3 activity and IL-6 production [50].

The manifestations of PAPS and SLE in the placenta itself have been described in numerous studies. A recent systematic review [51] was limited by difficulties in comparing the findings between different studies, as described generally in the introduction to this chapter, but nevertheless suggested a possible pattern of five features associated with aaPLs: placental infarction, increased syncytial knots, a reduced number of vasculosyncytial membranes, impaired spiral artery remodeling, and decidual inflammation. However, it is apparent that the first four features are associated with all forms of uteroplacental malperfusion, and the decidual inflammation is significant only when compared to uncomplicated control pregnancies. Indeed, decidual perivascular chronic inflammatory infiltrates are part of the spectrum of decidual vasculopathic lesions and there is, to date, no clear comparison of decidual inflammatory infiltrates in placental bed biopsies from cases with uteroplacental malperfusion according to antiphospholipid antibody status.

Placental Histopathological Findings Associated with Umbilical Artery Doppler Abnormalities

Abnormal umbilical artery (UA) Doppler indices are associated with increased rates of fetal hypoxia and perinatal mortality [52]. In most cases, the UA Doppler changes are progressive and are accompanied by abnormal uterine artery Doppler velocimetry, which typically develops well before the umbilical arterial abnormality [53]. Abnormal UA Doppler indices represent increased fetoplacental circulation resistance and histologically, the UA Doppler resistance is related to several factors, including stem villous fetal vessel wall thickening, narrowed lumina and luminal herniation, and terminal villi that are smaller, fibrotic, and hypovascular [54]. Furthermore, particularly in association with absent or reversed end-diastolic umbilical artery flow (and preterm delivery), the pattern of "distal villous hypoplasia" has been described, in which the centers of placental lobules have reduced numbers of terminal villi, with remaining villi having smaller diameters, fewer branches, reduced vascularity, and, in some, syncytial knots [23,55,56]. The available evidence suggests that these changes in the stem and terminal villi are most likely secondary to uteroplacental malperfusion in the majority of cases, rather than a primary defect, for the following reasons [53]: first, the changes in the stem villus arteries are strongly suggestive of a response to chronic vasoconstriction, and develop in parallel with a progressive umbilical artery Doppler abnormality; second, similar changes in terminal villi also occur in the territory of an upstream fetal vascular occlusion; third, in most cases there is defective uteroplacental perfusion secondary to defective trophoblast invasion, with associated uterine artery Doppler abnormality in advance of the umbilical artery Doppler abnormality; and finally, experimental evidence from animal studies demonstrates a rapid increase in umbilical artery resistance upon reducing the maternal placental perfusion [57].

Furthermore, there is experimental evidence of rapid and reversible fetal vasoconstriction in the human placenta in response to hypoxia [58], which involves inhibition of K+ channels in isolated placental cotyledons, analogous to the lung [59]. This activity is localized to vessels distal to the chorionic plate. In both lungs and placenta, hypoxic vasoconstriction allows for deoxygenated blood to perfuse regions where it will be most efficiently oxygenated, given that the distribution of highly oxygenated gas (pulmonary ventilation) or blood (maternal placental perfusion) is not uniform. In the setting of global placental hypoxia due to impaired maternal perfusion, as seen in typical FGR, reactive fetal vasoconstriction would gradually increase the global resistance to flow through the fetoplacental circulation. Similar to the pulmonary circulation, hypoxia-induced and K+ channel mediated depolarization of vascular smooth muscle cells activates voltage-gated L-type gated Ca2+ channels,

which provides cytosolic Ca2+ for activating the contractile apparatus [60].

One should point out, however, that experimental demonstrations of possible fetal hypoxic vasoconstriction in the placenta have been made with oxygen tensions that are greater than those in the placenta *in vivo* [52]. To the best of our knowledge, no studies have reported the effect of hypoxia, at levels approximating those in the placenta, on preparations including the entire fetal subchorionic vasculature. There have been reports studying placental levels of hypoxia on isolated chorionic plate arteries and veins with diameters of 268 ± 13 μm (arteries) and 266 ± 19 μm (veins), reporting increased chorionic vessel vasodilatation in response to NO, but no convincing hypoxic chorionic artery vasoconstriction. However, the isolated vessels used in these studies were too large to represent stem villus vessels, whose diameter is typically in the range of 10–100 μm in both normal and FGR pregnancies [61].

Separately, a similar role for hypoxic fetal vasoconstriction in FGR was hypothesized and suggested as the most likely explanation of the fetal vascular and villous tree abnormalities identified in FGR with umbilical artery Doppler abnormalities. It is likely that there is also a capacity to regulate fetal stem venous tone, subject to autocrine/paracrine signaling, to maintain water balance against fluctuations in capillary pressure driven by changes in intervillous pressure (from maternal uteroplacental perfusion) and fetal arterial perfusion pressure; such mechanisms appear feasible based on iterative mathematical models for homeostasis in response to placental hypoxia and other fluctuations in uteroplacental blood flow [62–64].

To adequately test these hypotheses, one would need an experimental system that can maintain placental cotyledons at physiological levels of oxygenation and also truly representative levels of hypoxia, while allowing for independent variation of intervillous perfusion pressure, while measuring vascular tone across all the different vessel types (arterial, venous, different calibers). To date, such a system has not been reported.

More recently, the similarity of the changes in the stem villus arteries between severe FGR and preterm preeclampsia was further highlighted by the report that in both clinical situations smooth muscle cells in the stem villus arteries show markedly reduced expression of cystathione-lyase (CSE), an enzyme responsible for synthesis of the potent vasodilator hydrogen sulphide (H2S). Its reduced expression in the fetal villous resistance vessels supports the view that there is vasoconstriction in the fetal stem villi in association with an abnormal umbilical Doppler profile [65].

Placental Histopathological Features of FGR at Term

The classic placental histological phenotype of uteroplacental malperfusion occurs in association with preterm FGR and/or preeclampsia. Nevertheless, a proportion of fetuses delivered at term is growth restricted, and may or may not also be SGA. These cases have significantly increased frequencies of typical uteroplacental vascular lesions (especially infarcts) when compared to normal fetuses delivered at term, but the actual frequencies are much less than those described in preterm SGA fetuses [3,16]. Therefore, there are at least two groups of small fetuses at term, in addition to those that are constitutionally small. First are those with a similar uteroplacental perfusion defect to classical preterm FGR, but with a milder phenotype; study of this group may provide insights into how the same mechanism can have such variable impact on fetal growth and perinatal outcome. Second are those that are FGR at term due to other (currently unknown) causes; importantly, this group does not appear to overlap with late-onset term preeclampsia, which, unlike preterm preeclampsia, is typically not associated with FGR regardless of clinical phenotype severity.

Distal villous immaturity and distal villous hypoplasia have recently been reported as placental histological phenotypes that may be seen in some cases of term FGR. The patterns are not well studied, and it is not clear if this represents the cases of FGR with distal villous hypoplasia that continue to term or alternative late primary villous maldevelopment [66].

Fetal Growth Restriction and Villitis of Unknown Etiology (VUE)

VUE is characterized by chorionic villous infiltration by chronic inflammatory cells, particularly histiocytes, and to a lesser extent, lymphocytes, especially in basal/maternal floor villi, in the absence of a known, typically infective cause. These changes may be accompanied by fibrin deposition and villous destruction.

Despite this detailed description, there is considerable variation among placental pathologists in recognizing this lesion on routine histological evaluation, particularly in cases in which the inflammatory infiltrate is mild, the diagnosis often being subjective [67]. Furthermore, the reports of different rates of VUE are based on varied sampling methods and studies of different populations. VUE frequency ranges from 8–90%! [32] It is not appropriate, therefore, to simply combine the published reports into one meta-analysis. Nevertheless, there does appear to be a consistently increased frequency of VUE in SGA/FGR series, with one published notable exception being a series containing 38 placentas from SGA pregnancies and 175 from appropriate-for-gestational age (AGA) pregnancies, in which the overall rate of VUE was relatively high (31%), but not significantly different between SGA and AGA placentas [68].

The frequency of VUE is reported as increased in cases of in vitro fertilization (IVF) with donor oocytes vs. cases with native oocytes [69]. In addition, there is an increased risk of VUE recurrence in women with affected pregnancies (from approximately 5–11% to 17–20%) [70]; VUE is approximately twice as common and more diffuse in multi-gravid patients [71], and there is a greater-than-expected concordance in twin pregnancies [72]. Taken together, these data suggest that VUE represents a possible maternal immune reaction against tissue of fetal origin, but the mechanism by which it results in FGR in some cases remains uncertain. Note that although there is an association with FGR and PET, since VUE is relatively common, the vast majority of placentas in which it is detected in an unselected population are not associated with FGR, or indeed any other significant complication, it representing a clinically incidental finding [73].

Fetal Growth Restriction and Other Specific Pathologies

Other specific histological patterns are also described more frequently with FGR/SGA pregnancies. A relatively rare placental histological phenotype is chronic histiocytic intervillositis, characterized by an intervillous infiltrate rich in histiocytes, in the absence of villitis and without evidence of infection. This condition is recognized as an important association of recurrent pregnancy loss, since it has a high recurrence risk, with a probable immune pathogenesis, and while it more commonly leads to pregnancy loss in the first trimester, the majority of cases lost in the second or third trimesters are severely growth-restricted [74].

Another rare lesion with a possible immune-related pathogenesis is massive perivillous fibrin deposition: while this may occur in conjunction with features of uteroplacental malperfusion, it may also be the only placental histopathological lesion identified in a small number of FGR cases [17]. Such cases are typified by extensive areas of fibrin deposition in the intervillous space hence reducing villous oxygen delivery, associated with trophoblast proliferation into the surrounding fibrin. Perivillous fibrin of some degree is a normal finding in uncomplicated control placentas and hence the distinction between normal and "increased" perivillous fibrin is somewhat arbitrary and prone to sampling effects.

In some cases of FGR, the only abnormal placental findings are of diffusely "avascular" villi (in which the vessels are collapsed and difficult to visualize on standard hematoxylin- and eosin-stained sections), with or without detectable thrombotic occlusion of upstream fetal vessels. Excluding avascular villi secondary to intrauterine fetal demise, this pattern, known as fetal thrombotic vasculopathy or fetal vascular occlusion, is observed at greater frequency in FGR and other major pregnancy complications, but is also found in placentas from apparently uncomplicated pregnancies [73,75].

Conclusion

While certain specific placental lesions, or patterns of histological findings, are reported more frequently in FGR cases than in controls, in unselected populations, the positive and negative predictive values of these findings are typically low. In general, more marked histological changes are identified in cases presenting with FGR at earlier gestational ages and in association with preeclampsia. Uteroplacental malperfusion is the dominant underlying mechanism in which associated placental parenchymal changes may be identified. This mechanism may be a final common pathway for a number of underlying predisposition states.

Fetal circulatory compromise, detected by abnormal umbilical artery Doppler abnormalities, is associated with placental findings suggestive of chronic vasoconstriction of stem vessels with secondary villous morphological changes. In a minority of cases,

other specific histological findings are present, some associated with significantly increased recurrence risk. Despite these findings, many cases of FGR, especially at term, may be associated with minimal morphological changes in the delivered placenta and objective determination of the significance of any such findings in an individual case remains unreliable.

Future studies are required to recruit well-defined patient populations, with blinded, objective histological assessment and evaluation of future novel laboratory approaches, in order to develop standardized and objective criteria to identify lesions and evaluate their significance in clinical practice.

Key Points

- Specific placental lesions, or patterns of histological findings, are reported more frequently in FGR cases than in controls.
- In unselected populations, the positive and negative predictive values of placental features for FGR are poor.
- FGR at earlier gestational ages are more likely to demonstrate typical features of uteroplacental malperfusion/maternal vascular malperfusion.
- Abnormal umbilical artery Doppler abnormalities are associated with chronic vasoconstriction of stem vessels and secondary villous changes.
- Rarely, other specific pathologies are associated with FGR, such as villitis, intervillositis, and perivillous fibrin deposition.
- Some cases of FGR, especially at term, may show minimal morphological changes in the placenta.
- Future studies require well-defined populations, with blinded, objective histological assessment.
- Novel laboratory approaches are required to provide standardized and objective criteria for lesions and their significance.

References

1. Fox H, Sebire NJ. The placenta in abnormalities and disorders of the fetus. In Fox H, Sebire NJ,

editors. *Pathology of the Placenta* (Major Problems in Pathology 7). Philadelphia, PA: Saunders Elsevier.

2. Bjoro K. Gross pathology of the placenta in intrauterine growth restriction. *Ann Chir Gynaecol* 1981;70(6):316–22.

3. Salafia CM, Vintzileos AM, Silberman L, Bantham KF, Vogel CA. Placental pathology of idiopathic intrauterine growth retardation at term. *Am J Perinatol*. Department of Laboratory Medicine, Danbury Hospital, Connecticut; 1992;9(3):179–84.

4. Biswas S, Ghosh SK. Gross morphological changes of placentas associated with intrauterine growth restriction of fetuses: A case control study. *Early Hum Dev* 2008;84(6):357–62.

5. Tomas SZ, Roje D, Prusac IK, Tadin I, Capkun V. Morphological characteristics of placentas associated with idiopathic intrauterine growth retardation: A clinicopathologic study. *Eur J Obstet Gynecol Reprod Biol*. School of Medicine University Split, Soltanska 2, 21000 Split, Croatia. sandrazt@online.hr; 2010;152(1):39–43.

6. Harris RD, Simpson WA, Pet LR, Marin-Padilla M, Crow HC. Placental hypoechoic-anechoic areas and infarction: Sonographic-pathologic correlation. *Radiology* 1990;176(1):75–80.

7. Sebire NJ. Pathophysiological significance of abnormal umbilical cord coiling index. *Ultrasound Obstet Gynecol* 2007;30(6):804–6.

8. Gerretsen GG, Huisjes HJ, Elema JD. Morphological changes of the spiral arteries in the placental bed in relation to pre-eclampsia and fetal growth retardation. *BJOG* 1981;88(9):876–81.

9. Olofsson P, Laurini RN, Marsál K. A high uterine artery pulsatility index reflects a defective development of placental bed spiral arteries in pregnancies complicated by hypertension and fetal growth retardation. *Eur J Obstet Gynecol Reprod Biol*. Department of Obstetrics and Gynecology, University of Lund, Malmö General Hospital, Sweden; 1993;49(3):161–8.

10. Lin S, Shimizu I, Suehara N, Nakayama M, Aono T. Uterine artery Doppler velocimetry in relation to trophoblast migration into the myometrium of the placental bed. *Obstet Gynecol*. Department of Obstetrics and Pathology, Osaka Medical Center, Japan; 1995;85(5 Pt 1):760–5.

11. Khong TY, Chambers HM. Alternative method of sampling placentas for the assessment of uteroplacental vasculature. *J Clin Pathol*. Department of Pathology, Adelaide Medical Centre for Women and Children, Queen Victoria Hospital, Australia: BMJ Group; 1992;45(10):925–7.

12. Wigglesworth JS. The gross and microscopic pathology of the prematurely delivered placenta. *J Obstet Gynaecol Br Emp* 1962;69:934–43.

13. Wigglesworth JS. Morphological variations in the insufficient placenta. *J Obstet Gynaecol Br Commonw* 1964;71:871–84.

14. Altshuler G, Russell P, Ermocilla R. The placental pathology of small-for-gestational age infants. *Am J Obstet Gynecol*. Elsevier Inc; 1975;121(3):351–9.

15. Garcia AG. Placental morphology of low-birth-weight infants born at term. *Contrib Gynecol Obstet* 1982;9:100–12.

16. Salafia CM, Minior VK, Pezzullo JC, Popek EJ, Rosenkrantz TS, Vintzileos AM. Intrauterine growth restriction in infants of less than thirty-two weeks' gestation: Associated placental pathologic features. *Am J Obstet Gynecol*. Division of Anatomic Pathology, University of Connecticut Health Center, Farmington, USA: Elsevier Inc; 1995;173(4):1049–57.

17. Oliveira LH, Xavier CC, Lana AMA. [Changes in placental morphology of small for gestational age newborns]. *J Pediatr* (Rio J). Universidade Federal de Juiz de Fora, MG. lucio@icb.ufjf.br; 2002;78(5):397–402.

18. Labarrere CC, Althabe OO, Telenta MM. Chronic villitis of unknown aetiology in placentae of idiopathic small for gestational age infants. *Placenta*. Elsevier Ltd.; 1982;3(3):309–17.

19. Van der Veen F, Fox H. The human placenta in idiopathic intrauterine growth retardation: A light and electron microscopic study. *Placenta*. Elsevier Ltd.; 1983;4(1):65–77.

20. Boyd PA, Scott A. Quantitative structural studies on human placentas associated with pre-eclampsia, essential hypertension and intrauterine growth retardation. *BJOG* 1985;92(7):714–21.

21. Macara L, Kingdom JC, Kaufmann P, Kohnen G, Hair J, More IA, et al. Structural analysis of placental terminal villi from growth-restricted pregnancies with abnormal umbilical artery Doppler waveforms. *Placenta*. Department of Obstetrics and Gynaecology, University of Glasgow, Scotland, UK: Elsevier Ltd.; 1996;17(1):37–48.

22. Krebs C, Macara LM, Leiser R, Bowman AW, Greer IA, Kingdom JC. Intrauterine growth restriction with absent end-diastolic flow velocity in the umbilical artery is associated with maldevelopment of the placental terminal villous tree. *Am J Obstet Gynecol*. Department of Veterinary Anatomy, Justus Liebig University, Giessen, Germany: Elsevier Inc; 1996;175(6):1534–42.

23. Todros T, Sciarrone A, Piccoli E, Guiot C, Kaufmann P, Kingdom J. Umbilical Doppler

waveforms and placental villous angiogenesis in pregnancies complicated by fetal growth restriction. *Obstet Gynecol*. Department of Obstetrics and Gynaecology, University of Torino, Italy. todros@iol.it; 1999;93(4):499–503.

24. Mayhew TM, Ohadike C, Baker PN, Crocker IP, Mitchell C, Ong SS. Stereological investigation of placental morphology in pregnancies complicated by pre-eclampsia with and without intrauterine growth restriction. *Placenta*. Elsevier Ltd.; 2003;24(2–3):219–26.

25. Sheppard BL, Bonnar JJ. An ultrastructural study of utero-placental spiral arteries in hypertensive and normotensive pregnancy and fetal growth retardation. *BJOG* 1981;88(7):695–705.

26. Brosens IA, Robertson WB, Dixon HG. The role of the spiral arteries in the pathogenesis of preeclampsia. *Obstet Gynecol Annu* 1972;1:177–91.

27. De Wolf F, Brosens I, Renaer M. Fetal growth retardation and the maternal arterial supply of the human placenta in the absence of sustained hypertension. *BJOG* 1980;87(8):678–85.

28. Khong TY, De Wolf F, Robertson WB, Brosens I. Inadequate maternal vascular response to placentation in pregnancies complicated by pre-eclampsia and by small-for-gestational age infants. *BJOG* 1986;93(10):1049–59.

29. Voigt HJ, Becker V. Doppler flow measurements and histomorphology of the placental bed in uteroplacental insufficiency. *J Perinat Med*. Department of Obstetrics and Gynecology, University of Erlangen-Nuernberg, Fed. Rep. of Germany; 1992;20(2):139–47.

30. Roberts JM, Redman CW. Pre-eclampsia: More than pregnancy-induced hypertension. *Lancet*. Department of Obstetrics, Gynecology, and Reproductive Sciences, Magee Women's Hospital, University of Pittsburgh, Pennsylvania 15213; 1993;341(8858):1447–51.

31. Salafia CM, Pezzullo JC, López-Zeno JA, Simmens S, Minior VK, Vintzileos AM. Placental pathologic features of preterm preeclampsia. *Am J Obstet Gynecol*. Division of Anatomic Pathology, University of Connecticut Health Center, Farmington, USA: Elsevier Inc.; 1995;173(4):1097–105.

32. Mifsud W, Sebire NJ. Placental pathology in early-onset and late-onset fetal growth restriction. *Fetal Diagn Ther* 2014.

33. Sağol S, Sağol O, Ozdemir N. Stereological quantification of placental villus vascularization and its relation to umbilical artery Doppler flow in intrauterine growth restriction. *Prenat Diagn*. Department of Obstetrics and Gynaecology, Medical Faculty, Ege University, Turkey. sagol@med.ege.edu.tr; 2002;22(5):398–403.

34. Aardema MW, Oosterhof H, Timmer A, Van Rooy I, Aarnoudse JG. Uterine artery Doppler flow and uteroplacental vascular pathology in normal pregnancies and pregnancies complicated by pre-eclampsia and small for gestational age fetuses. *Placenta* 2001;22(5):405–11.

35. Madazli R, Somunkiran A, Calay Z, Ilvan S, Aksu MF. Histomorphology of the placenta and the placental bed of growth restricted foetuses and correlation with the Doppler velocimetries of the urine and umbilical arteries. *Placenta* 2003;24(5):510–16.

36. McFadyen IR, Price a B, Geirsson RT. The relation of birthweight to histological appearances in vessels of the placental bed. *BJOG* 1986;93(5):476–81.

37. Frusca T, Morassi L, Pecorelli S, Grigolato P, Gastaldi A. Histological features of uteroplacental vessels in normal and hypertensive patients in relation to birthweight. *BJOG* 1989;96(7):835–9.

38. Kupferminc MJ, Fait G, Many A, Gordon D, Eldor A, Lessing JB. Severe preeclampsia and high frequency of genetic thrombophilic mutations. *Obstet Gynecol* 2000;96(1):45–9.

39. Driul L, Damante G, D'Elia A, Ianni A, Springolo F, Marchesoni D. Genetic thrombophilias and uterine artery Doppler velocimetry and preeclampsia. *Int J Gynecol Obstet* 2005;88(3):265–70.

40. Mousa HA, Alfirevic l Z. Do placental lesions reflect thrombophilia state in women with adverse pregnancy outcome? *Hum Reprod* 2000;15(8):1830–3.

41. Many A, Schreiber L, Rosner S, Lessing JB, Eldor A, Kupferminc MJ. Pathologic features of the placenta in women with severe pregnancy complications and thrombophilia. *Obstet Gynecol* 2001;98(6):1041–4.

42. Sikkema JM, Franx A, Bruinse HW, Van Der Wijk NG, De Valk HW, Nikkels PGJ. Placental pathology in early onset pre-eclampsia and intra-uterine growth restriction in women with and without thrombophilia. *Placenta*. Department of Obstetrics, University Medical Center, Utrecht, The Netherlands. J.M.Sikkema@azu.nl: Elsevier Ltd.; 2002;23(4):337–42.

43. Lockwood CJ, Romero R, Feinberg RF, Clyne LP, Coster B, Hobbins JC. The prevalence and biologic significance of lupus anticoagulant and anticardiolipin antibodies in a general obstetric population. *Am J Obstet Gynecol* 1989;161(2):369–73.

44. Branch DW, Andres R, Digre KB, Rote NS, Scott JR. The association of antiphospholipid antibodies with severe preeclampsia. *Obstet Gynecol* 1989;541–5.

45. Hayslett JP. The effect of systemic lupus erythematosus on pregnancy and pregnancy outcome. *Am J Reprod Immunol* 28(3–4):199–204.

46. Venkat-Raman N, Backos M, Teoh TG, Lo WT, Regan L. Uterine artery Doppler in predicting pregnancy outcome in women with antiphospholipid syndrome. *Obstet Gynecol* 2001;98(2):235–42.

47. Abramowsky CR, Vegas ME, Swinehart G, Gyves MT. Decidual vasculopathy of the placenta in lupus erythematosus. *N Engl J Med* 1980;303(12):668–72.

48. Sebire NJ, Fox H, Backos M, Rai R, Paterson C, Regan L. Defective endovascular trophoblast invasion in primary antiphospholipid antibody syndrome-associated early pregnancy failure. *Hum Reprod* 2002;17(4):1067–71.

49. Stone S, Pijnenborg R, Vercruysse L, Poston R, Khamashta MA, Hunt BJ, et al. The placental bed in pregnancies complicated by primary antiphospholipid syndrome. *Placenta* 2006;27(4–5):457–67.

50. Mulla MJ, Myrtolli K, Brosens JJ, Chamley LW, Kwak-Kim JY, Paidas MJ, et al. Antiphospholipid antibodies limit trophoblast migration by reducing IL-6 production and STAT3 activity. *Am J Reprod Immunol*. Department of Obstetrics, Gynecology & Reproductive Sciences, Yale University School of Medicine, New Haven, CT 06510, USA; 2010;63(5):339–48.

51. Viall CA, Chamley LW. Histopathology in the placentae of women with antiphospholipid antibodies: A systematic review of the literature. *Autoimmun Rev*. Elsevier B.V.; 2015;14(5):1–20.

52. Nicolaides KH, Bilardo CM, Soothill PW, Campbell S. Absence of end diastolic frequencies in umbilical artery: A sign of fetal hypoxia and acidosis. *BMJ*. Harris Birthright Research Centre for Fetal Medicine, King's College School of Medicine and Dentistry, London; 1988;297(6655):1026–7.

53. Sebire NJ. Umbilical artery Doppler revisited: Pathophysiology of changes in intrauterine growth restriction revealed. *Ultrasound Obstet Gynecol* 2003;21(5):419–22.

54. Fok RY, Pavlova Z, Benirschke K, Paul RH, Platt LD. The correlation of arterial lesions with umbilical artery Doppler velocimetry in the placentas of small-for-dates pregnancies. *Obstet Gynecol*. Department of Obstetrics-Gynecology, Los Angeles County/University of Southern California Medical Center; 1990;75(4):578–83.

55. Redline RW, Boyd T, Campbell V, Hyde S, Kaplan C, Khong TY, et al. Maternal vascular underperfusion: Nosology and reproducibility of placental reaction patterns. *Pediatr Dev Pathol*. Department of Pathology, University Hospitals of Cleveland and Case Western Reserve University, 1100 Euclid Avenue, 44106, USA. raymond.redline@uhhs.com; 2004;7(3):237–49.

56. Fitzgerald B, Kingdom J, Keating S. Distal villous hypoplasia. *Diagnostic Histopathol*. Elsevier Ltd.; 2012;18(5):195–200.

57. Lang U, Baker RS, Khoury J, Clark KE. Fetal umbilical vascular response to chronic reductions in uteroplacental blood flow in late-term sheep. *Am J Obstet Gynecol*. Department of Obstetrics and Gynecology, Justus-Liebig University Giessen, Germany: Elsevier Inc.; 2002;187(1):178–86.

58. Howard RB, Hosokawa T, Maguire MH. Hypoxia-induced fetoplacental vasoconstriction in perfused human placental cotyledons. *Am J Obstet Gynecol*. Department of Pharmacology, Toxicology, and Therapeutics, University of Kansas Medical Center, Kansas City 66103: Elsevier Inc; 1987;157(5):1261–6.

59. Hampl V, Bíbová J, Straňák Z, Wu X, Michelakis ED, Hashimoto K, et al. Hypoxic fetoplacental vasoconstriction in humans is mediated by potassium channel inhibition. *Am J Physiol Heart Circ Physiol*. Department of Physiology, Charles University Second Medical School, 15000 Prague 5, Czech Republic. vaclav.hampl@lfmotol.cuni.cz; 2002;283(6):H2440–9.

60. Jakoubek V, Bíbová J, Hampl V. Voltage-gated calcium channels mediate hypoxic vasoconstriction in the human placenta. *Placenta*. Department of Physiology, Charles University Second Medical School, Prague, Czech Republic: Elsevier Ltd.; 2006;27(9–10):1030–3.

61. Wareing M, Greenwood SL, Baker PN. Reactivity of human placental chorionic plate vessels is modified by level of oxygenation: Differences between arteries and veins. *Placenta*. Maternal and Fetal Health Research Centre, University of Manchester, St. Mary's Hospital, Hathersage Road, Manchester M13 0JH, UK. mark.wareing@man.ac.uk: Elsevier Ltd.; 2006;27(1):42–8.

62. Sebire NJ, Talbert D. The role of intraplacental vascular smooth muscle in the dynamic placenta: A conceptual framework for understanding uteroplacental disease. *Med Hypotheses*. Department of Histopathology, Great Ormond Street Hospital, London, UK. 2002;58(4):347–51.

63. Talbert D, Sebire NJ. The dynamic placenta: I. Hypothetical model of a placental mechanism matching local fetal blood flow to local intervillus oxygen delivery. *Med Hypotheses*. Institute of Reproduction and Developmental Biology, ICSM, Hammersmith Hospital, Du Cane Road, London, UK; 2004;62(4):511–19.

64. Sebire NJ, Talbert D. The dynamic placenta: II. Hypothetical model of a fetus driven transplacental water balance mechanism producing low apparent

permeability in a highly permeable placenta. *Med Hypotheses*. Department of Histopathology, Camelia Botnar Laboratories, Great Ormond Street Hospital, Great Ormond Street, London WC1N 3JH, UK. SebirN@gosh.nhs.uk; 2004;62(4):520–8.

65. Cindrova-Davies T, Herrera EA, Niu Y, Kingdom J, Giussani DA, Burton GJ. Reduced cystathionine γ-lyase and increased miR-21 expression are associated with increased vascular resistance in growth-restricted pregnancies. *Am J Pathol*. American Society for Investigative Pathology; 2013;182(4):1448–58.

66. Redline RW. Distal villous immaturity. *Diagnostic Histopathol*. Elsevier Ltd.; 2012;18(5):189–94.

67. Khong TY, Staples A, Moore L, Byard RW. Observer reliability in assessing villitis of unknown aetiology. *J Clin Pathol*. Department of Pathology, Queen Victoria Hospital, Australia: BMJ Group; 1993;46(3):208–10.

68. Altemani AM, Gonzatti AR. [Villitis of unknown etiology in placentas of pregnancies with hypertensive disorders and of small-for-gestational-age infants]. *Rev Assoc Med Bras*. Departamento de Anatomia Patológica, Faculdade de Ciências Mêdicas, UNICAMP, Campinas, SP, Brasil; 2003;49(1):67–71.

69. Styer AK, Parker HJ, Roberts DJ, Palmer-Toy D, Toth TL, Ecker JL. Placental villitis of unclear etiology during ovum donor in vitro fertilization pregnancy. *Am J Obstet Gynecol*. Department of Obstetrics and Gynecology, Vincent Center for Reproductive Biology, Boston, MA, USA: Elsevier Inc.; 2003;189(4):1184–6.

70. Redline RW, Abramowsky CR. Clinical and pathologic aspects of recurrent placental villitis. *Hum Pathol*. 1985;16(7):727–31.

71. Becroft DM, Thompson JM, Mitchell EA. Placental villitis of unknown origin: Epidemiologic associations. *Am J Obstet Gynecol*. Department of Obstetrics and Gynaecology, University of Auckland, New Zealand: Elsevier Inc.; 2005;192(1):264–71.

72. Jacques SM, Qureshi F. Chronic villitis of unknown etiology in twin gestations. *Pediatr Pathol*. Department of Pathology, Hutzel Hospital, Detroit, Michigan 48201; 1994;14(4):575–84.

73. Pathak S, Lees CC, Hackett G, Jessop F, Sebire NJ. Frequency and clinical significance of placental histological lesions in an unselected population at or near term. *Virchows Arch* 2011;459(6):565–72.

74. Boyd TK, Redline RW. Chronic histiocytic intervillositis: A placental lesion associated with recurrent reproductive loss. *Hum Pathol* 2000;31(11):1389–96.

75. Gruenwald P. Abnormalities of placental vascularity in relation to intrauterine deprivation and retardation of fetal growth. Significance of avascular chorionic villi. *N Y State J Med* 1961;61:1508–13.

Chapter

10

Maternal Volume Homeostasis in Fetal Growth Restriction

Johannes J. Duvekot

Introduction

Uncomplicated pregnancies show an increase of more than 40% in total blood volume since both plasma volume and to a lesser extent erythrocyte volume show large increments. There is a distinct relationship with the relative increase in total blood volume and fetal weight. It is not clear whether a decreased or attenuated augmentation of the blood volume is a sign or a cause of inadequate fetal growth. Pregnancy is also characterized by large changes in cardiovascular parameters. These changes arise simultaneously with the changes in volume homeostasis. An important question is how volume homeostasis precedes or follows the changes in cardiovascular parameters.

History

The first report on the increase in blood volume during pregnancy dates back to the middle of the 19th century [1]. The German scientist Welcker measured total blood volume in pregnant mice. The animals were exsanguinated and their vascular systems washed out. The conclusion of Welcker's experiments was that during pregnancy, blood volume was 7.6 grams per 100 grams body weight, which was decreased in relation to the 8 grams per 100 grams body weight in non-pregnant mice, but he was not taking into account the increase in total body weight of the pregnant mice wrought by the litter. In rabbits and dogs, investigators showed an increase of, respectively, 20% and 34% in total blood volume during pregnancy [2].

The German scientist Zuntz was the first to measure blood volume during pregnancy in humans [3]. He used a carbon monoxide method in six pregnant women near term and compared that to the values after delivery. In the first half of the 20th century, more investigators using different methods examined the increase in blood volume during pregnancy. Their results were rather undetermined, but the general conclusion of all studies was that the increased blood volume during pregnancy could be characterized as "the plethora of pregnancy," which can be translated as that a woman is able to lose more blood during delivery than a non-pregnant woman could.

Measurement Techniques of Blood Volume

One of the most important points in studying blood volume during pregnancy is the selection of the subjects. Basic measurements should be performed in healthy, non-smoking, lean, young, and preferably nulliparous women experiencing uncomplicated singleton pregnancies. All these mentioned factors might influence the amount of blood volume by several different mechanisms. Blood volume is composed of primarily plasma volume and to a lesser extent red blood cell mass. Less than 1% of blood volume consists of other components like platelets and white blood cells. In most studies, only plasma volume or red blood cell mass is measured.

It is without any doubt that the most optimal determination of the changes in total blood volume would be in a longitudinal way in healthy, pregnant subjects with a normally growing child and without hypertensive complications. For obvious reasons, most studies, however, use transversal data. So far, only a few studies have measured total blood volume longitudinally during pregnancy [4–6]. Caton was the first to measure simultaneously plasma volume and red cell mass on a monthly basis during pregnancy and the puerperium.

Plasma Volume

The methods used to measure plasma volume are indicator dilution methods [7]. Commonly used indicators to measure plasma volume are albumin, labeled with a dye, indocyanine green, T-1824 or Evans blue dye, or a radioactive isotope like 131I or 125I. Because of their size and hydrophilic nature, the transplacental transfer of these indicators is probably negligible. A disadvantage of these techniques is the large measurement error. This may be caused by dilution of the dye bound to albumin in the extravascular and interstitial space and the position of the pregnant women. Albumin metabolism makes this molecule not ideal for determining plasma volume. Every hour, 5% of intravascular albumin is lost to the extravascular space in healthy subjects. Vascular permeability for albumin is also influenced by different pathological circumstances. Especially in pregnancies at term, in supine position the mixing of the dye may be suboptimal and takes more time due to stasis in the lower extremities.

It is obvious that the amount of plasma volume also depends on the length and weight of the woman. An example of an indirect method to determine plasma volume during the latter half of pregnancy was described by Smith using the following equation [8]:

Plasma volume = 673 + 32.9 (weeks of pregnancy*) + 1,857.2 x body surface area (BSA)

* weeks of pregnancy are defined as follows: 20 and 21 weeks = 1, 22 and 23 weeks = 2 and so on

Red Cell Mass

The total volume of red cell mass may be measured by dilution techniques by tagging an aliquot of the subject's own erythrocytes with usually a radioactive isotope like iron or chromium. After reinfusion, the red cell mass can be calculated from the degree of dilution.

To calculate total blood volume from a known plasma volume, whole-body hematocrit can be used. However, whole-body hematocrit cannot be determined from a simple blood collection from a large vessel like the antecubital vein. Hematocrit in smaller vessels is substantially higher than in the larger vessels. In non-pregnant subjects, whole-body hematocrit is 0.91% of the hematocrit in large vessels and 0.88–0.89% of that during pregnancy. This is called the f cell ratio.

Blood Volume Changes in Uncomplicated Pregnancies

Studies using the aforementioned techniques supported the presence of a larger blood volume during pregnancy. The magnitude of the rise of the blood volume varied widely in several reports until 1972. By "correcting" as much as possible for confounding factors, Chesley calculated an average increase in plasma volume of 42% (21–66%) [9]. He reviewed the literature of 31 studies so far and only used the higher limits of the calculations in these studies. For non-pregnant women, mean plasma volume was 2,580 mL. During pregnancy, this increased to 3,655 mL. Per kg/body weight plasma volume during pregnancy increased from 48.3 mL to 62.2 mL. No subdivision was made between nulliparous and multiparous women, singleton and multiple pregnancies, or magnitude of the fetal growth or race. Two studies that tried to select patients more properly found a maximal increase of 1,230 mL and 1,246 mL [10,11].

Plasma Volume Changes in Early Pregnancy

A first significant increase in plasma volume compared to preconceptional values is not seen but after the sixth week of pregnancy [4,12]. Plasma volume, measured by the Evans blue dye dilator technique, was preconceptionally 2,378 mL (95% CI 2,296–2,460 mL) [4]. Plasma volume rose significantly between the 7th and 12th weeks of gestation with 190 mL to 310 mL in these three studies constituting an increase of 8–14% during the first 12 weeks of pregnancy.

Plasma Volume Changes after 12 Weeks of Pregnancy

After a steep rise between 12 and 28 weeks of 854 mL, only a small increase was seen into 36 weeks of 139 mL, plateauing after this period, 3,646 mL (95% CI 3,508–3,784 mL) [4]. After 36 weeks, most other studies even see a decrease in plasma volume. The latter is possibly the result of technical problems with the measurement techniques as mentioned before.

After delivery plasma volume returns toward preconceptional values at least by 12 weeks postpartum.

It can be concluded that the total amount of increase in plasma volume is 1,250 mL; this constitutes 50% of the preconceptional amount of plasma volume in subjects who had singleton pregnancies that developed uneventfully. Perhaps not very surprisingly, these data are almost identical to the earlier and much older reports by Chesley, Hytten, and Pirani.

Parity also influences the increase in plasma volume. In subsequent pregnancies, plasma volume increases even more than in first pregnancies, which

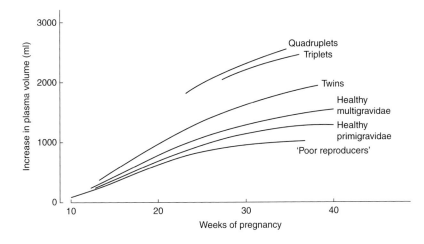

Figure 10.1 Plasma volume in single and multiple pregnancies.
Source: Letzky E. The haematological system. In *Clinical Physiology in Obstetrics*. Blackwell Scientific Publications, London, 1991, page 41.

coincides with the increased fetal weight in subsequent pregnancies [13]. Despite the fact that in the study by Campbell the measurements were performed in a different maternal position in the first and second pregnancies, plasma volume shows a 500 mL more increase than in the first pregnancy. Later studies could not confirm this large increase and found only a nonsignificant increase of 100 mL in parous women [4].

Considerably larger increases in plasma volume can be seen in multiple pregnancies [14].

In conclusion, in uncomplicated pregnancies, the rise in plasma volume is proportional to the number of fetuses, parity, and the intrauterine growth of the conceptus (Figure 10.1) [14].

Red Cell Mass Changes during Pregnancy

Chesley found an average increase in red cell mass of on average 24% (17–49%) in 11 different studies [9]. For non-pregnant women, red cell mass was 1,353 mL; during pregnancy, this increased to 1,677 mL. Other authors measured an increase of 18% with 250 mL. The increase in red cell mass during pregnancy is thought to be linear. Whether erythropoietin, human placental lactogen, or other hormones play a role in this increase is not known. This increase is highly dependent on the concomitant use of iron medication during pregnancy. When iron supplement is given, the absolute increase goes up to 400 to 450 mL. In multiple pregnancies, red cell mass increases even more.

It is unclear whether red cell mass decreases slightly in early pregnancy. This might be the result of the exaggerated renal blood flow leading to diminished production of erythropoietin. It is obvious that the concomitant steep rise in plasma volume leads first to a hemodilution and a lowering of the hematocrit followed by an increase after 30 weeks when plasma volume increases more slowly. In this study, all women were iron and folate supplemented, ruling out these deficiencies.

The Initiation of Blood Volume Changes

The events that lead to volume expansion, although not completely understood, are most likely triggered by an early primary fall in systemic vascular tone [15]. This acute fall in vascular tone of the arterial and venous system takes place at the time of or shortly after nidation. The "underfill state" that results from this vasodilatation leads to an activation of several volume-retaining mechanisms. The old concept of shunting in the placental bed is not very likely in this first stage of volume increase since during the first weeks of pregnancy, when relatively large hemodynamic changes occur, there is only a small placental unit present yet. Later in pregnancy, this second mechanism is more likely to influence the increase in plasma volume.

Although many factors are likely candidates, the hormone most probably responsible for this onset of the hemodynamic changes in pregnancy is the corpus luteal hormone relaxin [16]. Administration of this hormone to non-pregnant animals and men leads to similar changes in hemodynamics as seen in pregnancy. Women receiving donor eggs lack this hormone and are more prone to develop complications during

87

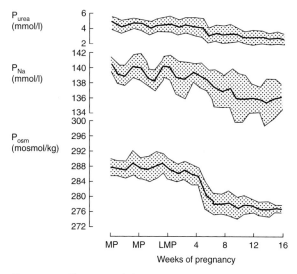

Figure 10.2 The course of plasma ureum, sodium, and osmolality during menstrual cycle and early pregnancy.
Source: Davison JM, Vallotton MB, Lindheimer MD. Plasma osmolality and urinary concentration and dilution during and after pregnancy: Evidence that lateral recumbency inhibits maximal urinary concentrating ability. *BJOG* 1981; **88**:472–9.

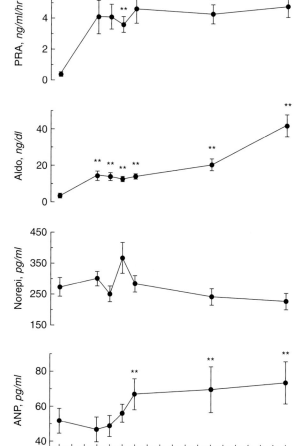

Figure 10.3 Vasopressor hormone profiles throughout early human pregnancy.
Source: Chapman AB, Abraham WT, Zamudio S, Coffin C, Merouani A, Young D, Johnson A, Osorio F, Goldberg C, Moore LG, Dahms T, Schrier RW. Temporal relationships between hormonal and hemodynamic changes in early human pregnancy. *Kidney Int* 1998; **54**:2056–63.

their pregnancies. Relaxin produces short- and long-term effects on hemodynamics by different molecular mechanisms. A final common pathway is most probably endothelial nitric oxide. Since pregnancy can be established in the absence of relaxin-producing ovaries, relaxin was also found to be produced by endometrial cells, but this production does not lead to measurable circulating relaxin.

The most striking phenomenon soon after nidation is the decrease in plasma osmolality (Figure 10.2) [17]. In this classical study, women were followed during their menstrual cycles until they conceived. Plasma osmolality decreased abruptly with 10 mosmol/L when pregnancy occurred. This resetting of the osmoreceptors remains throughout pregnancy. Other volume-retaining mechanisms are the activation of the renin-angiotensin-aldosterone system and the diuretic effects of natriuretic peptides in response to atrial and ventricular wall stretch [15]. Atrial natriuretic peptide tends to decrease in very early pregnancy and rises after weeks 10 to 12 of pregnancy, suggesting an early underfill that slowly abates in the following weeks (Figure 10.3) [15,18]. All these mechanisms eventually result in renal sodium and water retention and an increase in plasma volume.

The vascular volume to fill is primarily the maternal vasculature that as a result of the generalized vasodilatation, especially of the venous system, may accommodate more volume. The cardiovascular changes in early pregnancy follow the changes in intravascular volume and filling state. At first the decrease of vascular tone and the "underfill state" induce a maternal rise in heart rate, which is followed by an increase in stroke volume due to the effects of the volume-retaining mechanisms that refill the vascular tree [15].

Besides this volume capacity, the total capacity of the vascular system will also increase. This takes place mostly in the second half of pregnancy. The expansion of the blood volume serves to fill the greatly increased vasculature of the pregnant uterus and breasts, especially the large veins. In this second part of pregnancy, total blood volume keeps increasing, but cardiovascular changes change only slightly.

Blood Volume in the Preconceptional Phase

During the spontaneous menstrual cycle, the amount of plasma volume is influenced by the fluctuations of the sex hormones. During the midfollicular and the midluteal phases, plasma volume is lower than during the menstrual period and probably the late luteal phase [12,19]. The small but distinct changes in plasma volume during the menstrual cycle follow more or less the concentration of serum estrogen. There is no additional increase in plasma volume during the second half of a conceiving menstrual cycle [12].

According to some investigators, blood volume is different outside pregnancy between women experiencing complicated and uncomplicated pregnancies. In women, after unexplained first trimester recurrent pregnancy loss, plasma volume is 9–14% lower than in healthy controls [20]. After preeclampsia and FGR, women also have a lower plasma volume [21]. However, the cyclic variation of the plasma volume during the menstrual cycle was preserved even in these formerly preeclamptic patients [22]. Furthermore, formerly preeclamptic women who develop preeclamptic pregnancies again had even lower plasma volumes outside pregnancy [23]. The chance to develop a recurrence of preeclampsia is inversely related to a lower preconceptional plasma volume, OR 0,6 (95% CI 0,5-0,8) per 100 mL difference in plasma volume. The same equation could be made for development of pregnancies complicated by fetal growth restriction, OR 0,8 (95% CI 0,5-0,9) per 100 mL difference in plasma volume. For women prone to develop preeclampsia on behalf of their genetic predisposition, plasma volume is also reduced outside pregnancy. When predisposing factors like hypertension and smoking are present, this is also accompanied by decreased non-pregnant plasma volumes.

The lower plasma volume in non-pregnant women who are prone to experience complications of pregnancy is probably due to a lower unstressed volume since the arterial hemodynamic function of these subjects is equal to control women [20]. Arterial compliance is also lower in this group of women.

Blood Volume Changes in Complicated Pregnancies

Chesley, in his classical work on this subject, already found that preeclamptic patients had a decreased plasma volume as compared to normotensive pregnant women [9]. Plasma volume decreased by 9% (-5–29%) from 3,620 mL to 3,295 mL. This was the combined result from 11 studies. These studies, except one, concluded that red cell mass remained stable, leading to the concept of "contracted blood volume" during preeclamptic pregnancies as a result of the decrease in plasma volume.

Circulating blood volume is an important, but not often measured or known variable in pregnant women. Severe volume depletion leads to clinically overt shock; minor volume depletion does not lead to clinical features since vasoconstriction supports arterial pressure and leads to redistribution to vital organs. The placental perfusion is not one of those vital organs and is severely compromised by sudden, but probably also by chronic hypovolemia.

So-called placental fetal growth restriction may be the result of inadequate placental blood flow. That the increase in plasma volume is related to the development of the conceptus and especially fetal weight has already been shown for a long time [10,11,13,24,25]. Gibson prospectively studied the increments of plasma volume in pregnancies of "poor reproducers" and found a distinct correlation with the fetal weight [24]. However, it is difficult to determine whether this is result or cause of the fetal growth retardation. Actually, these two variables probably interact. The increase in plasma volume proved to be more related to the weight of the fetus than to the mother's weight or height. The correlation coefficient relating plasma volume increment and birth weight was shown to be 0.43–0.44. The regression equation is: birth weight = 0,275 x plasma volume + 2250,6.

Most studies show that plasma volume is already decreased weeks before the clinical onset of preeclampsia or fetal growth restriction. A serial study between 10–13 week' gestation and term showed a constantly decreased increment of plasma volume with 100–150 mL both for women who developed preeclampsia or fetal growth restriction (Figure 10.4) [5].

Other investigators show that already in early pregnancy plasma volume increments in pregnancies that eventually develop fetal growth restriction are attenuated. An indirect measure to detect plasma

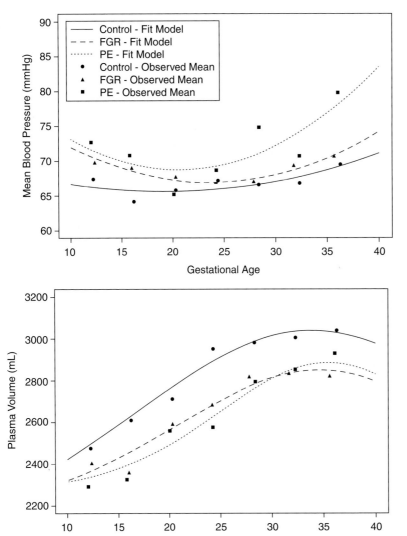

Figure 10.4 Mean blood pressure and plasma volume in uncomplicated pregnancies and pregnancies complicated by preeclampsia or fetal growth restriction.
Source: Salas SP, Marshall G, Gutiérrez BL, Rosso P. Time course of maternal plasma volume and hormonal changes in women with preeclampsia or fetal growth restriction. *Hypertension* 2006; **47**:203–8.

volume expansion in early pregnancy is an increase in left atrial diameter. Left atrial diameter increases significantly during the first weeks of pregnancy in uncomplicated pregnancies. In pregnancies later complicated by fetal growth restriction, this increase is attenuated [26].

Hematocrit

The disproportionate increase in plasma volume and red cell mass during pregnancy results in the so-called physiologic anemia of pregnancy. This results in a decrease in the hematocrit. The most important result of this hemodilution is the decrease of whole-blood viscosity by almost 20%. This lower whole-blood viscosity enhances blood flow in the low-pressure

intervillous space and ameliorates the placental perfusion. Also the maternal blood circulation is enhanced by this decrease.

Fetal growth restriction is increased at both edges of the normal values for this parameter. This is the so-called U-shaped relationship of hematocrit and fetal growth restriction. On both sides a different pathophysiologic mechanism causing fetal growth restriction may be operational.

A high hematocrit may be considered an indirect measure of decreased plasma volume. Many studies have found that high values for the hematocrit in the first half of pregnancy predispose for complications like fetal growth restriction, preterm delivery, and preeclampsia. Higher hematocrit values before

20 weeks' gestation are significantly correlated with fetal growth restriction. Hematocrits above 40% show ORs between 1.2 and 1.4. Above 30 weeks hematocrits above 40% are more strongly associated (OR 1.5–2.5) with fetal growth restriction [27]. It is likely that the poor outcome is related to a failure of the plasma volume to expand. The pathophysiological mechanism of fetal growth restriction from a high hematocrit may be related to a change in rheological properties, especially an increase in whole-blood viscosity. The increase in viscosity might hamper the diffusion processes within the placental circulation and the low pressure intervillous space, leading to worsening of fetal nutrition. However, probably due to the large inter-individual variation of hematocrit values in the third trimester, the hematocrit value is clinically not useful to predict fetal growth restriction.

On the other hand, a decreased hematocrit, below 80 mg/dL, is predictive of the development of fetal growth restriction, according to a recent meta-analysis [28]. Below this value, fetal growth restriction is also increased with an OR of 1.53 (95% CI 1.24–1.87). It seems that the pathophysiologic mechanism for this finding is an impaired or reduced oxygen supply to the fetoplacental unit. Furthermore, the results of this meta-analysis have to be treated with caution because of the heterogeneity across the included studies.

Regulation of Blood Volume: Role of the Kidney

The kidney plays in both non-pregnant and pregnant individuals an important role in the regulation of blood volume by controlling both the plasma volume and red cell mass. In this concept, it is supposed that the kidney coordinates the relative volumes of these two blood components and in so doing regulates the hematocrit [29]. Red cell mass is governed by the need to transport oxygen; plasma volume is governed by the need to fill the vascular space and maintain blood pressure. Erythropoiesis is regulated by the hormone erythropoietin produced by the kidney under influence of blood oxygen tension. Renal function determines body sodium and water content under influence of arterial pressure and urinary sodium or volume excretion. Excretion or retention of water and sodium is sharply regulated when plasma volume changes only slightly. Besides this, the sympathetic regulation of vascular tone plays a role in volume homeostasis. Plasma volume is thus regulated by hormonal and neural mechanisms [7].

Renal function undergoes large changes early in pregnancy in uncomplicated pregnancies. The course in early pregnancy of glomerular filtration rate (GFR) measured with the 24-hour creatinine clearance in the first weeks of pregnancy was first described in 1981 [30]. The course of the 24-hour creatinine clearance in 11 uncomplicated pregnancies and two pregnancies with spontaneous miscarriages were described. In the latter, the rise in GFR was attenuated. GFR displays a cyclic pattern during the menstrual cycle with a 20% higher value during the luteal phase. During the first weeks of pregnancy GFR increases to 45% above the level at the follicular phase. This level is maintained throughout pregnancy. This presents clinically as a decrease in serum creatinine.

GFR is determined by three factors: the hydrostatic and oncotic pressure gradients across the glomerular membrane, the glomerular plasma flow, and the glomerular permeability [15]. Only the first two factors are known to change during early pregnancy. Hyperfiltration appears to be almost completely due to the increase in renal plasma flow resulting from profound reductions in both the renal afferent and efferent arteriolar resistances. Relaxine has an important role in this concept of vasodilatation.

In pregnancies complicated by placental syndromes, the increase in GFR is also attenuated during the clinical phase of the disease. How renal function behaves in cases of fetal growth restriction before the clinical onset is not clear, but probably the decrease of GFR is attenuated from the early beginning of pregnancy [26].

To result in an uncomplicated pregnancy, normal renal function is necessary to enable optimal plasma volume expansion. The kidneys increase their production of erythropoietin, vitamin D, and renin. The inability of diseased kidneys to produce these hormones leads to anemia, reduced plasma volume increment, and vitamin D deficiency. The increment in plasma volume is blunted in moderate renal insufficiency and is absent in severe renal insufficiency. This results more often in placental syndromes like preeclampsia and fetal growth restriction in women with chronic kidney dysfunction (CKD). CKD is fortunately a rather uncommon disease during pregnancy. The occurrence of placental syndromes is dependent on the severity of the clinical disease. Consequently, increasing renal failure with worsening creatinine

Mean (SD) prepregnancy serum creatinine value (μmol/l)	Effects on pregnancy outcome				Loss of >25% renal function		
	Fetal growth restriction	Preterm delivery	Pre-eclampsia	Perinatal deaths	During pregnancy	Persists postpartum	End stage renal failure after 1 year
<125	25	30	22	1	2	0	0
125-180	40	60	40	5	40	20	2
>180	65	>90	60	10	70	50	35
On dialysis	>90	>90	75	50*	N/A	N/A	N/A

N/A=not applicable.
Estimates are based on literature from 1985-2007, with all pregnancies attaining at least 24 weeks' gestation. [1-4 7 B w8-w16]
*If conceived on dialysis, 50% of infants survive; if conceived before introduction of dialysis, 75% of infants survive.

Figure 10.5
Source: Williams D, Davison J. Chronic kidney disease in pregnancy. *BMJ* 2008; **336**:211–15.

values leads to an increase in fetal growth restriction (Figure 10.5). In women with severe CKD this results in fetal growth restriction in 75% of the cases. The influence of comorbidities like maternal hypertension and/or proteinuria is difficult to discern separately and has probably cumulative influence on the occurrence of fetal growth restriction [31].

Another important aspect is that maternal renal function in women with CKD often deteriorates after pregnancy. In women with severe renal insufficiency 35% of these women develop end-stage renal failure within 1 year after delivery as shown in Figure 10.5.

Conclusions

During pregnancy total blood volume shows an increase in plasma volume of 1,250 mL and in red blood cell mass of 250 mL. The increments in plasma volume are proportional to the number of fetuses, parity, and the intrauterine growth of the fetus. The trigger to increase blood volume arises from a generalized vascular relaxation in very early pregnancy. Together with the increase in blood volume cardiovascular parameters start to increase. In the second part of pregnancy the growth of the vascular tree results in a further increase in blood volume but less in cardiovascular parameters.

In pregnancies complicated by fetal growth restriction this increment in, primarily, plasma volume is substantially lower from the early stages of pregnancy. Besides of this, women prone to have complicated pregnancies already have a diminished total blood volume due to a lower amount of unstressed volume.

The kidney may be considered the regulator of total blood volume. Inability to increase plasma volume during pregnancy, as is the case in women with CKD, makes these women more prone to develop pregnancy complications like preeclampsia and fetal growth restriction.

Key Points

- During pregnancy, total blood volume shows a large increase of more than 40%.
- The increment of plasma volume and to lesser extent of red cell volume causes the increase in blood volume.
- The increase in blood volume is triggered by an early systemic fall in vascular tone.
- The relative increase in plasma volume strongly correlates with the increase in fetal weight.
- Women with pregnancies complicated by fetal growth restriction (FGR) have reduced increases in plasma volume throughout pregnancy.
- Women with impaired renal function are prone to develop pregnancy complications.

References

1. Welcker H. Blutkorperzahlung und farbeprüfende Methode. *Prag Vierteljahrschr prakt Heilk* 1854;4:11–80.

2. Spiegelberg O, Gescheidlen H. Untersuchungen über die Blutmenge trächtiger Hunde. *Arch Gynäk* 1872;4:112–20.

3. Zuntz L. Untersuchungen über die Gesamtblutmenge in der Gravidität und im Wochenbett. *Zbl Gynäk* 1911;35:1365–9.

4. Whittaker PG, Lind T. The intravascular mass of albumin during human pregnancy: A serial study in normal and diabetic women. *BJOG* 1993;100:587–92.

5. Salas SP, Marshall G, Gutiérrez BL, Rosso P. Time course of maternal plasma volume and hormonal

changes in women with preeclampsia or fetal growth restriction. *Hypertension* 2006;47:203–8.

6. Caton WL, Roby CC, Reid DE, Caswell R, Maletskos CJ, Fluharty RG, Gibson JG, 2nd. The circulating red cell volume and body hematocrit in normal pregnancy and the puerperium by direct measurement using radioactive red cells. *Am J Obstet Gynecol* 1951;61:1207–17.

7. Jones JG, Wardrop CAJ. Measurement of blood volume in surgical and intensive care practice. *Br J Anaesth* 2000;84:224–35.

8. Smith RW, Yarbrough CJ. Plasma volume prediction in normal pregnancy. *Am J Obstet Gynecol* 1967;99:18–20.

9. Chesley LC. Plasma and red cell volumes during pregnancy. *Am J Obstet Gynecol* 1972;112:440–50.

10. Hytten FE, Paintin DB. Increase in plasma volume during normal pregnancy. *J Obstet Gynaecol Br Commonw* 1963;70:402–7.

11. Pirani BBK, Campbell DM. Plasma volume in normal first pregnancy. *J Obstet Gynaecol Br Commonw* 1973;80:884–7.

12. Bernstein IM, Ziegler W, Badger GJ. Plasma volume expansion in early pregnancy. *Obstet Gynecol* 2001; 97(5 Pt 1):669–72.

13. Campbell DM, MacGillivray I. Comparison of maternal response in first and second pregnancies in relation to baby weight. *J Obstet Gynaecol Br Commonw* 1972;79:684–93.

14. Letzky E. The haematological system. In *Clinical Physiology in Obstetrics*. Blackwell Scientific Publications, London, 1991, page 41.

15. Duvekot JJ. Early pregnancy changes in hemodynamics and volume homeostasis are consecutive adjustments triggered by a primary fall in systemic vascular tone. *Am J Obstet Gynecol* 1993; 169:1382–92.

16. Conrad KP, Davison JM. The renal circulation in normal pregnancy and preeclampsia: Is there a place for relaxin? *Am J Physiol Renal Physiol* 2014;306:F1121–35.

17. Davison JM, Vallotton MB, Lindheimer MD. Plasma osmolality and urinary concentration and dilution during and after pregnancy: Evidence that lateral recumbency inhibits maximal urinary concentrating ability. *BJOG* 1981;88:472–9.

18. Chapman AB, Abraham WT, Zamudio S, Coffin C, Merouani A, Young D, Johnson A, Osorio F, Goldberg C, Moore LG, Dahms T, Schrier RW. Temporal relationships between hormonal and hemodynamic changes in early human pregnancy. *Kidney Int* 1998;54:2056–63.

19. Fortney SM, Turner C, Steinmann RN, Driscoll CNMT, Alfrey C. Blood volume responses of men and women to bed rest. *J Clin Pharmacol* 1994;34:434–9.

20. Donckers J, Scholten RR, Oyen WJG, Hopman MTE, Lotgering FK, Spaanderman MEA. Unexplained first trimester recurrent pregnancy loss and low venous reserves. *Human Reprod* 2012;27:2613–18.

21. Spaanderman ME, Willekes C, Hoeks AP, Ekhart TH, Aardenburg R, Courtar DA, Van Eijndhoven HW, Peeters LL. Maternal nonpregnant vascular function correlates with subsequent fetal growth. *Am J Obstet Gynecol* 2005;192:504–12.

22. Spaanderman ME, Van Beek E, Ekhart TH, Van Eyck J, Cheriex EC, De Leeuw PW, Peeters LL. Changes in hemodynamic parameters and volume homeostasis with the menstrual cycle among women with a history of preeclampsia. *Am J Obstet Gynecol* 2000;182:1127–34.

23. Scholten RR, Sep S, Peeters L, Hopman MT, Lotgering FK, Spaanderman ME. Prepregnancy low-plasma volume and predisposition to preeclampsia and fetal growth restriction. *Obstet Gynecol* 2011;117:1085–93.

24. Gibson HM. Plasma volume and glomerular filtration rate in pregnancy and their relation to differences in fetal growth. *J Obstet Gynaecol Br Commonw* 1973;80:1067–74.

25. Sibai BM, Abdella TN, Anderson GD, McCubbin JH. Plasma volume determination in pregnancies complicated by chronic hypertension and intrauterine fetal demise. *Obstet Gynecol* 1982;60:174–8.

26. Duvekot JJ, Cheriex EC, Pieters FA, Menheere PP, Schouten HJ, Peeters LL. Maternal volume homeostasis in early pregnancy in relation to fetal growth restriction. *Obstet Gynecol* 1995;85:361–7.

27. Scanlon KS, Ray YIP, Schieve LA, Cogswell ME. High and low hemoglobin levels during pregnancy: Differential risks for preterm birth and small for gestational age. *Obstet Gynecol* 2000;96:741–8.

28. Kozuki N, Lee AC, Katz J; Child Health Epidemiology Reference Group. Moderate to severe, but not mild, maternal anemia is associated with increased risk of small-for-gestational-age outcomes. *J Nutr* 2012;142:358–62.

29. Dunn A, Donnelly S. The role of the kidney in blood volume regulation: The kidney as a regulator of the hematocrit. *Am J Med Sci* 2007;334:65–71.

30. Davison JM, Noble MC. Serial changes in 24 hour creatinine clearance during normal menstrual cycles and the first trimester of pregnancy. *BJOG* 1981;88:10–17.

31. Williams D, Davison J. Chronic kidney disease in pregnancy. *BMJ* 2008;336:211–15.

Chapter

11

First Trimester Combined Screening Algorithms for Fetal Growth Restriction

Rosemary Townsend and Asma Khalil

Screening in obstetrics is well established, with pregnancies routinely risk-classified from the time of the first booking visit. Traditionally, more care is directed at women classified as high risk, although of course the risk categorization is a spectrum rather than a binary classification, and no pregnancy is known to be entirely uncomplicated until it has ended. Although many relevant conditions may be identified at the beginning of pregnancy, such as preexisting maternal disease, obesity, or previous obstetric complications, the real challenge is how to identify those women who, while healthy at the outset of pregnancy, are destined to develop serious complications, maternal or fetal, in later pregnancy. Equally, it is essential to avoid unnecessary intervention in the majority of women who will progress through their pregnancies uneventfully.

Screening for fetal anomalies is the archetype of modern obstetric screening. Screening for aneuploidy and fetal anomaly in two visits typically forms the basis of routine fetal anomaly screening in most antenatal care protocols. This pattern provides a possible model for screening for preeclampsia and fetal growth restriction (FGR) that could easily be included in current care pathways.

The first visit at 11–14 weeks takes the form of ultrasound assessment for accurate dating and screening for major anomalies and markers of aneuploidy, as well as measurement of biochemical markers. Since no single non-invasive diagnostic test for aneuploidy is currently widely available, several markers are combined to provide an individualized risk for the pregnancy. In the combined test in common use in the United Kingdom today, the nuchal thickness (NT) together with the maternal age, and measurements of serum beta human chorionic gonadotrophin (bHCG) and pregnancy-associated plasma protein A (PAPP-A) are used to determine a first trimester risk of aneuploidy.

Several of the markers routinely measured in the first trimester have been associated with preeclampsia and FGR, so offer the possibility of developing a similar combined screening tool for these conditions, incorporating maternal factors, biochemical markers, and ultrasound indices. The advent of circulating free fetal DNA (cffDNA) in screening for aneuploidy raises the possibility that the early combined test may one day be discarded, but given that outcomes other than aneuploidy (including FGR) may also be detected by the combined test [1], it would seem preferable to adopt a two stage-screening approach, using cffDNA only for high-risk women after the combined test [2].

Screening for fetuses that will be small for gestational age (SGA) at delivery currently takes the form of noting maternal risk factors at booking and increasing surveillance accordingly. In the United Kingdom, current guidance recommends that maternal characteristics and history are used to identify a high-risk group that undergoes screening for SGA at 20–24 weeks by measurement of the uterine artery pulsatility index (UtA PI) [3]. This approach is better at predicting preeclampsia than FGR and has significant false negative and positive rates [4]. Late-onset FGR is often not predicted by screening with UtA PI, while a large proportion of fetuses is subject to unnecessary additional surveillance [5].

FGR is a condition associated with significant perinatal morbidity and mortality, often associated with preeclampsia, preterm birth, Caesarean section, intrauterine and neonatal death, and long-term health sequelae for the surviving preterm child. The primary intervention for FGR detected from the second trimester is increased ultrasound and cardiotocograph (CTG) surveillance, with timely delivery of a compromised fetus. Antenatal identification of FGR is associated with a reduction in the risk of stillbirth [7]. In a UK population study, the risk of stillbirth was

Table 11.1 Factors predisposing to fetal growth restriction (after Mayer et al.) [6]

Placental factors	Maternal factors	Drugs	Fetal factors
Preeclampsia	High body mass index	Tobacco	Aneuploidy
Placenta previa	Diabetes	Cocaine	Gene deletions/duplications
Velamentous cord insertion	Auto immune disease	Alcohol	Congenital infections
Twin-twin transfusion syndrome	Chronic illness	Anticonvulsants	Congenital malformations
	Chronic infection	Heparin	Multiple gestation
	Uterine anomaly	Methotrexate	
	Malnutrition		

five times lower when FGR was detected antenatally (6.2% vs. 32.0% in those not detected antenatally) [7]. Identification of growth-restricted fetuses does improve outcomes, but these babies are still at four times higher risk of perinatal morbidity [8].

Since the primary known and modifiable pathological process is poor placental implantation and angiogenesis in the first trimester, any potential intervention aimed at preventing FGR is more likely to be successful if implemented at this early stage. The earlier a pregnancy at risk of FGR is identified, the greater the potential to modify progression to disease in later pregnancy. This can be seen in the significant difference in risk reduction of FGR with low-dose aspirin when started before or after 16 weeks' gestation [9]. As the pathophysiology of growth restriction becomes better understood, novel therapeutic options may become available, but they are all likely to be of greatest benefit if initiated in the first trimester. A screening test that could be performed at the time of the early combined test for aneuploidy screening would be ideal.

Since a large proportion of growth-restricted fetuses is affected by placental pathology, screening for growth restriction is closely related to screening for preeclampsia and faces many of the same challenges. Screening for preeclampsia is problematic because it is a heterogeneous condition with considerable differences in etiology and patient characteristics between the most common presentation of late-onset preeclampsia without evidence of placental insufficiency and the less common (but more commonly associated with fetal and maternal morbidity) preterm-onset presentation, which is often associated with FGR. Individual tests for screening for preeclampsia by maternal characteristics or biochemical markers or ultrasound indices tend to favor one form of the

disease or another and detection rates are inadequate for use in general screening of all pregnant women.

Screening for growth restriction faces an even wider array of pathophysiological processes that may lead to a growth-restricted fetus and that should ideally be addressed in any combined screening model. Although inadequate placentation is a leading cause of growth restriction, models that predict placental insufficiency alone will never predict all cases of FGR. In particular, while early-onset FGR fetuses are a homogenous group where the pathology is closely associated with placental insufficiency, late-onset FGR fetuses present a diverse range of features. Late-onset FGR may be associated with placental insufficiency and preeclampsia, but also includes a number of babies that are constitutionally small or are affected by a heterogeneous array of conditions. The outcomes of late-onset FGR fetuses are worse than average-size fetuses, but there are subgroups within the late onset FGR cohort that have similar outcomes to their appropriately grown companions [10]. Screening should be targeted at those fetuses at greater risk of adverse outcomes within the late-onset FGR cohort, but in order for this to occur a greater understanding of the mechanism of late-onset FGR is required.

As many as one quarter of placentas from FGR pregnancies have no abnormality detected on histopathological assessment [11]. In late-onset FGR, placentae may be normal, may demonstrate the maternal vascular lesions typical of early-onset preeclampsia/FGR to a lesser degree, or may show other changes not associated with preeclampsia such as evidence of fetal thrombotic events or villitis of uncertain etiology (VUE) [12]. Screening tests currently available target maternal vascular changes and impaired placentation, but late-onset FGR without PE is associated with other pathologies that need to be addressed.

Biochemical Markers Evaluated for First Trimester Screening for FGR

A number of biochemical factors have been evaluated for potential as first trimester screening tests for FGR. The choice of markers has largely been driven either by those features known to be associated with impaired trophoblast invasion, preeclampsia, or those analytes already commonly tested in early pregnancy. Markers broadly fall into three groups: placental proteins and hormones, promoters and inhibitors of angiogenesis, and immune-modulating factors.

Placental Protein 13 (PP13)

PP13 is a galectin expressed by the placenta and involved in placental implantation [13]. Its level is reduced in pregnancies that subsequently develop preeclampsia [14] and seems likely to also be associated with FGR. However, a number of studies have found no association with SGA [13,15] or limited sensitivity [16]. Meta-analysis shows that for SGA alone, the sensitivity of PP13 is only 26% for a false positive rate (FPR) of 5% [15]. There is evidence that the assay used to determine the PP13 level affects the accuracy of the test [17], but even with the best-performing assay it seems unlikely that PP13 will contribute usefully to a combined screening algorithm for FGR.

Pregnancy-Associated Plasma Protein A (PAPP-A)

PAPP-A is already routinely measured as part of the first trimester aneuploidy screening and low levels have long been known to be associated with adverse pregnancy outcomes in euploid fetuses. PAPP-A is closely associated with placental mass [18]. PAPP-A is particularly associated with the risk of developing SGA [1,15,19,20], but is probably not sensitive enough to be clinically useful [21]. The RCOG guideline states that a level of <0.42 MoM should be included as a major risk factor for SGA, and should prompt fetal surveillance with serial growth scans in later pregnancy [3]. However, this level has a sensitivity of only 12.2% [22]. The serum level of PAPP-A alone for FGR has been shown to have a detection rate of 13% (95% confidence interval 7.9–21.2%) for a false positive rate of 10% [23]. Maternal characteristics (height, weight, parity, and ethnic origin) combined with PAPP-A

provide a detection rate of 29.5% (95% CI 21.5–39.1) with an FPR of 10% [18].

Beta Human Chorionic Gonadotrophin (b-hCG)

Beta hCG is a hormone produced by the syncytiotrophoblast, and low levels in the first trimester have been associated with adverse pregnancy outcomes, including FGR [22]. It is easily and cheaply measured and already incorporated into first trimester aneuploidy screening, but reported sensitivity in screening is variable. In comparison to PAPP-A, b-hCG is not significantly associated with SGA pregnancies [20].

A-Disintegrin and Metalloproteinase 12 (ADAM 12)

ADAM 12 is a metalloproteinase highly expressed in placental tissue and known to be involved in placental development, as well as associated with a number of cancers, as well as with SGA [24]. Low levels have been shown to predict early pregnancy failure [25] and are significantly associated with PAPP-A levels [26]. Individually, however, ADAM 12 performs poorly in the prediction of SGA.

Placental Growth Hormone (PGH)

PGH is a product of the syncytiotrophoblast involved in regulating the maternal metabolic adaptation to pregnancy, associated with levels of IGF1 and trophoblast invasion. Low serum levels have previously been linked to pregnancies affected by FGR [27]. A recent case control study demonstrated no association between first trimester PGH and birth-weight centile, and thus PGH is unlikely to be of value in first trimester screening for SGA [28].

Placental Growth Factor (PlGF)

Low levels of PlGF, a proangiogenic factor, particularly in association with increased levels of the anti-angiogenic soluble fms like tyrosine kinase 1 (sFlt1), are strongly associated with early-onset preeclampsia [29]. Low PlGF has been shown to be significantly associated with vascular placental lesions on postpartum examination [19]. PlGF is also associated with SGA and first trimester PAPP-A, and can contribute significantly to combined screening algorithms for prediction of SGA fetuses [30].

Metabolomics Applied to Screening for FGR

Rather than testing for known markers of placental or immune function, metabolomics provides an alternative approach to providing mechanistic understanding of fetal growth restriction and identifying potentially valuable screening markers. Metabolomics refers to non-targeted metabolic profiling of the collective metabolic response to physiological or pathological stress. The metabolome represents the sum of the metabolites present and is dynamic in response to environmental changes. Changes in the maternal, fetal, and neonatal metabolic profiles have been observed in relation to FGR pregnancies and offer potential novel tests that could be developed for screening in the future [31].

Neonatal Metabolomics

It is demonstrable that there is a difference in the urinary metabolome of neonates affected by fetal growth restriction [32], which may provide a mechanistic explanation of the observed phenomenon of fetal programming, where neonates who have been affected by fetal growth restriction are more likely to develop cardiovascular disease and the metabolic syndrome in adult life [33]. Both large- and small-for-gestational-age neonates have altered urinary metabolic profiles with significantly increased inositol in neonatal urine samples [34]. Altered metabolism persists into adult life and is still detectable in those adults who were affected by FGR in intrauterine life.

Fetal Metabolomics

Blood sampled from the umbilical cord provides a source for direct assessment of the fetal metabolism. Umbilical vein blood metabolomics assessment in the pig FGR model demonstrates significant change in lipid, glucose, and protein metabolism and highlights deficient placental transport as a potential cause for FGR [35].

Human umbilical cord blood sampled at birth has also been observed to have significant differences in the abundance of amino acids phenylalanine and tryptophan in FGR fetuses compared to controls [36]. Differences in amino acid patterns can be detected

between the early- and late-onset FGR groups; however, both groups exhibit altered lipid metabolism in a pro-atherogenic pattern. This implies that differences in physiology leading to the disease exist, while the metabolic consequences of disease are consistent [10].

Fetal Brain Metabolism

Induction of FGR in rabbit models has been shown to induce metabolic change in all brain regions [37]. The changes affected the frontal regions of the brain most, which is in keeping with the clinical and behavioral observations of children affected by FGR. MRI spectroscopy offers the potential for non-invasive metabolic assessment of the brain tissue, which could be usefully incorporated into screening. Alteration in the brain metabolism may be related to clinically important outcomes in neurodevelopment and provide important prognostic information for counseling parents. This remains a theoretical approach, but this rabbit model identified aspargine, ornithine, N-acetylaspartylglutamate (NAAG), N-acetyl aspartate (NAA), and palmitoleic acid as possible new markers of metabolic derangement secondary to FGR that could be assessed further.

Placental Metabolomics

Metabolomic investigation of the placenta assists in understanding the mechanism of growth restriction. It has been shown that the metabolic profile differs between placental cell cultures of pregnancies affected by preeclampsia compared to pregnancies not affected by preeclampsia or growth restriction. More importantly, the same changes in metabolic profile can be induced by culturing the normal placental cells in a hypoxic environment, demonstrating that the preeclamptic phenotype can be provoked by chronic hypoxia and suggesting that this could be further investigated in relation to growth restriction [38]. Placental tissue is of course obtainable in pregnancy by chorionic villus sampling; however, an invasive test is not likely to offer a viable screening tool.

Maternal Urine Metabolomics

The maternal urine metabolic profile has been shown to be altered in pregnancies affected by central nervous system (CNS) malformations, trisomy 21, preterm delivery, gestational diabetes mellitus, preeclampsia, and FGR [31].

Maternal urine tested in the second trimester can identify metabolic changes associated with neural tube defects and trisomy 21 [39], but changes in the maternal urinary metabolic profile associated with FGR are detectable as early as the first trimester. Maternal urine tested between 11–13 weeks has been shown to provide a distinct metabolic signature for FGR pregnancies (decreased urinary acetate, citrate, formate, glycine, tyrosine, and trimethylamine) [40]. The study that demonstrated this was not designed to look at FGR pregnancies, but the abnormal metabolites coincide with a number of other metabolomic studies. Since women already attend a screening test at 11–13 weeks in most models of antenatal care, the addition of a urinary screening test is a feasible and low-cost potential screening test.

Maternal Hair

Hair provides a stable metabolome that is consistent over time and less variable than the results of testing blood or urine. Metabolomic assessment of maternal hair sampled between 26 and 28 weeks' gestation has been shown to discriminate between FGR and normal growth pregnancies. Combining the five most discriminating metabolites (lactate, levulinate, 2-methyloctadecanate, tyrosine, margarate) provided an AUC of 0.998 for prediction of FGR in this small preliminary study [41]. Further investigation is necessary to determine if testing in the first trimester could be informative, given that the metabolic profile of the maternal hair reflects the metabolic activity over the preceding months.

Ultrasound Markers for First Trimester Screening for FGR

Ultrasound examination allows assessment of resistance in maternal and fetal blood vessels, and direct measurement of placental size and depth. A number of different measurements can be made, requiring varying degrees of skills to assess the placental function, and could potentially usefully be included in screening for FGR.

Uterine Artery Doppler

High resistance flow in the maternal compartment of the uteroplacental unit is associated with villous hypoperfusion and incomplete trophoblastic invasion that may predispose to preeclampsia and FGR. Uterine artery Doppler is commonly included in screening models for both conditions. UtA PI may be taken as the mean of the two uterine artery measurements or as the greater of the two values, and the presence of notching in the waveform is also associated with placental insufficiency [4]. Guidance on how to record the uterine artery Doppler in the first trimester is illustrated in Figure 11.1. Uterine artery pulsatility index measured at 18–23+6 weeks gestation is strongly correlated with birth weight [5].

In the second trimester, a combined model using UtA PI, mean arterial pressure (MAP), and maternal risk factors can achieve a detection rate for small fetuses of 27% for a FPR of 10%. Although the same model reports a 100% detection rate for early-onset preeclampsia [42], the detection rate for SGA using

Figure 11.1 Uterine artery Doppler recorded at 11+0–13+6 weeks' gestation.

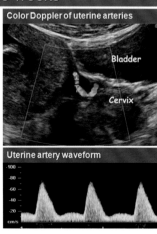

Uterine artery Doppler at 11–13 weeks

- The uterine arteries are at the level of the internal cervical os

- Set the sampling gate to 2 mm so as to cover whole vessel

- Angle of insonation should be less than 30°

- The peak systolic velocity should be more than 60 cm/s

- Obtain three similar consecutive waveforms

- The mean pulsatility index (PI) is obtained as the average of the left PI and right PI

Color Doppler of uterine arteries

Bladder

Cervix

Uterine artery waveform

second trimester UtA PI alone is only 22% with a 10% FPR. First trimester UtA PI is also associated with the risk of SGA, but to a lesser degree [4]. After adjusting for confounding factors, the UtA PI in the first trimester may not contribute significantly to improved detection rates in first trimester screening [13]. However, the predictive performance of uterine Doppler recorded in the first trimester is far better for the early FGR (<34 weeks), which is related to placental insufficiency, compared to the term SGA.

Placental Volume Measurements

With the advent of 3D ultrasound, it is now possible to measure the volume of the placenta indirectly, and a number of measurements have been shown to be associated with later FGR. Mean placental volume (MPV) is the best-performing individual 3D parameter, but interestingly mean chorionic diameter (MCD), a measurement that is obtainable on 2D scanning, is also strongly associated with later placental insufficiency [13]. Since a wider, flatter placenta has been shown to be associated with SGA, the mean diameter is logically also associated with SGA, as is an assessment of placental depth. The placental quotient (PQ) relates placental volume to fetal size using the crown-rump length (CRL) measurement and has been shown to have a similar predictive value for small fetuses to first trimester UtA PI [43].

Umbilical Artery (UA) Pulsatility Index

Since the Ut PI is an established factor associated with later placental pathology and it primarily assesses resistance in the maternal compartment of the uteroplacental unit, it is reasonable to propose that including UA Dopplers, a fetal measure, in screening for a fetal condition, growth restriction, could add value to the screening model. So far, however, this has not been shown, possibly because of the wider prevalence of high resistance flow in the UA at very early gestations. Combining UA PI with UtA PI in the first trimester provides an AUC of 0.56, and is of limited value in screening [44].

Maternal Hemodynamics in Screening for FGR

Early changes in maternal hemodynamics are detectable in pregnancies destined to develop both preeclampsia and FGR. Increased uterine artery Doppler resistance indices reflect impaired placentation, and this positive finding increases the risk of both preeclampsia and FGR. In women destined to develop preeclampsia with FGR, the central systolic blood pressure and augmentation index (a measure of arterial stiffness) are elevated in the first trimester (11–13 weeks) [45], whereas in women destined to deliver an SGA fetus without developing PE, these markers are normal.

Similarly, maternal cardiac output measured in the first trimester may help to discriminate between women destined to develop PE with FGR and those who will have FGR alone. Although in the third trimester both groups show reduced cardiac output compared to normal pregnant women, in the first trimester women who will develop PE have a greater increase in cardiac output than that normally seen in pregnancy, whereas women who will be affected by FGR alone are noted to have a blunting of the pregnancy-associated increase in cardiac output [46].

These findings offer the possibility of adding maternal hemodynamic assessment to first trimester screening models for preeclampsia or FGR.

Combined First Trimester Screening Algorithms

Several combined screening algorithms incorporating a number of these measurements with maternal risk factors have been proposed. Table 11.2 summarizes the proposed algorithms. The best-performing algorithm can detect 73% of early SGA (those requiring delivery before 37 weeks) [23], but this model includes a number of markers not routinely collected in the first trimester – PlGF, PP13, and ADAM 12. A less complex algorithm reported by the same group achieves a detection rate of 55.5% for early SGA and 44.3% for late SGA, including maternal factors, UtA PI, MAP, PAPP-A, and PlGF [47]. Similar models for the prediction of early preeclampsia have undergone external validation [48], and it is now necessary to evaluate the screening algorithms for SGA in a variety of populations to test their utility in general clinical use.

No algorithms have been reported with FGR with evidence of placental dysfunction as the outcome. It would be a practical challenge, requiring large-scale ultrasound assessment in later pregnancy, which is not practicable in most resource settings. Although FGR is associated with greater morbidity, the outcome of SGA is clinically relevant and includes most severely

Table 11.2 First trimester screening algorithms for small for gestational age (SGA) or fetal growth restriction (FGR)

Study	Gestation at screening	Participants	Definition of SGA/FGR	Maternal characteristics	Biochemical markers	Ultrasound markers	Accuracy
Poon 2013 [47]	11–13+6 weeks	3168 cases 57458 controls	SGA: Birth weight <5th centile Early requiring delivery <37 weeks; late delivering after 37 weeks	Age, BMI, ethnicity, prior SGA, smoking, hypertension, type 2 diabetes, APS, assisted conception, MAP	PAPP-A PlGF	UtAPI (mean)	Early SGA: DR 55.5% (FPR 10.9%) Late SGA: DR 44.3% (FPR 10.9%)
Plasencia 2011 [18]	11–13+6 weeks	3104 participants 144 cases	SGA: Birth weight <5th centile	Weight, height, parity, ethnicity.	PAPP-A	MPV	Maternal factors + PAPP-A: DR 32.6% (24.2–42.3) (FPR 10%) Maternal factors + MPV DR 29.2% (21.2–38.8) (FPR 10%) Maternal factors + MPV + PAPP-A DR: 34.7 (26.1–44.4) (FPR 10%)
Karagiannis 2011 [23]	11–13+6 weeks	1536 cases 31314 controls	SGA: Birth weight <5th centile Early requiring delivery <37 weeks; late delivering after 37 weeks	Age, weight, ethnicity, previous SGA, parity, assisted conception, smoking, hypertension, type 2 diabetes, SLE or APS, MAP	PAPP-A bHCG PlGF ADAM 12 PP13	UtAPI (mean) NT	All SGA: DR 47.3% (FPR 10%) Early SGA: DR 73.2% (FPR 10%) Late SGA: DR 45.8% (FPR 10%)
Poon 2008 [30]	11–13+6 weeks	296 cases 609 controls	SGA: Birth weight <5th centile	Maternal factors	PAPP-A PlGF	UtAPI	DR 27% (FPR 10%)
Crovetto 2014 [49]	11–13+6 weeks	4970 participants	Early SGA: birth weight < 10th centile (requiring delivery <34 weeks) Late SGA: birth weight <10th centile (delivered >34 wks)	Ethnicity, hypertension, renal disease, previous PE/SGA MAP	PAPP-A bHCG	UtAPI	With PE DR 90% (FPR 15%) Without PE DR 40% (FPR 15%)
Schwartz 2014 [13]	11–14 weeks		SGA: estimated fetal weight less than 5th centile	Ethnicity, smoking		MCD	AUC = 0.804
Seravalli 2014 [44]	11–14 weeks	2267 participants 191 cases	Birth weight <10th centile		PAPP-A bHCG	UtAPI UAPI	AUC=0.558

The "Autoimmune disease, age, parity, smoking, diabetes MAP" row appears under Crovetto 2014 Maternal characteristics for the Late SGA line.

BMI: body mass index; APS: antiphospholipid syndrome; MAP: mean arterial pressure; PAPP-A: pregnancy-associated plasma protein A; PlGF: placental growth factor; UtAPI: uterine artery pulsatility index; MPV: mean placenta volume; systemic lupus erythematosus; b-hCG: beta human chorionic gonadotrophin; ADAM 12: a-disintegrin and metalloproteinase 12; PP13: placental protein 13; NT: nuchal translucency; PE: preeclampsia; MCD: mean chorionic diameter; UAPI: umbilical artery Doppler growth-restricted fetuses. A group of significant concern is those fetuses that fail to achieve their growth potential because of placental insufficiency but still fall within the 5th–95th centiles for birth weight and may not be identified as FGR. These fetuses are also at risk of perinatal and lifelong morbidity and are not detected with current screening protocols.

Future Challenges

It is not surprising that better detection rates are achieved for early SGA, a group that presumably incorporates a greater percentage of FGR babies secondary to placental insufficiency. The diagnosis of late SGA remains an important clinical problem if the rate of intrauterine deaths at term is to be reduced. Late SGA is vastly more common, more heterogeneous and yet still significantly associated with increased perinatal morbidity. A combination of novel ultrasound markers and biomarkers identified through metabolomics offers hope for screening successfully for late as well as early onset FGR.

Key Points

- Screening algorithms in the first trimester enable the identification of fetuses at risk of being delivered small for gestational age before 37 weeks' gestation.

- The best performing algorithms incorporate maternal factors, biochemical markers, and ultrasound assessment of placental function either by UtAPI or placental volume.

- Priorities for future research include identifying effective interventions for preventing growth restriction that can be started in the first trimester, and improving screening for late-onset FGR.

References

1. Dukhovny S, Zera C, Little SE, McElrath T, Wilkins-Haug L. Eliminating first trimester markers: Will replacing PAPP-A and βhCG miss women at risk for small for gestational age? *J Matern Fetal Neonatal Med* 2014.

2. Nicolaides KH, Wright D, Poon LC, Syngelaki A, Gil MM. First-trimester contingent screening for trisomy 21 by biomarkers and maternal blood cell-free DNA testing. *Ultrasound Obstet Gynecol* 2013 Jul;42(1):41–50.

3. The Investigation and Management of the Small-for-Gestational-Age Fetus: Greentop Guideline 31. Royal College of Obstetricians and Gynaecologists, London, UK; 2013.

4. Cnossen JS, Morris RK, Ter Riet G, Mol BWJ, Van der Post JAM, Coomarasamy A, et al. Use of uterine artery Doppler ultrasonography to predict pre-eclampsia and intrauterine growth restriction: A systematic review and bivariable meta-analysis. *CMAJ* 2008 Mar 11;178(6):701–11.

5. Verlohren S, Melchiorre K, Khalil A, Thilaganathan B. Uterine artery Doppler, birth weight and timing of onset of pre-eclampsia: Providing insights into the dual etiology of late-onset pre-eclampsia. *Ultrasound Obstet Gynecol* 2014 Oct;44(3):293–8.

6. Mayer C, Joseph KS. Fetal growth: A review of terms, concepts and issues relevant to obstetrics. *Ultrasound Obstet Gynecol* 2013 Feb;41(2):136–45.

7. Gardosi J, Madurasinghe V, Williams M, Malik A, Francis A. Maternal and fetal risk factors for stillbirth: Population based study. *BMJ* 2013;346:f108.

8. Lindqvist PG, Molin J. Does antenatal identification of small-for-gestational age fetuses significantly improve their outcome? *Ultrasound Obstet Gynecol* 2005 Mar;25(3):258–64.

9. Roberge S, Nicolaides KH, Demers S, Villa P, Bujold E. Prevention of perinatal death and adverse perinatal outcome using low-dose aspirin: A meta-analysis. *Ultrasound Obstet Gynecol* 2013;41:491–9.

10. Sanz-Cortés M, Carbajo RJ, Crispi F, Figueras F, Pineda-Lucena A, Gratacós E. Metabolomic profile of umbilical cord blood plasma from early and late intrauterine growth restricted (IUGR) neonates with and without signs of brain vasodilation. *PLoS One* 2013 Jan;8(12):e801217.

11. Mifsud W, Sebire NJ. Placental pathology in early-onset and late-onset fetal growth restriction. *Fetal Diagn Ther* 2014 Jan;36(2):117–28.

12. Kovo M, Schreiber L, Ben-Haroush A, Wand S, Golan A, Bar J. Placental vascular lesion differences in pregnancy-induced hypertension and normotensive fetal growth restriction. *Am J Obstet Gynecol* 2010 Jul;202(6):561.e1–5.

13. Schwartz N, Sammel MD, Leite R, Parry S. First-trimester placental ultrasound and maternal serum markers as predictors of small-for-gestational-age infants. *Am J Obstet Gynecol* Elsevier; 2014 Sep 9;211(3):253.e1–8.

14. Romero R, Kusanovic JP, Than NG, Erez O, Gotsch F, Espinoza J, et al. First-trimester maternal serum PP13 in the risk assessment for preeclampsia. *Am J Obstet Gynecol* Elsevier; 2008 Aug 8;199(2):122.e1–122.e11.

15. Stamatopoulou A, Cowans NJ, Matwejew E, Von Kaisenberg C, Spencer K. Placental protein-13 and pregnancy-associated plasma protein-A as first trimester screening markers for hypertensive disorders and small for gestational age outcomes. *Hypertens Pregnancy* 2011:384–95.

16. Schneuer FJ, Nassar N, Khambalia AZ, Tasevski V, Ashton AW, Morris JM, et al. First trimester screening of maternal placental protein 13 for predicting preeclampsia and small for gestational age: In-house study and systematic review. *Placenta* 2012;33:735–40.

17. Cowans NJ, Stamatopoulou A, Khalil A, Spencer K. PP13 as a marker of pre-eclampsia: A two platform comparison study. *Placenta* 2011;32.

18. Plasencia W, Akolekar R, Dagklis T, Veduta A, Nicolaides KH. Placental volume at 11–13 weeks' gestation in the prediction of birth weight percentile. *Fetal Diagn Ther* 2011;30:23–8.

19. Odibo AO, Patel KR, Spitalnik A, Odibo L, Huettner P. Placental pathology, first-trimester biomarkers and adverse pregnancy outcomes. *J Perinatol* 2014;34:186–91.

20. Spencer K, Cowans NJ, Avgidou K, Molina F, Nicolaides KH. First-trimester biochemical markers of aneuploidy and the prediction of small-for-gestational age fetuses. *Ultrasound Obstet Gynecol* 2008;31:15–19.

21. D'Antonio F, Rijo C, Thilaganathan B, Akolekar R, Khalil A, Papageourgiou A, et al. Association between first-trimester maternal serum pregnancy-associated plasma protein-A and obstetric complications. *Prenat Diagn* 2013 Sep;33(9):839–47.

22. Dugoff L, Hobbins JC, Malone FD, Porter TF, Luthy D, Comstock CH, et al. First-trimester maternal serum PAPP-A and free-beta subunit human chorionic gonadotropin concentrations and nuchal translucency are associated with obstetric complications: A population-based screening study (The FASTER Trial). *Am J Obstet Gynecol* 2004:1446–51.

23. Karagiannis G, Akolekar R, Sarquis R, Wright D, Nicolaides KH. Prediction of small-for-gestation neonates from biophysical and biochemical markers at 11–13 weeks. *Fetal Diagn Ther* 2011;29:148–54.

24. Wortelboer EJ, Koster MPH, Kuc S, Eijkemans MJC, Bilardo CM, Schielen PCJI, et al. Longitudinal trends in fetoplacental biochemical markers, uterine artery pulsatility index and maternal blood pressure during the first trimester of pregnancy. *Ultrasound Obstet Gynecol* 2011 Oct;38(4):383–8.

25. Yang J, Wu J, Guo F, Wang D, Chen K, Li J, et al. Maternal serum disintegrin and metalloproteinase protein-12 in early pregnancy as a potential marker of adverse pregnancy outcomes. *PLoS One* 2014 Jan 15;9(5):e97284.

26. Poon LCY, Chelemen T, Granvillano O, Pandeva I, Nicolaides KH. First-trimester maternal serum a disintegrin and metalloprotease 12 (ADAM12) and adverse pregnancy outcome. *Obstet Gynecol* 2008 Nov;112(5):1082–90.

27. Lacroix MC, Guibourdenche J, Frendo JL, Muller F, Evain-Brion D. Human placental growth hormone – a review. *Placenta* 2002 Apr;23 Suppl A:S87–94.

28. Sifakis S, Akolekar R, Kappou D, Mantas N, Nicolaides KH. Maternal serum placental growth hormone at 11–13 weeks' gestation in pregnancies delivering small for gestational age neonates. *J Matern Fetal Neonatal Med* 2012:1796–9.

29. Romero R, Nien JK, Espinoza J, Todem D, Fu W, Chung H, et al. A longitudinal study of angiogenic (placental growth factor) and anti-angiogenic (soluble endoglin and soluble vascular endothelial growth factor receptor-1) factors in normal pregnancy and patients destined to develop preeclampsia and deliver a small for. *J Matern Fetal Neonatal Med* 2008 Jan;21(1):9–23.

30. Poon L, Zaragoza E, Akolekar R, Anagnostopoulos E, Nicolaides KH. Maternal serum placental growth factor (PlGF) in small for gestational age pregnancy at 11 + 0 to 13 + 6 weeks of gestation. *Prenat Diagn* 2008;28:1110–15.

31. Dessì A, Marincola F, Fanos V. Metabolomics and the great obstetrical syndromes – GDM, PET, and IUGR. *Best Pract Res Clin Obstet Gynaecol* 2014 Aug 21;29(2):156–64.

32. Dessì A, Atzori L, Noto A, Visser GHA, Gazzolo D, Zanardo V, et al. Metabolomics in newborns with intrauterine growth retardation (IUGR): Urine reveals markers of metabolic syndrome. *J Matern Fetal Neonatal Med* 2011 Oct;24 Suppl 2:35–9.

33. Barker DJ, Gluckman PD, Godfrey KM, Harding JE, Owens JA, Robinson JS. Fetal nutrition and cardiovascular disease in adult life. *Lancet* 1993 Apr 10;341(8850):938–41.

34. Barberini L, Noto A, Fattuoni C, Grapov D, Casanova A, Fenu G, et al. Urinary metabolomics (GC-MS) reveals that low and high birth weight infants share elevated inositol concentrations at birth. *J Matern Fetal Neonatal Med* 2014 Oct;27 Suppl 2:20–6.

35. Lin G, Liu C, Feng C, Fan Z, Dai Z, Lai C, et al. Metabolomic analysis reveals differences in umbilical vein plasma metabolites between normal and growth-restricted fetal pigs during late gestation. *J Nutr* 2012 Jun;142(6):990–8.

36. Favretto D, Cosmi E, Ragazzi E, Visentin S, Tucci M, Fais P, et al. Cord blood metabolomic profiling in intrauterine growth restriction. *Anal Bioanal Chem* 2012 Jan;402(3):1109–21.

37. Van Vliet E, Eixarch E, Illa M, Arbat-Plana A, González-Tendero A, Hogberg HT, et al. Metabolomics reveals metabolic alterations by intrauterine growth restriction in the fetal rabbit brain. *PLoS One* 2013 Jan;8(5):e64545.

38. Heazell AEP, Brown M, Worton SA, Dunn WB. Review: The effects of oxygen on normal and pre-eclamptic placental tissue – insights from metabolomics. *Placenta* 2011 Mar 32 Suppl 2:S119–24.

39. Diaz SO, Barros AS, Goodfellow BJ, Duarte IF, Galhano E, Pita C, et al. Second trimester maternal urine for the diagnosis of trisomy 21 and prediction of poor pregnancy outcomes. *J Proteome Res American Chemical Society* 2013 Jun 7;12(6):2946–57.

40. Maitre L, Fthenou E, Athersuch T, Coen M, Toledano MB, Holmes E, et al. Urinary metabolic profiles in early pregnancy are associated with preterm birth and fetal growth restriction in the Rhea mother-child cohort study. *BMC Med* 2014 Jan;12:110.

41. Sulek K, Han T-L, Villas-Boas SG, Wishart DS, Soh S-E, Kwek K, et al. Hair metabolomics: Identification of fetal compromise provides proof of concept for biomarker discovery. *Theranostics* 2014 Jan;4(9):953–9.

42. Onwudiwe N, Yu CKH, Poon LCY, Spiliopoulos I, Nicolaides KH. Prediction of pre-eclampsia by a combination of maternal history, uterine artery Doppler and mean arterial pressure. *Ultrasound Obstet Gynecol* 2008 Dec;32(7):877–83.

43. Hafner E, Metzenbauer M, Höfinger D, Stonek F, Schuchter K, Waldhör T, et al. Comparison between three-dimensional placental volume at 12 weeks and uterine artery impedance/notching at 22 weeks in screening for pregnancy-induced hypertension, pre-eclampsia and fetal growth restriction in a low-risk population. *Ultrasound Obstet Gynecol* 2006 Jun;27(6):652–7.

44. Seravalli V, Block-Abraham DM, Turan OM, Doyle LE, Kopelman JN, Atlas RO, et al. First-trimester prediction of small-for-gestational age neonates incorporating fetal Doppler parameters and maternal characteristics. *Am J Obstet Gynecol* Elsevier; 2014 Sep 9;211(3):261.e1–8.

45. Khalil A, Sodre D, Syngelaki A, Akolekar R, Nicolaides KH. Maternal hemodynamics at 11–13 weeks of gestation in pregnancies delivering small for gestational age neonates. *Fetal Diagn Ther* 2012 Jan;32(4):231–8.

46. De Paco C, Kametas N, Rencoret G, Strobl I, Nicolaides KH. Maternal cardiac output between 11 and 13 weeks of gestation in the prediction of preeclampsia and small for gestational age. *Obstet Gynecol* 2008;111:292–300.

47. Poon LCY, Syngelaki A, Akolekar R, Lai J, Nicolaides KH. Combined screening for preeclampsia and small for gestational age at 11–13 weeks. *Fetal Diagn Ther* 2013;33:16–27.

48. Kane S, da Silva Costa B. First trimester biomarkers in the prediction of later pregnancy complications. *Biomed Res Int* 2014 (Article ID 807196).

49. Crovetto F, Crispi F, Scazzocchio E, Mercade I, Meler E, Figueras F, et al. First-trimester screening for early and late small-for-gestational-age neonates using maternal serum biochemistry, blood pressure and uterine artery Doppler. *Ultrasound Obstet Gynecol* 2014;43:34–40.

Chapter

12

Second Trimester and Late-Pregnancy Screening for Fetal Growth Restriction

Raffaele Napolitano and Pasquale Martinelli

Introduction

Several second and third trimester screening strategies for fetal growth restriction (FGR) have been proposed.

The effectiveness of screening tests has been evaluated in association with dedicated monitoring or intervention. Screening tests used are based on the evaluation of maternal risks factors, symphysial fundal height (SFH), uterine artery Doppler (UtA), maternal biochemical markers, and serial growth scans.

The efficacy of each screening test is reported in literature, with variable results [1]. The lack of type A evidence in screening and monitoring growth-restricted fetuses led to variable and inconsistent practice worldwide. Uterine artery Doppler velocimetry is associated with promising results in observational studies and in randomized trials (RCT) when used in combination with preventive treatment or dedicated monitoring strategies. Nevertheless, to date, the only monitoring strategy that has been associated with an improvement in the perinatal outcome is the umbilical artery Doppler velocimetry performed in "high-risk" pregnancies.

The World Health Organization recommends that a screening test should satisfy specific conditions known as the Wilson's criteria [2,3]. The Wilson's criteria are difficult to apply to the screening for FGR. Specifically, doubts remain about the most appropriate time to intervene, in this context, with delivery, and making the diagnosis of growth restriction can be difficult as it may become apparent only with repeated observations of a fetus [4]. Furthermore, cost-effective analysis has not shown encouraging results. No screening strategies have been considered cost-effective if used in isolation [5].

A key methodological issue in evaluating screening performances is the definition of FGR used in different studies.

Fetal growth restriction is defined as a pathological inhibition of fetal growth and failure of the fetus to attain its growth potential [1]. There are however, no standard defined criteria of FGR; therefore, it is referred to in this chapter according with the definition reported in each study. Small for gestational age (SGA) is defined as a newborn having a birth weight below the 10th percentile of an accepted reference standard. To establish whether a fetus is SGA or FGR, fetal biometry, as a single or repeated observation, and the evaluation of the fetal Doppler velocimetry are required (umbilical artery, middle cerebral artery, etc.). It is beyond the scope of this chapter to compare screening test performances according with one or the other definition of FGR reported.

For the purpose of this chapter, "mid trimester" or "second trimester" is defined as the gestational age between 16+0 and 24+0. The reported cut-offs are used for two main reasons. Preventive treatments for FGR have been reported to be effective in low-risk or unselected populations if adopted before 16 completed weeks (for example, aspirin) (see Chapter 13) [6]. Therefore, any screening policy tested beyond 16 weeks should be referred to as a "late" screening policy and only enables the identification of fetuses who would benefit from a more intense surveillance as the chance for a preventive treatment to be effective is reduced. There is general consensus that a fetus with FGR developed before 24 weeks should be managed as being at the borderline of viability due to the very guarded outlook in case of iatrogenic delivery [7], and therefore any screening policy after 24 weeks is referred to in this chapter as "third trimester" or "late pregnancy."

Patient History

Several maternal risks factors are associated with delivering a fetus with SGA or FGR as reported in numerous observational studies. A most recent summary of pooled data is available from the Royal College of Obstetricians and Gynaecologists (RCOG) guidelines (Table 12.1) [8]. There are maternal conditions

Table 12.1 Risk factors for small for gestational age

	Risk Index	LR	95% CI
Maternal medical conditions:			
Antiphospholipid syndrome	RR	6.22	(2.43, 16.0)
Maternal diabetes	OR	6	(1.5, 2.3)
Renal disease	OR	5.3	(2.8, 10)
Chronic hypertension	RR	2.5	(2.1, 2.9)
Maternal risk factors:			
Vigorous exercise	OR	3.3	(1.5, 7.2)
Cocaine abuse	OR	3.23	(2.43, 4.3)
Maternal age > 40	OR	3.2	(1.9, 5.4)
Smoking (more than 11 cigarettes per day)	OR	2.21	(2.03, 2.4)
Previous pregnancy risk factors:			
Previous stillbirth	OR	6.4	(0.78, 52.56)
Previous small for gestational age	OR	3.9	(2.14, 7.12)
Current pregnancy:			
Antepartum hemorrhage	OR	5.6	(2.5, 12.2)
Low maternal weight gain	OR	4.9	(1.9, 12.6)
Pregnancy hypertensive disorders	OR	2.26	(1.22, 4.18)
Echogenic bowel	OR	2.1	(1.5, 2.9)

Modified from RCOG green top guidelines 2013, risk factors reported showing a LR > 2.
LR: likelihood ratio, RR: risk ratio, OR: odds ratio, CI: confidence intervals.

preexisting pregnancy that carry a well-demonstrated increased risk for SGA and FGR as associated with placental insufficiency. Chronic hypertension, maternal diabetes, renal disease, and antiphospholipid syndrome have risk ratio (RR) and odds radio (OR) between 2.5 and 6.2 with 95% confidence intervals (95% CI) between 1.5–2.8 and 2.3–16.0, representing the highest reported for FGR risk. These syndromes are in fact absolute indications for aspirin prophylaxis, according to the National Institute of Clinical Excellence guidelines [9].

Some maternal characteristics are more associated with FGR than others (maternal age >40 years, smoking, cocaine abuse, or vigorous exercise) with OR between 2.2 and 3.3 (95% CI between 1.9–2.43 and 2.4–7.2). Previous pregnancy history of SGA and stillbirth represent the most severe obstetric history risk factors with OR of 6.4 and 3.9. Complications occurring in pregnancy would put the fetus at risk of being SGA or growth restricted and therefore these also require further investigation (antepartum hemorrhage, maternal preeclampsia, and echogenic bowel).

The RCOG guidance on Doppler screening recommendation varies depending on whether one or more risk factor is present. In all cases of RR or OR greater than 2.0 (Table 12.1) serial ultrasound scans are recommended from 28 weeks onward. There are no RCT comparing the difference in detection rate of SGA and FGR using UtA Doppler or serial growth scans. In case of moderate/mild risk factors (for example: BMI > 30, maternal or paternal SGA, assisted reproduction), the RCOG guidelines recommend UtA Doppler screening with serial growth scans only in cases of abnormal UtA Doppler results.

American and Canadian guidelines do not recommend any specific policy other than the use of UtA Doppler and/or serial growth scans in case of any risk factors [10,11]. UtA Doppler findings might be of value in high-risk women even if serial growth scans are due to be performed due to the management of late FGR.

It is therefore reasonable to recommend UtA Doppler screening along with serial ultrasound scans to all the women with risk factors (Table 12.1).

Women with moderate-mild risk factors can undergo UtA Doppler screening and in case of normal result only one dedicated scan in the late third trimester is required at 34–36 weeks.

Symphysial Fundal Height

SFH is commonly practiced primarily to screen other than to detect FGR. The method involves using a tape measure to take a measurement in centimeters from the fundus (variable point) to the mother's symphysis pubis (fixed point). The measurement is then applied to the gestation by a simple rule of thumb and compared with normal growth [12]. Currently there is no RCT reported, comparing the SFH with ultrasound in screening or detection of FGR. SFH has been compared in one RCT to abdominal palpation recruiting more than 1,600 women. There was no difference in the perinatal outcome or the detection of SGA between the two groups [12].

Measuring the SFH is the method of assessing FGR that is the easiest to perform and the least costly. SFH has been mainly studied as a surveillance tool for prediction of SGA rather than a screening tool to be integrated in more comprehensive strategies, for example in association with maternal or fetal Doppler. The sensitivity rate of SGA detection at birth reported in systematic reviews is variable, between 20% and 90%. The heterogeneity of the studies reported reflects this result [9,13]. The comparison of SFH and fetal ultrasound biometry in prediction of SGA or FGR shows controversial results. In an era when an ultrasound biometrical evaluation of fetal growth is available, it appears more sensible to evaluate the effectiveness of the SFH in screening for growth restriction *in association with* rather *in comparison* to other tests, as the ultrasound biometry. This suggested strategy has not been used and it can explain the lack of evidence in using the SFH as an isolated screening test.

SFH is still recommended as the practice of choice to screen for FGR in low-risk women [8,10,11]. In an observational study recruiting more than 600 women, the use of customized centile charts and the recommendation of plotting the SFH measurements onto the customized chart showed to reduce the false positive rate and increase the detection rate of SGA. The authors argued that the study was not adequately powered to show an improvement in the perinatal outcome. The concept underlying customization is still a matter of debate.

Large prospective studies are yet to demonstrate its usefulness in reducing perinatal morbidity and mortality as part of a comprehensive screening strategy.

There is consensus between the authors of this book that the definition of a "low-risk" woman should include normal placentation in the second trimester, i.e., the SFH should be used as the only screening tool for FGR in case there are no maternal risk factors and the UtA Doppler screening is normal (see following section).

Uterine Artery Doppler

Uterine spiral arteries undergo a physiological transformation in pregnancy that reduces the resistance in the vessel and increases the blood flow to the uterus [14]. This placentation process can be affected if there is a poor conversion of the spiral arteries, and it will be reflected in increased UtA Doppler resistance [15].

Uterine artery Doppler has been investigated in RCTs. In a meta-analysis including two studies, women were randomized to undergo or not UtA Doppler screening in the second trimester. There was no difference in the perinatal outcome between the two groups. The two studies recruited more than 5,000 women from a mixed-risk population, and they were clearly not sufficiently powered to show any difference in the incidence of SGA (defined as a birth weight below the 10th or the 3rd centiles) [14]. Fox and colleagues elegantly demonstrated how the ideal design of RCT should be in testing both the test and the intervention (aspirin in this case). The "test-treatment" design involves randomizing women to undergo or not UtA screening and subsequently treating the women positive on the test [16]. This approach was used in the two studies reported in the meta-analysis [17,18]. The need to recruit an even larger number of women would make such study difficult to reproduce, and therefore it is unlikely that such effectiveness will be reported in the future. Otherwise most of the studies evaluating UtA Doppler and either the prediction of FGR or the improvement in the perinatal outcome are performed in populations with mixed low- and high-risk women. They are not randomized to undergo the screening test (UtA Doppler), but they are rather randomized to receive the treatment (aspirin) after they have *all* been screened [19,20]. Such design would answer a different question, i.e., is the intervention effective in selected cases?

In a meta-analysis published in 2008 recruiting more than 30,000 women, both in high- and in low-risk populations, UtA Doppler screening was analyzed in prediction of SGA [21]. The authors report a positive likelihood ratio (LR) of 9.1 (95% CI 5.0, 16.7) and a negative LR of 0.89 (95% CI 0.85, 0.93) in predicting SGA in low-risk women. Due to the incidence of SGA and FGR (< 8%) in Western countries, the sensitivity of this test can be considered acceptable in terms of predictive power (positive LR >10 and negative LR <0.1) [22].

Sensitivity was reported to be between 12% and 53%, according to different Doppler parameter used, 95% CI between 7–42 the lower, and 18–64 the higher, with a specificity higher than 80% in all the cases. No Doppler parameter used was considered consistently better than the others. A mean pulsatility index greater than the 95th centile, a mean resistance index greater than the 95th centile (>0.58 in most of the studies), or the presence of bilateral notching should be considered abnormal results [21].

A selection of studies reporting the predictive value of UtA Doppler for FGR in the second trimester where an LR and a defined outcome are reported is listed in Table 12.2.

In a cost-effective analysis, Morris and colleagues estimated that it would be more cost-effective to treat all the women with aspirin (£5 per woman) rather than screening all the women with UtA Doppler and treating only the women positive on the screening test (estimated £20 per woman) [5]. To date UtA Doppler screening in the second trimester is the screening test for FGR with the best performance used in isolation. Nevertheless, the lack of evidence from screening studies using the "test-treatment" approach and the lack of cost-effectiveness influenced the decision to not recommend the test in low-risk populations [8–11].

As a result of consultation of the authors of this volume, there is consensus in recommending UtA screening test in all the high-risk pregnancies [8]. Further research is needed to evaluate test-treatment-designed studies in unselected or low-risk women to implement UtA in routine clinical practice. It is difficult to justify a screening policy in low-risk multiparous women due to the poor performance of the test [23], but in absence of a best screening test, a policy recommending UtA Doppler screening to all the nulliparous low-risk women is advisable.

Serum and Other Biochemical Markers

Several biomarkers have been proposed as predictors of FGR in the second trimester. All of those have been tested in case-control or cohort studies.

Second trimester screening markers for Down syndrome have been extensively reported due to large amounts of retrospective data. Even if there is a correlation between their values and FGR, the pathophysiologic hypotheses remain dubious [24].

In a large meta-analysis published in 2008, Morris and colleagues report 53 studies in prediction of SGA defined as SGA below the 10th centile, SGA below the 5th centile, or birth weight below 2.5kg. Alpha fetoprotein (AFP), unconjugated Estradiol, human chorionic gonadotrophin (HCG), pregnancy-associated plasma protein A (PAPP-A), and Inhibin A were tested in the second trimester. Different cut-off and different FGR definitions were used to test the screening performance (Table 12.3).

The results showed low predictive accuracy overall. For SGA, the best predictor overall for birth weight <10th centile was AFP <10th centile.

None of the markers reported a LR >10 as recommended cut-off for a test to be implemented in clinical practice, due to the average SGA incidence. No cost-effective analysis was reported, but the authors hazarded a possibility of using a screening test (testing all the women) in association with a preventive treatment (aspirin). The use of markers for Down syndrome would reduce the number of women necessary to treat. Serum markers for aneuploidy have been analyzed in combination. A meta-analysis recruiting unselected women and testing the screening performance of AFP, unconjugated Estradiol, and HCG reports a positive LR or 15 for SGA detection. Despite this promising result, the negative LR crossed 1 [25].

In a meta-analysis of 2013 investigating the predictive value of novel serum markers, other than those used for chromosomal abnormality screening, the criteria for inclusion in the study were more selective in favor of detecting true growth-restricted fetuses [26]. Criteria for inclusion were SGA below the 10th centile in addition to other findings suggestive of FGR as: abnormal fetal or maternal Doppler velocimetry, abnormal placental pathology or olygohydramnios, and SGA below the 5th centile. Using such settings, it

Table 12.2 Uterine artery Doppler screening studies in prediction of fetal growth restriction in both high-risk and unselected populations

Study	Abnormal result	Birth weight outcome	Positive LR Absolute value (95% CI)	Negative LR Absolute value (95% CI)	Sensitivity %	Specificity %	Positive Predictive value %	Negative predictive value %
Campbell et al., 1986	RI >0.58	<10th centile	/	/	67	65	24	92
Hanretty et al., 1989	RI >0.52	<5th centile	/	/	6	93	5	95
Newnham et al., 1990	S/D ratio > 2.18	<10th centile	1.32 (0.42, 3.87)	0.98 (0.87, 1.03)	6	95	13	90
Steel et al., 1990	RI >0.58	<5th centile	4.26 (2.86, 6.02)	0.64 (0.48, 0.78)	43	90	18	97
		<10th centile	3.52 (2.46, 4.91)	0.74 (0.63, 0.84)	33	91	27	93
Bewley et al., 1991	mean RI >95th centile	<3rd centile	3.84 (1.74, 7.67)	0.74 (0.63, 0.84)	20	95	12	97
		<5th centile	3.84 (1.74, 7.67)	0.84 (0.66, 0.96)	19	95	19	95
		<10th centile	3.57 (2.08, 6.01)	0.89 (0.81, 0.94)	15	96	35	88
Bower et al., 1993	RI >95th centile or notches	<3rd centile	3.13 (2.35, 4.00)	0.63 (0.49, 0.76)	47	85	10	98
		<5th centile	3.22 (2.52, 4.01)	0.63 (0.52, 0.74)	46	86	15	97
		<10th centile	2.79 (2.26, 3.41)	0.72 (0.65, 0.79)	37	87	26	92
Valensise et al., 1993	mean RI >0.58	<10th centile	13.94 (7.33, 25.69)	0.35 (0.18, 0.57)	67	95	54	97
North et al., 1994	RI >0.57	<10th centile	5.21 (3.18, 7.98)	0.55 (0.37, 0.74)	50	90	27	96
Todros et al., 1995	S/D ratio >2.7	<10th centile	1.93 (0.81, 4.24)	0.94 (0.80, 1.01)	12	94	8	96
Harrington et al., 1996	RI >95th centile or notches	<10th centile	5.06 (3.58, 7.04)	0.73 (0.64, 0.81)	32	94	38	92

(continued)

Table 12.2 (continued)

Study	Abnormal result	Birth weight outcome	Positive LR Absolute value (95% CI)	Negative LR Absolute value (95% CI)	Sensitivity %	Specificity %	Positive Predictive value %	Negative predictive value %
Frusca et al., 1997	mean RI >0.58	<3rd centile	7.42 (3.54, 12.71)	0.49 (0.23, 0.78)	55	93	17	99
		<10th centile	7.33 (4.05, 12.56)	0.60 (0.42, 0.77)	43	94	36	96
Irion et al., 1998	mean RI >0.57	<10th centile	2.68 (1.93, 3.67)	0.80 0.70, 0.88	29	89	25	91
Kurdi et al., 1998	mean RI >0.55 and bilateral notches	<5th centile	3.38 (2.82, 4.00)	0.71 (0.65, 0.77)	37	89	18	95
		<10th centile	2.43 (1.92, 3.03)	0.68 (0.58, 0.77)	45	82	32	88
Albaiges et al., 2000	mean PI >95th centile or bilateral notches	<3rd centile	4.68 (2.93, 7.06)	0.74 (0.60, 0.86)	30	93	13	98
		<10th centile	3.76 (2.60, 5.34)	0.83 (0.75, 0.89)	22	94	25	93
Papageorghiou et al., 2001	mean PI >95th centile	<10th centile	4.15 (3.40, 5.06)	087 (0.84, 0.90)	16	96	30	92

Modified from Papageorghiou et al., 2002 and Fayyad et al., 2005.
LR: likelihood ratio, SD: standard deviations, CI: confidence intervals, RI: resistance index, S/D: systolic to diastolic ratio, PI: pulsatility index.

Table 12.3 Second trimester maternal serum and urine biomarkers in prediction of SGA and FGR reported in studies with cohort greater than 100 women

Marker	Cut-off	Outcome	Positive LR Absolute value (95% CI)	Negative LR Absolute value (95% CI)	Sensitivity % (95% CI)	Specificity % (95% CI)
AFP	<10th centile	BW <10th centile	8.80 (5.57,13.91)	0.02 (0.00,0.34)	/	/
HCG	>2.0 MoM	BW <10th centile	1.74 (1.48,2.04)	0.95 (0.93,0.96)	/	/
	>2.0 MoM	BW <5th centile	2.08 (1.78, 2.42)	0.94 (0.92, 0.95)	0.12 (0.10, 0.14)	0.94 (0.94, 0.95)
	<10th centile	BW <10th centile	2.35 (0.80, 6.92)	0.90 (0.76, 1.08)	0.16 (0.05, 0.36)	0.93 (0.88, 0.97)
	>90th centile	BW <10th centile	1.68 (0.37, 7.63)	0.97 (0.86, 1.09)	0.08 (0.01, 0.26)	0.95 (0.90, 0.98)
Estradiol	<0.75 MoM	BW <10th centile	2.54 (1.54, 4.19,)	0.75 (0.63, 0.89)	/	/
PAPP-A	<10th centile	BW <10th centile	1.82 (0.95, 3.50)	0.91 (0.75, 1.05)	0.20 (0.10, 0.33)	0.89 (0.85, 0.92)
	<1st centile	BW <10th centile	3.50 (2.53, 4.82)	0.98 (0.97, 0.99)	/	/
Inibin A	>2.0 MoM	BW <10th centile	4.45 (3.92, 5.06,)	0.92 (0.91, 0.93)	/	/
Triple test†	>1:190	BW <10th centile	1.07 (0.60, 1.91,)	0.98 (0.82, 1.17)	/	/
PlGF	<152 or 280 pg/ml‡	BW <10th centile*	1.4 (1.2, 1.6)	0.8 (0.7, 0.9)	46 (41, 51)	68 (66, 69)
sFlt-1	>1,230 pg/ml	BW <5th centile	1.4 (1.1, 1.8)	0.8 (0.7, 0.9)	48 (40, 56)	67 (61, 72)
VEGF	(unreported)	BW <2 SD	4.4 (1.6, 12.2)	0.5 (0.2, 1.1)	56 (27, 81)	88 (74, 95)
Endoglin	>6.20 ng/ml	BW <5th centile	1.8 (1.4, 2.3)	0.6 (0.5, 0.7)	61 (52, 69)	67 (60, 73)
Homocysteine	>90th centile	BW <10th centile*	2.3 (1.7, 3.1)	0.8 (0.8, 0.9)	26 (19, 33)	89 (87, 90)
sVCAM-1	>790 µg/l	BW <10th centile*	9.0 (3.9, 20.7)	0.9 (0.7, 1.0)	16 (7, 30)	98 (97, 99)

(continued)

Table 12.3 (continued)

Marker	Cut-off	Outcome	Positive LR	Negative LR	Sensitivity	Specificity
sICAM-1	>350 µg/l	BW <10th centile*	19.2 (11.5, 32.1)	0.6 (0.5, 0.8)	42 (28, 58)	98 (97, 99)
8-OHdG	>38.9 ng/mg creatinine	BW <10th centile*	1.7 (1.3, 2.4)	0.8 (0.7, 0.9)	38 (28, 48)	78 (74, 81)
Isoprostane	>21.39 ng/mg creatinine	BW <10th centile*	0.8 (0.3, 1.8)	1.1 (0.9, 1.2)	16 (7, 32)	80 (76, 83)
Fibronectin	>475 mg/l	BW <10th centile*	13.3 (5.0, 35.0)	0.5 (0.2, 0.8)	57 (33, 79)	96 (90, 98)
IGFBP-1	>90th centile	BW <10th centile*	2.7 (1.1, 6.5)	0.8 (0.7, 1.0)	24 (12, 43)	91 (85, 95)
SP1	(unreported)	Any FGR	2.5 (1.9, 3.3)	0.8 (0.7, 0.9)	32 (26, 38)	87 (85, 90)
Urinary albumin: Creatinine ratio	>34.5 mg/mmol	BW <10th centile*	1.9 (1.3, 2.8)	0.4 (0.1, 1.3)	78 (45, 94)	59 (53, 65)

LR: likelihood ratio, SD: standard deviations, CI: confidence intervals, AFP: alpha feto-protein, HCG: human chorionic gonadotrophin, BW: birth weight, MoM: multiple of median, PAPP-A: pregnancy-associated plasma protein A, PlGF: placental growth factor, SP1: pregnancy-specific beta-1-glycoprotein, VEGF: vascular endothelial growth factor, sFlt-1: soluble fms-like tyrosine kinase-1, sVCAM: soluble vascular cell adhesion molecule, sICAM: soluble intercellular adhesion molecule; 8-OHdG: 8-oxo-7,8 dihydro-2-deoxyguanosine, IGFBP: insulin-like growth factor binding protein.

* Newborns with additional findings suggestive of FGR (abnormal feto-maternal Doppler, olygohydramnios, BW below the 5th centile, abnormal placental pathology)

† (AFP, HCG, Estriol)

‡ Range of cut-off used according to different studies

Modified from Morris et al. 2008 and Conde-Agudelo et al. 2013 was more likely to not include constitutionally small babies and to investigate screening performances of tests potentially more predictive of FGR.

Second trimester biomarkers evaluation is reported in 49 studies (less than 22 weeks' gestation). None of the 37 novel biomarkers evaluated in the review showed a high predictive accuracy for FGR. In Table 12.3 are reported only second or third trimester markers analyzed in cohort studies including more than 100 women (Table 12.3). The biomarker most extensively reported was the placental growth factor (PlGF). Other biomarkers were: angiogenesis-related biomarkers (SP1: pregnancy-specific beta-1-glycoprotein, VEGF: vascular endothelial growth factor, sFlt-1: soluble fms-like tyrosine kinase-1); endothelial function/oxidative stress-related biomarkers (sVCAM: soluble vascular cell adhesion molecule, sICAM: soluble intercellular adhesion molecule; 8-OHdG: 8-oxo-7,8 dihydro-2-deoxyguanosine, IGFBP: insulin-like growth factor binding protein, fibronectin); placental proteins/hormone-related biomarkers (IGFBP-1).

The higher the severity of the FGR, the higher the performance of almost each single marker. No marker other than fibronectin has an LR greater than 10 and therefore their use in clinical practice in isolation should be discouraged. No cost-effective analysis was reported.

The potential use of second trimester or late-pregnancy markers predictive of FGR can be of any use only in association with other screening tests (UtA Doppler). This can optimize resources and allocate appropriate founding to serial growth scans in order to diagnose early any FGR and improve the outcome. Such studies have not been performed so far.

Combined Screening Test

Since no single screening test has yet been shown to meet all the requirements of a clinically useful predictive test for FGR in women with a singleton gestation, there is growing interest in the use of combinations of tests in a multiparameter test approach.

Most of the multiparameter screening tests for pregnancy complications have been evaluated to detect preeclampsia [27]. It can be argued that the FGR does not necessarily have the same pathophysiology, but the two syndromes have numerous findings in common. Obvious limitations in the late screening test for preeclampsia and FGR are related to the absence of a safe, effective, and affordable intervention to prevent the syndrome in high-risk women; furthermore, the benefit of intensive monitoring has not been proven to improve the outcome in the second half of pregnancy [28]. As highlighted earlier, this raises questions regarding the potential effectiveness of a screen-and-treat strategy in the second trimester. In an individual patient data meta-analysis recruiting more than 6,700 nulliparous women, the added value of screening in the second trimester with UtA Doppler to maternal characteristics was to reduce the false positive rate only [29]. In other words, women with high risk of developing preeclampsia due to their characteristics have a lower chance to falsely be considered high risk after 20 weeks of pregnancy if UtA Doppler are normal. It can be argued that the same would apply in the screening for FGR.

In an observational study recruiting more than 2,500 women, UtA Doppler were obtained between 18 and 26 weeks, whereas HCG and AFP were obtained between 14 and 18 weeks' gestation to screen for Down syndrome [30]. The screening performance for SGA detection was tested combining the serum markers and the Doppler parameters. The presence of at least one UtA notch was associated with the highest test sensitivity (23%) with a specificity of 89%. The combination of serum markers and the UtA did not increase the screening performance (sensitivity: between 2% and 20%). Nevertheless, the positive predictive value in case of presence of bilateral UtA Doppler notches in combination with either HCG <0,5 MoMs or AFP >1,5 MoMs increases to 42–50% compared with bilateral notches alone (positive predictive value: 26%).

Most of the combined tests for FGR are based on second trimester UtA Doppler combined with first trimester serum markers. As no substantial improvement to the UtA Doppler alone in FGR detection has been demonstrated, the use of a combined screening test for FGR in the second trimester is not recommended.

Serial Growth Scans

The screening for FGR in the third trimester is mainly based on the evaluation of the fetal biometry. Due to the limitation of the antenatal diagnosis of FGR, there is therefore an overlap between fetuses considered at risk of having FGR later in pregnancy and fetuses who show already signs of growth impairment. The purpose of using ultrasound in discerning between a screening test and a diagnostic test is beyond the scope of this chapter. Its use will be therefore discussed as a screening tool to identify fetuses who will have FGR phenotype after birth.

The routine use of ultrasound as either a fetal biometry tool or a maternal and fetal Doppler tool in the general population is controversial beyond 24 weeks of pregnancy. In a meta-analysis recruiting more than 10,000 women randomized in four trials to have a dedicated third trimester scan compared with women having only selective scan (required by the clinician or following local protocols), there was no difference in the detection of birth weight below the 10th centile (RR 0.98; CI 0.74–1.28) [31].

The two main reasons why ultrasound has poor performance are the lack of defined thresholds for normality versus abnormality (related also to which referring growth chart to use) and the absence of a useful demonstrated policy in employing ultrasound in the third trimester.

First, there is substantial heterogeneity in the study quality reporting dating and fetal growth charts [32,33]. In a systematic review of the charts developed to compute a craw-rump-length equation for pregnancy dating, 29 studies were selected. Out of all, four studies were considered to have the best methodology design and the discrepancy in gestational age estimation can be as high as 4 days on average [32]. In a systematic review aimed to report the quality and results of studies where fetal population-based growth charts (reference charts) were developed, the heterogeneity of the results was even higher. Out of 83 studies selected, 7 had the highest methodology quality and the reported centiles were analyzed. The value of the 10th abdominal circumference centile at 32 and 36 weeks' gestation, according to one study, was similar to the value of the 50th abdominal circumference centile, according to another study [33].

Many authors have proposed different solutions to improve the accuracy of the growth charts. Gardosi and colleagues proposed a model using "customized" growth charts where specific maternal characteristics should be considered in the definition of SGA fetuses [34]. The proposed approach can improve significantly the detection rate of FGR fetuses antenatally (SGA associated with abnormal perinatal outcome and stillbirth) [35], but it has not been tested in randomized trials.

Owen and Ogston proposed a model to improve the detection rate of SGA fetuses using longitudinal observations. This approach is defined as "conditional," and it consists of establishing predicted range of growth based on previous measurements [36].

In practical terms, a fetus with an estimated weight at the 30th centile cannot expect the next measurement to be distributed somewhere in the entire range for the reference population, nor is it true that the 30th centile of the reference chart is the expected growth trajectory for this fetus.

Both methods (customized and conditional) are developed to monitor the growth in pregnancies at risk of growth deviations without crossing the 10th centile, and show their advantage particularly in growth alterations in fetuses that are within normal ranges.

In order to correct the issues associated with population-based fetal growth charts, Villar and colleagues proposed the adoption of international prescriptive (how the fetus "should" grow) standards selecting women worldwide without risk factors for FGR. This should remove the bias introduced by the use of descriptive growth charts (how the fetus grows at a specific time), which are the population-based charts currently in use. International standards based on a multiethnic, multicenter study are now available. Their accuracy has not been validated by prospective studies, but the authors demonstrate that the growth data from the eight sites were similar enough to be pooled for construction of international standards designed for use as a screening method worldwide [37,38].

Regarding the second issue, the use of a single dedicated ultrasound biometry in the third trimester, as part of a not-specified management protocol, has been investigated in observational studies. A single measurement of the abdominal circumference or the estimated fetal weight is associated with a detection rate of SGA at term of 53–75% for a false positive rate of 20–25% [39–42]. A large Swedish population-based study comparing 56,000 women who had a single ultrasound at 34 weeks versus 153,000 women who did not have any other investigation other than the SFH found no significant difference in perinatal mortality, even if the authors do not report the SGA rate [43]. Nevertheless, the identification of SGA fetuses antenatally remains essential as it improves significantly the outcome at birth in observational retrospective studies [40]. Studies powered to demonstrate an improvement in perinatal mortality are difficult to perform in view of the sample required. Another approach is to compare different screening or diagnostic strategies to predict a composite neonatal outcome associated with FGR. Such approach has been studied by Sovio and colleagues in the POP observational study, which reflects more contemporaneous practice [44]. Unselected women underwent either a selected scan policy (according with clinical indication) or universal scan policy (at 28 and 36 weeks). The managing clinicians were blinded to the universal scan results. The latter group reported a higher detection rate of SGA (57% versus 20%). Furthermore, as a marker of FGR, an abdominal circumference centile drop from 20 weeks was associated with significant neonatal morbidity. Promising results are coming from multiparameter tests where the association of maternal history and a dedicated single ultrasound at 35–37 weeks could identify more than 70% of SGA delivering in the next 2 weeks [45].

Prospective interventional trials on how to improve the outcome are needed to demonstrate the benefit of introducing a policy of either a universal scan or a multiparameter test. Those should include an ultrasound evaluation at around 36 weeks. In fact, another study reports on the best timing to perform a single ultrasound in low-risk women. In this RCT, women were randomized to have a dedicated ultrasound at 32 or at 36 weeks. The sensitivity rate of customized SGA at birth below the 10th and the 3rd centiles was 22.5% and 32.5% at 32 weeks versus 32.5% and 61.4% at 36 weeks, respectively [46].

The change in fetal size between two time points is a direct measure of fetal growth and hence serial measurement of abdominal circumference or estimated fetal weight (growth velocities) should allow the diagnosis of FGR, rather than a 'spot' measurement being assumed to screen for the condition.

In an interventional trial, 2,700 unselected women were randomized to have an ultrasound every 4 weeks from 18 weeks of pregnancy versus having an ultrasound only if requested by the clinician. There were no differences between screened and control groups in any obstetric interventions, perinatal outcome, and childhood development outcomes even if data on antenatal FGR detection are not reported [47].

No other interventional trial is reported on investigating if serial ultrasound measurements can be used as a valid screening test or even as a diagnostic test of FGR.

Several attempts have been considered in order to identify the fetus at risk of abnormal perinatal outcome associated with FGR using the "eyeballing" of a chart, conditional centiles (previously described), or abdominal circumference growth velocity drop expressed in standard deviation changes [8,48,49]. No study has been demonstrated to be clinically feasible and effective. The previously cited POP study is encouraging in identifying fetuses at high risk of morbidity out of the antenatal SGA cohort using abdominal circumference centile drop.

In the absence of any other effective tool, the authors would suggest that serial growth scans should be recommended every 4 weeks from 24 weeks of pregnancy in case of presence of significant risk factors (Table 12.1) or abnormal UtA Doppler.

If UtA Doppler is normal, a single ultrasound should be performed at 36 weeks of pregnancy in low-risk women, acknowledging the current paucity of evidence for this strategy.

Any impression of growth velocity impairment should require further investigation (serial biometry or fetal Doppler) especially in order to identify the FGR fetus in absence of SGA. Further studies are needed to compare SFH and ultrasound in the prediction of FGR after improvement in the design and the standardization of the technique are adopted to reduce the variability [50,51].

Conclusion

Several second and third trimester screening strategies for FGR have been proposed. WHO essential criteria to evaluate and adopt a screening test are difficult to apply to the screening for FGR due to limitations in the antenatal diagnosis and the difficulty in estimating the cost-effectiveness. To date, no screening test has been demonstrated to be effective in the second trimester or in late pregnancy for FGR. Any screening policy tested beyond the first trimester enables the identification of fetuses who would benefit from a more intense surveillance as the chance for effective preventive treatments is reduced. The association of a screening policy with a specific monitoring strategy to identify fetuses who would benefit from delivery has not been evaluated in RCTs. Maternal characteristics should be evaluated from the first trimester in order to plan UtA Doppler screening and possible serial growth scan in the third trimester. If women are in their second pregnancy without any risk factor for FGR, SFH can be used as the main screening tool. SFH sensitivity rate in FGR prediction is between 20 and 90% confirming the heterogeneity of the studies performed. The use of customized centiles may improve the detection rate for FGR, but they have not been tested in RCTs. More detailed analysis of the placental function should be performed in order to rely on the SFH as the only screening tool in nulliparous low-risk women. Equally, UtA Doppler has not been demonstrated to be effective in improving the outcome of FGR fetuses in RCTs when unselected women were recruited. This evidence is coming from two studies evaluating the "test-treatment" approach, i.e., randomizing unselected women to undergo UtA Doppler or not, prior to any prophylactic treatment initiation. This study design is not ideal in our view, and it is unlikely to be performed in an adequately powered study. Sensitivity rate between 12 and 56% in unselected women with a LR of 9 would confirm the UtA to be the screening test of choice in low-risk/unselected women rather than in high-risk women. Routine third trimester fetal biometry has not been demonstrated to improve the pregnancy outcome. There are issues in terms of variability associated with which reference chart to use. The use of international prescriptive charts can be adopted to exclude any possible effect of referring to different reference charts but prospective validating studies are needed.

SFH should be compared to ultrasound in studies where strategies to minimize the variability of the technique are part of the protocol.

Nevertheless, UtA Doppler has low sensitivity in detecting milder FGR phenotypes and therefore an ultrasound at 36 weeks should be performed in moderate-risk/unselected women in addition to UtA Doppler (RR or OR for FGR between 2 and 4). Otherwise, serial growth scan should be recommended every 4 weeks from 24 weeks of pregnancy in case of presence of significant risk factors or abnormal UtA Doppler. If growth velocity is impaired further, investigation is required (serial biometry or fetal Doppler) especially to identify the FGR fetus in absence of SGA.

Key Points

- No screening test has been demonstrated to be effective in the second trimester or in late pregnancy for fetal growth restriction.
- The conventional essential criteria for a screening test to be considered effective are difficult to apply to fetal growth restriction.

- Maternal characteristics should drive the screening policy
- SFH can be used as the policy of screening for FGR in low-risk women especially if there is normal uterine artery Doppler flow.
- Uterine artery Doppler should be recommended to all high-risk women and all nulliparous low-risk women.
- Serial growth scan should be recommended every 4 weeks from 24 weeks of pregnancy in case of presence of significant risk factors or abnormal UtA Doppler.
- Any impression of growth velocity impairment requires further investigation (serial biometry and fetal Doppler) especially to identify the FGR fetus in absence of SGA.
- There is a strong rationale for a dedicated fetal growth scan at 36 weeks to be performed in all women.

References

1. Imdad A, Yakoob MY, Siddiqui S, Bhutta ZA. Screening and triage of intrauterine growth restriction (IUGR) in general population and high risk pregnancies: A systematic review with a focus on reduction of IUGR related stillbirths. *BMC Public Health* 2011;11 Suppl 3:S1. DOI 10.1186/1471-2458-11-S3-S1.

2. Wilson JMG, Jungner G. *Principles and Practice of Screening for Disease.* World Health Organization: Geneva, 1968.

3. Cetin I, Huppertz B, Burton G, Cuckle H, Gonen R, Lapaire O, Mandia L, Nicolaides K, Redman C, Soothill P, Spencer K, Thilaganathan B, Williams D, Meiri H. Pregenesys pre-eclampsia markers consensus meeting: What do we require from markers, risk assessment and model systems to tailor preventive strategies? *Placenta* 2011;32 Suppl:S4–16. DOI 10.1016/j.placenta.2010.11.022.

4. Breeze AC, Lees CC. Prediction and perinatal outcomes of fetal growth restriction. *Semin Fetal Neonatal Med* 2007;12:383–97. DOI 10.1016/j.siny.2007.07.002.

5. Morris RK, Malin GL, Tsourapas A, Roberts TE, Khan KS. An economic evaluation of alternative test-intervention strategies to prevent fetal growth restriction in singleton pregnancies. *Arch Dis Child Fetal Neonatal Ed* 2010;95:F12.

6. Bujold E, Roberge S, Lacasse Y, Bureau M, Audibert F, Marcoux S, Forest JC, Giguere Y. Prevention of

preeclampsia and intrauterine growth restriction with aspirin started in early pregnancy: A meta-analysis. *Obstet Gynecol* 2010;116:402–14. DOI 10.1097/AOG.0b013e3181e9322a.

7. Baschat AA, Cosmi E, Bilardo CM, Wolf H, Berg C, Rigano S, Germer U, Moyano D, Turan S, Hartung J, Bhide A, Muller T, Bower S, Nicolaides KH, Thilaganathan B, Gembruch U, Ferrazzi E, Hecher K, Galan HL, Harman CR. Predictors of neonatal outcome in early-onset placental dysfunction. *Obstet Gynecol* 2007;109:253–61. DOI 10.1097/01.AOG.0000253215.79121.75.

8. Royal College of Obstetricans and Gynaecologists (2013). Green-top guidelines No. 31. The investigation and management of the Small-for-Gestational-Age Fetus. London: Royal College of Obstetricans and Gynaecologists. Available at www.rcog.org.uk/en/guidelines-research-services/guidelines/gtg31 (accessed 11/10/2014).

9. NICE. In *Antenatal Care: Routine Care for the Healthy Pregnant Woman*. London, 2008.

10. Lausman A, Kingdom J, Gagnon CR, Basso M, Bos H, Crane J, Davies G, Delisle MF, Hudon L, Menticoglou S, Mundle W, Ouellet A, Pressey T, Pylypjuk C, Roggensack A, Sanderson F. Intrauterine growth restriction: Screening, diagnosis, and management. *JOGC* 2013;35:741–57.

11. American College of Obstetrics and Gynecologists. ACOG Practice bulletin no. 134: fetal growth restriction. *Obstet Gynecol* 2013;121:1122–33. DOI 10.1097/01.AOG.0000429658.85846.f9.

12. Robert Peter J, Ho JJ, Valliapan J, Sivasangari S. Symphysial fundal height (SFH) measurement in pregnancy for detecting abnormal fetal growth. *Cochrane Database Syst Rev* 2012;7:CD008136. DOI 10.1002/14651858.CD008136.pub2.

13. Morse K, Williams A, Gardosi J. Fetal growth screening by fundal height measurement. *Best Pract Res Clin Obstet Gynaecol* 2009;23:809–18. DOI 10.1016/j.bpobgyn.2009.09.004.

14. Stampalija T, Gyte GM, Alfirevic Z. Utero-placental Doppler ultrasound for improving pregnancy outcome. *Cochrane Database Syst Rev* 2010:CD008363. DOI 10.1002/14651858.CD008363.pub2.

15. Napolitano R, Melchiorre K, Arcangeli T, Dias T, Bhide A, Thilaganathan B. Thilaganathan. Screening for pre-eclampsia by using changes in uterine artery Doppler indices with advancing gestation. *Prenat Diagn* 2012;32:180–4. DOI 10.1002/pd.2930.

16. Fox C, Khan KS, Coomarasamy A. How to interpret randomised trials of test-treatment combinations: A critical evaluation of research on uterine Doppler test to predict, and aspirin to prevent, pre-eclampsia. *BJOG* 2010;117:801–8. DOI 10.1111/j.1471-0528.2010.02577.x.

17. Goffinet F, Aboulker D, Paris-Llado J, Bucourt M, Uzan M, Papiernik E, Breart G. Screening with a uterine Doppler in low risk pregnant women followed by low dose aspirin in women with abnormal results: A multicenter randomised controlled trial. *BJOG* 2001;108:510–18.

18. Subtil D, Goeusse P, Houfflin-Debarge V, Puech F, Lequien P, Breart G, Uzan S, Quandalle F, Delcourt YM, Malek YM, Essai G, Regional Aspirine Mere-Enfant Collaborative. Randomised comparison of uterine artery Doppler and aspirin (100 mg) with placebo in nulliparous women: The Essai Regional Aspirine Mere-Enfant study (Part 2). *BJOG* 2003;110:485–91.

19. Papageorghiou AT, Yu CK, Cicero S, Bower S, Nicolaides KH. Second-trimester uterine artery Doppler screening in unselected populations: A review. *J Matern Fetal Neonatal Med* 2002;12:78–88. DOI 10.1080/jmf.12.2.78.88.

20. Papageorghiou AT, Leslie K. Uterine artery Doppler in the prediction of adverse pregnancy outcome. *Curr Opin Obstet Gynecol* 2007;19:103–9. DOI 10.1097/GCO.0b013e32809bd964.

21. Cnossen JS, Morris RK, ter Riet G, Mol BW, van der Post JA, Coomarasamy A, Zwinderman AH, Robson SC, Bindels PJ, Kleijnen J, Khan KS. Use of uterine artery Doppler ultrasonography to predict pre-eclampsia and intrauterine growth restriction: A systematic review and bivariable meta-analysis. *CMAJ* 2008;178:701–11. DOI 10.1503/cmaj.070430.

22. Deeks JJ, Altman DG. Diagnostic tests 4: Likelihood ratios. *BMJ* 2004;329:168–9. DOI 10.1136/bmj.329.7458.168.

23. Fayyad AM, Harrington KF. Prediction and prevention of preeclampsia and IUGR. *Early Hum Dev* 2005;81:865–76. DOI 10.1016/j.earlhumdev.2005.09.005.

24. Morris RK, Cnossen JS, Langejans M, Robson SC, Kleijnen J, Ter Riet G, Mol BW, van der Post JA, Khan KS. Serum screening with Down's syndrome markers to predict pre-eclampsia and small for gestational age: Systematic review and meta-analysis. *BMC Pregnancy Childbirth* 2008;8:33. DOI 10.1186/1471-2393-8-33.

25. Hui D, Okun N, Murphy K, Kingdom J, Uleryk E, Shah PS. Combinations of maternal serum markers

to predict preeclampsia, small for gestational age, and stillbirth: A systematic review. *JOGC* 2012;34:142–53.

26. Conde-Agudelo A, Papageorghiou AT, Kennedy SH, Villar J. Novel biomarkers for predicting intrauterine growth restriction: A systematic review and meta-analysis. *BJOG* 2013;120:681–94. DOI 10.1111/1471-0528.12172.

27. Napolitano R, Santo S, D'Souza R, Bhide A, Thilaganathan B. Sensitivity of higher, lower and mean second-trimester uterine artery Doppler resistance indices in screening for pre-eclampsia. *Ultrasound Obstet Gynecol* 2010;36:573–6. DOI 10.1002/uog.7645.

28. Meads CA, Cnossen JS, Meher S, Juarez-Garcia A, ter Riet G, Duley L, Roberts TE, Mol BW, van der Post JA, Leeflang MM, Barton PM, Hyde CJ, Gupta JK, Khan KS. Methods of prediction and prevention of pre-eclampsia: Systematic reviews of accuracy and effectiveness literature with economic modelling. *Health Technol Assess* 2008;12:iii–iv, 1–270.

29. Kleinrouweler CE, Bossuyt PM, Thilaganathan B, Vollebregt KC, Arenas Ramirez J, Ohkuchi A, Deurloo KL, Macleod M, Diab AE, Wolf H, van der Post JA, Mol BW, Pajkrt E. Value of adding second-trimester uterine artery Doppler to patient characteristics in identification of nulliparous women at increased risk for pre-eclampsia: An individual patient data meta-analysis. *Ultrasound Obstet Gynecol* 2013;42:257–67. DOI 10.1002/uog.12435.

30. Audibert F, Benchimol Y, Benattar C, Champagne C, Frydman R. Prediction of preeclampsia or intrauterine growth restriction by second trimester serum screening and uterine Doppler velocimetry. *Fetal Diagn Ther* 2005;20:48–53. DOI 10.1159/000081369.

31. Bricker L, Neilson JP, Dowswell T. Routine ultrasound in late pregnancy (after 24 weeks' gestation). *Cochrane Database Syst Rev* 2008:CD001451. DOI 10.1002/14651858.CD001451.pub3.

32. Napolitano R, Dhami J, Ohuma EO, Ioannou C, Conde-Agudelo A, Kennedy SH, Villar J, Papageorghiou AT. Pregnancy dating by fetal crown-rump length: A systematic review of charts. *BJOG* 2014;121:556–65. DOI 10.1111/1471-0528.12478.

33. Ioannou C, Talbot K, Ohuma E, Sarris I, Villar J, Conde-Agudelo A, Papageorghiou A. Systematic review of methodology used in ultrasound studies aimed at creating charts of fetal size. *BJOG* 2012;119:1425–39.

34. Gardosi J, Chang A, Kalyan B, Sahota D, Symonds EM. Customised antenatal growth charts. *Lancet* 1992;339:283–7.

35. Gardosi J, Francis A. Adverse pregnancy outcome and association with small for gestational age birthweight by customized and population-based percentiles. *Am J Obstet Gynecol* 2009;201:28 e21-28. DOI 10.1016/j.ajog.2009.04.034.

36. Owen P, Ogston S. Conditional centiles for the quantification of fetal growth. *Ultrasound Obstet Gynecol* 1998;11:110–17. DOI 10.1046/j.1469-0705.1998.11020110.x.

37. Papageorghiou AT, Kennedy SH, Salomon LJ, Ohuma EO, Cheikh Ismail L, Barros FC, Lambert A, Carvalho M, Jaffer YA, Bertino E, Gravett MG, Altman DG, Purwar M, Noble JA, Pang R, Victora CG, Bhutta ZA, Villar J, International and Newborn Growth Consortium for the 21st Century. International standards for early fetal size and pregnancy dating based on ultrasound measurement of crown-rump length in the first trimester of pregnancy. *Ultrasound Obstet Gynecol* 2014;44:641–8. DOI 10.1002/uog.13448.

38. Papageorghiou AT, Ohuma EO, Altman DG, Todros T, Cheikh Ismail L, Lambert A, Jaffer YA, Bertino E, Gravett MG, Purwar M, Noble JA, Pang R, Victora CG, Barros FC, Carvalho M, Salomon LJ, Bhutta ZA, Kennedy SH, Villar J, International and Newborn Growth Consortium for the 21st Century. International standards for fetal growth based on serial ultrasound measurements: The Fetal Growth Longitudinal Study of the INTERGROWTH-21st Project. *Lancet* 2014;384:869–79. DOI 10.1016/S0140-6736(14)61490-2.

39. Souka AP, Papastefanou I, Pilalis A, Michalitsi V, Kassanos D. Performance of third-trimester ultrasound for prediction of small-for-gestational-age neonates and evaluation of contingency screening policies. *Ultrasound Obstet Gynecol* 2012; 39:535–42. DOI 10.1002/uog.10078.

40. Lindqvist PG, Molin J. Does antenatal identification of small-for-gestational age fetuses significantly improve their outcome? *Ultrasound Obstet Gynecol* 2005;25:258–64. DOI 10.1002/uog.1806.

41. Ben-Haroush A, Yogev Y, Hod M, Bar J. Predictive value of a single early fetal weight estimate in normal pregnancies. *Eur J Obstet Gynecol Reprod Biol* 2007;130:187–92. DOI 10.1016/j.ejogrb.2006.04.018.

42. De Reu PA, Smits LJ, Oosterbaan HP, and Nijhuis JG. Value of a single early third trimester fetal biometry for the prediction of birth weight deviations in a low risk population. *J Perinat Med* 2008;36:324–9. DOI 10.1515/JPM.2008.057.

43. Sylvan K, Ryding EL, Rydhstroem H. Routine ultrasound screening in the third trimester: A population-based study. *Acta Obstet Gynecol*

Scand 2005;84:1154–8. DOI 10.1111/j.0001-6349.2005.00649.x.

44. Sovio U, White IR, Dacey A, Pasupathy D, Smith GC. Screening for fetal growth restriction with universal third trimester ultrasonography in nulliparous women in the Pregnancy Outcome Prediction (POP) study: A prospective cohort study. *Lancet* 2015;386:2089–97. DOI 10.1016/S0140-6736(15)00131-2.

45. CFadigas C, Saiid Y, Gonzalez R, Poon LC, Nicolaides KH. Prediction of small-for-gestational-age neonates: Screening by fetal biometry at 35–37 weeks. *Ultrasound Obstet Gynecol* 2015;45:559–65. DOI 10.1002/uog.14816.

46. Roma E, Arnau A, Berdala R, Bergos C, Montesinos J, Figueras F. Ultrasound screening for fetal growth restriction at 36 vs 32 weeks' gestation: A randomized trial (ROUTE). *Ultrasound Obstet Gynecol* 2015;46:391–7. DOI 10.1002/uog.14915.

47. Evans S, Newnham J, MacDonald W, Hall C. Characterisation of the possible effect on birthweight following frequent prenatal ultrasound examinations. *Early Hum Dev* 1996;45:203–14.

48. Chang TC, Robson SC, Spencer JA, Gallivan S. Identification of fetal growth retardation: Comparison of Doppler waveform indices and serial ultrasound measurements of abdominal circumference and fetal weight. *Obstet Gynecol* 1993;82:230–6.

49. Owen P, Khan KS. Fetal growth velocity in the prediction of intrauterine growth retardation in a low risk population. *BJOG* 1998;105:536–40.

50. Sarris I, Ohuma E, Roseman F, Hoch L, Altman DG, Papageorghiou AT. Sonographer standardisation of fetal biometry ultrasound measurements: An exercise to improve quality and consistency in a large, prospective, multi-centre study. *Ultrasound Obstet Gynecol* 2011;38:681–87.

51. Sarris I, Ioannou C, Chamberlain P, Ohuma E, Roseman F, Hoch L, Altman DG, Papageorghiou AT. Intra- and interobserver variability in fetal ultrasound measurements. *Ultrasound Obstet Gynecol* 2012;39:266–73. DOI 10.1002/uog.10082.

Chapter

13

Prophylaxis for Fetal Growth Restriction: Aspirin and Low-Molecular-Weight Heparins

Tiziana Frusca and Federico Prefumo

Introduction

Scholars have written a large amount of literature on the use of aspirin for the prevention of preeclampsia; to a smaller extent, prevention studies have also been conducted using low-molecular-weight heparins. Unfortunately, the evidence regarding the use of these medications for the prophylaxis of fetal growth restriction is mainly related to the presence of preeclampsia complicating the index pregnancy or a previous pregnancy. Therefore, it is difficult to deduce the role of aspirin and/or heparins in the prevention of fetal growth restriction not associated with preeclampsia.

Aspirin and the Placenta

Fetal growth restriction due to placental vascular disease shares a common etiological substrate with early-onset preeclampsia (see Chapter 9). Therefore, the mechanism of action of aspirin for the prophylaxis of fetal growth restriction may to some extent be the same as for preeclampsia. It is well known that low-dose aspirin has selective effects on cyclooxygenase that enhance prostacyclin production by the endothelial cells and inhibit thromboxane production, giving as a result an important antiplatelet aggregation effect in the circulation. This mechanism of action has been extensively studied and is closely linked to the clinical effect of aspirin [1,2]. However, it is controversial whether low-dose aspirin has any effect on trophoblast invasion or function, as assessed in in vitro models [3,4]; thus all the clinical trials that underline the positive effects of low-dose aspirin only when given in the first trimester of pregnancy, or at least before 16 weeks' gestation, remain to be explained from the pathophysiological point of view.

Low-dose aspirin is known to have some preventive effect in preeclampsia: when compared to placebo in high-risk women, it was associated with a reduction in the risk of preeclampsia (relative risk [RR] 0.76; 95% CI 0.62 to 0.95) and preterm delivery (RR 0.86; 95% CI 0.76 to 0.98) [5]. Most studies included women who were started on low-dose aspirin at variable gestation ages, very often in the mid-trimester.

Although physiological transformation is often not completed until 24 weeks, evidence from studies in high-risk pregnancies suggests that aspirin prevention aimed at optimizing placental function should be started before 16 weeks to be more effective (before 16 weeks RR of preeclampsia 0.47; 95% CI 0.34 to 0.65 – after 16 weeks RR 0.81; 95% CI 0.63 to 1.03) [6]. However, this evidence derives from the meta-analysis of relatively small studies in the subgroup treated before 16 weeks; these data should therefore be interpreted cautiously, given also the possible systematic differences between women treated before and after 16 weeks [7], and have not been replicated in other meta-analyses [8,9]. A recent robustly designed trial demonstrated a significant reduction in preterm pre-eclampsia in a cohort of women identified at first trimester screening from the general pregnant population and started on aspirin at 11-14 weeks, when compared to placebo (odds ratio 0.38; 95% confidence interval 0.20 -0.74) [10].

Aspirin for the Prevention of Fetal Growth Restriction

An individual patient data meta-analysis published in 2005 [11] was able to analyze the incidence of small for gestational age (SGA) in 20 trials with a total of 21,426 pregnancies. The incidence of SGA was 5.3% in pregnancies treated with aspirin and 5.9% in controls (RR 0.90; 95% confidence interval 0.81 to 1.01), confirming a 10% reduction in the relative risk of the newborn being SGA, although the 95% confidence interval crossed the point of no effect. Unfortunately, no mention was made of fetal growth restriction in this study.

A recent systematic review and meta-analysis [12] identified 27 trials investigating the effect of prophylactic low-dose aspirin on fetal growth restriction, involving a total of 8,260 participants. The incidence of fetal growth restriction was 10.7% in the aspirin-treated population and 12.3% in controls (RR 0.86; 95% confidence interval 0.75 to 0.99), suggesting a significant effect of aspirin prophylaxis in preventing fetal growth restriction. RRs were also separately calculated according to gestational age at initiation of aspirin (within 16 weeks' gestation or later): if aspirin prophylaxis was started before 16 weeks, the RR for fetal growth restriction was 0.46 (95% confidence interval 0.33 to 0.64); if aspirin was started after 16 weeks, the effect on the incidence of fetal growth restriction was non-significant (RR 0.98; 95% confidence interval 0.88 to 1.08). However, note that the studies included in the meta-analysis with aspirin started before 16 weeks were 10, with a total of 1,064 women enrolled: although the incidence of fetal growth restriction was 8.0% in the aspirin treatment arm, this was as high as 17.6% in controls, suggesting that the trials included in this subgroup analysis have a particularly high risk profile. This implies that the effect of aspirin can be important in a very selected population at high risk, and only if this drug is started before 16 weeks of pregnancy.

Another systematic review and meta-analysis [9] analyzed 13 studies reporting on a total of 12,054 pregnancies, all from populations considered to be at increased risk of preeclampsia. The authors found a significant reduction in the risk of fetal growth restriction/SGA with the use of aspirin (RR 0.80; 95% CI 0–65 to 0.99), but suggested that the magnitude of the estimated reduction could be exaggerated by small study effects. This analysis also suggested an advantage in starting aspirin treatment before 16 weeks.

The conclusions of these meta-analyses should be interpreted with caution. One of the most important issues to consider is that fetal growth restriction was defined in most primary studies only on the basis of a birth weight below the 10th, 5th, or 3rd percentiles: this clearly defines a group of small fetuses (SGA), but does not distinctively identify really growth-restricted fetuses. Moreover, most primary studies do not easily allow the identification of pregnancies where SGA was isolated or coexistent with preeclampsia. *It is also possible that, in analogy with what has been suggested for preeclampsia [9], aspirin prophylaxis may have a differential effect on the most severe forms of fetal growth restriction, reducing their severity and need for early preterm delivery, while it may be less effective on late-preterm or term SGA; however, this has not been consistently proven so far.*

Furthermore, published trials used aspirin dosages ranging from 60 to 150 mg daily: this could theoretically affect the outcome of the intervention, but most meta-analyses failed to demonstrate any dose-response effect. The timing of aspirin administration may also be important, as two trials from the same group suggested that aspirin taken later in the day rather than at awakening may have an increased effect [13]. Finally, the role of aspirin resistance has just started to be investigated [14].

The characteristics of the most relevant randomized trials reporting the effect of aspirin on the prevention of fetal growth restriction [1,2,10,13,15–24] are summarized in Table 13.1.

Low-Molecular-Weight Heparins and the Placenta

The mechanisms through which low-molecular-weight heparins may prevent placental vascular disease are not clear. The anticoagulant action of low-molecular-weight heparins could directly affect the placenta and intervillous circulation. However, there is no clear demonstration from pathological examination that placental vascular damage (perivascular fibrin deposition, fibrinoid necrosis, infarction, abruption) is reduced by treatment [25,26]. Heparins may decrease trophoblast apoptosis and improve trophoblastic invasion of the decidua; they also have anti-inflammatory and anti-complement effects that may contrast inflammatory damage to the placenta and the maternal endothelium [27,28].

Two recent meta-analyses addressed the issue of the effect of low-molecular-weight heparin prophylaxis in pregnancies considered to be at high risk of placental complications [29,30]. All the primary studies included in these meta-analyses enrolled women at particularly high risk of adverse pregnancy outcomes, mainly based on previous history (preeclampsia/eclampsia, abruption, chronic renal disease, fetal loss, fetal growth restriction). Some studies excluded women with known thrombophilia, others allowed them to be enrolled, some limited inclusion to thrombophilic women. Overall, it must be noted that women who participated in these studies have a higher risk profile that those participating in studies on aspirin prophylaxis. Heparin treatment was always started in early pregnancy. The Cochrane review [29], based on the analysis of six trials with a total of 653 pregnancies, was able to demonstrate that heparin is associated with a reduction in perinatal mortality (RR 0.40; 95% CI 0.20 to 0.78). The review from the Low-Molecular-Weight Heparin

Table 13.1 Characteristics of the most relevant randomized trials reporting the effect of aspirin on the prevention of fetal growth restriction

Study	Year	Treatment group	Type	N	Start of treatment (weeks)	Definition of FGR/SGA	FGR/SGA,n (%)
Wallenburg	1986	Aspirin	60 mg	21	28	Not defined	4(19.0)
		Controls	Placebo	23			6(26.0)
Benigni	1989	Aspirin	60 mg	17	12	Not defined	2(11.8)
		Controls	Placebo	16			6(37.5)
Schiff	1989	Aspirin	100 mg	34	28–29	Birthweight<10th percentile	2(5.9)
		Controls	Placebo	32			6(19.4)
McParland	1990	Aspirin	75 mg	48	24	Birthweight<5th percentile	7(14.0)
		Controls	Placebo	52			7(14.0)
Viinikka	1993	Aspirin	50 mg	97	15	Birthweight<2 SDs	4(4.1)
		Controls	Placebo	100			9(9.0)
Caspi	1994	Aspirin	100 mg	48	18	Birthweight<10th percentile	6(12.5)
		Controls	Placebo	46			11(23.9)
CLASP	1994	Aspirin	60 mg	4,810	20–32	Birthweight<3rd percentile	244(5.9)
		Controls	Placebo	4,821			272(6.6)
Hermida	1997	Aspirin	100 mg	50	12–16	Not defined	1(2.0)
		Controls	Placebo	50			2(4.0)
MFMU	1998	Aspirin	60 mg	1,254	13–26	Birthweight<10th percentile	129(10)
		Controls	Placebo	1,249			108(9)
Vainio	2002	Aspirin	0.5 mg/kg	43	12–14	Not defined	1(2.3)
		Controls	Placebo	43			3(7.0)
Yu	2003	Aspirin	150 mg	276	22–24	Birthweight<5th percentile	61(22.1)
		Controls	Placebo	278			68(24.4)
Villa	2012	Aspirin	100 mg	61	12–14	Birthweight<2 SDs	2(3.3)
		Controls	Placebo	60			6(10.0)
Ayala	2013	Aspirin	100 mg	176	12–16	Not defined	16(9.1)
		Controls	Placebo	174			32(18.4)

Source: Modified from [9].
FGR: fetal growth restriction; SGA: small for gestational age.

for Placenta-Mediated Pregnancy Complications Study Group [30] considered as the primary outcome a composite outcome of preeclampsia, SGA, abruption, or fetal loss >20 weeks. Such composite outcome was observed in 67/358 from six trials (18.7%) receiving low-molecular-weight heparins, and in 127/296 controls (42.9%; RR 0.52; 95% CI 0.32 to 0.86).

Low-Molecular-Weight Heparins for the Prevention of Fetal Growth Restriction

None of the published trials on the use of low-molecular-weight heparins was specifically designed to assess the effect of this treatment on fetal growth restriction. However, most studies reported data on birth weight and SGA. The Cochrane meta-analysis, based on the analysis of seven trials with a total of 710 pregnancies, suggests that heparin treatment significantly decreases the chances of birth weight below the 10th percentile (RR 0.41; 95% CI 0.27 to 0.61) [29]. In the Rodger and colleagues meta-analysis, low-molecular-weight heparins are associated with a similar reduction in birth weight below the 10th percentile (RR 0.42; 95% CI 0.29 to 0.59) and below the 5th percentile (RR 0.52; 95% CI 0.28 to 0.94) [30].

Neither meta-analysis included the TIPPS trial, a multinational trial whose results were published in late 2014 [31]: this study randomized women with thrombophilia at increased risk of venous thromboembolism or with previous placenta-mediated pregnancy complications to receive dalteparin (n = 146) or no treatment (n = 143). No significant differences between the two groups were observed in the prevalence of birth weight below the 10th, 5th, or 3rd percentiles.

The characteristics of the most relevant randomized trials reporting the effect of low-molecular-weight heparins on the prevention of fetal growth restriction [31–36] are summarized in Table 13.2. Note that many studies published on this preventive treatment enrolled women at very high risk of poor obstetric outcomes, such as those with antiphospholipid syndrome or with inherited thrombophilia.

Table 13.2 Characteristics of the most relevant randomized trials reporting the effect of low-molecular-weight heparins on the prevention of fetal growth restriction

Study	Year	Previous pregnancy outcome	Treatment group	Type	N	Definition of FGR/SGA	FGR/SGA, n (%)
Mello	2005	PE with deleted/deleted angiotensin-converting enzyme genotype	Dalteparin	5000 IU	41	Birthweight<10th percentile	4 (9.8)
			Controls	No Treatment	41		17 (41.5)
Rey	2009	Early PE, SGA, loss>12 weeks, abruption	Dalteparin	5000 IU	53	Birthweight<5th percentile	2 (3.8)
			Controls	No Treatment	52		4 (7.7)
NOH-PE	2011	Severe PE	Enoxaparin	4000 IU ± aspirin	112	Birthweight<10th percentile	3 (2.7)
			Controls	± aspirin	112		9 (8.0)
FRUIT	2012	Early-onset PE and/or SGA	Dalteparin	5000 IU + aspirin Placebo	66	Birthweight<10th percentile	12 (18.2)
			Controls	Aspirin	67		19 (28.4)
HAPPY	2012	PE, SGA, loss>15 weeks, abruption	Nadroparin	3800 IU	67	Birthweight<10th percentile	5 (7.5)
			Controls	No Treatment	68		7 (10.3)
TIPPS	2014	Early PE, SGA, pregnancy loss, abruption	Dalteparin	5000 IU < 20 weeks, 10,000 IU >20 weeks	146	Birthweight<10th percentile	9 (6.2)
			Controls	No Treatment	143		12 (8.4)

Source: Modified from [30].
PE: preeclampsia; SGA: small for gestational age; IU: international units.

Safety Issues

Adverse events related to the use of aspirin or low-molecular-weight heparins have been differently reported in the various trials or in observational studies. As for aspirin, an analysis based on data from 19 randomized controlled and two observational trials was unable to demonstrate any increase in placental abruption, postpartum hemorrhage, fetal intracranial bleeding or congenital anomalies [9].

The safety of low-molecular-weight heparins in pregnancy was evaluated in a systematic review of 2,777 pregnancies from 64 studies [37]: significant bleeding occurred in 52 pregnancies (2.0%; 95% CI 1.50 to 2.61%), of which 24 cases were associated with primary obstetric causes and 17 with wound complications; only two women developed thrombocytopenia, and in neither case was this heparin or thrombosis related; there were 48 pregnancies with allergic skin reactions (1.84%; 95% CI 1.36 to 2.44%); only one woman developed an osteoporotic fracture (0.04%; 95% CI 0.01 to 0.21%). Moreover, it has been suggested that not-significant changes in bone mineral density at the proximal femur occur when low-molecular-weight heparins are given to pregnant women in conjunction with calcium supplementation, which should therefore be considered when heparins are prescribed [38].

Conclusion

Scholars have produced a significant amount of literature on the role of aspirin and/or low-molecular-weight heparins for the prevention of adverse pregnancy outcomes. Although fetal growth restriction due to placental vascular disease shares a common etiological substrate with early-onset preeclampsia, most prevention studies concentrated mainly on preeclampsia.

Based on the available data, it is currently impossible to give evidence-based suggestions for the prevention of fetal growth restriction with aspirin or low-molecular-weight heparins, except for those forms of fetal growth restriction related to previous preeclampsia, chronic hypertension, antiphospholipid syndrome, or thrombophilic conditions. Pure isolated fetal growth restriction is still difficult to differentiate from SGA, and this is the case in almost all the studies published in the literature.

From a practical point of view, a patient *with a previous pregnancy complicated by conditions related to placental vascular disease* with elective delivery at less than 34 weeks' gestation, and no other comorbidities,

should be started on low-dose aspirin from the first trimester of pregnancy. *Such approach should also be considered in women with chronic hypertension or other comorbidities. Selected women with a very high risk profile could be treated with aspirin and low-molecular-weight heparin. The available data suggest that both treatments are essentially safe in these groups of women.*

These treatment suggestions are based on limited evidence for what specifically concerns fetal growth restriction, but preventive treatments appear to reduce the overall incidence of complications related to placental vascular disease, to which fetal growth restriction pertains. Recent evidence suggests that, in women without a previous medical or obstetric history warranting prophylaxis with aspirin or low-molecular-weight heparins, early pregnancy screening for pregnancy complications may identify pregnancies that will benefit from such interventions.

Key Points

- In high-risk pregnancies, prophylaxis with aspirin is associated with a reduction in the risk of delivering an SGA newborn.
- Aspirin is more likely to be effective in SGA reduction if started in early pregnancy.
- In pregnancies with an even higher risk profile, low-molecular-weight heparin prophylaxis also appears to reduce the prevalence of SGA.
- Most trials did not differentiate SGA from fetal growth restriction.
- Both aspirin and low-molecular-weight heparins have a good safety profile in high-risk pregnancies.

References

1. Schiff E, Peleg E, Goldenberg M, Rosenthal T, Ruppin E, Tamarkin M, Barkai G, Ben-Baruch G, Yahal I, Blankstein J, et al. The use of aspirin to prevent pregnancy-induced hypertension and lower the ratio of thromboxane A2 to prostacyclin in relatively high risk pregnancies. *N Engl J Med* 1989;321:351–6.

2. Benigni A, Gregorini G, Frusca T, Chiabrando C, Ballerini S, Valcamonico A, Orisio S, Piccinelli A, Pinciroli V, Fanelli R, et al. Effect of low-dose

aspirin on fetal and maternal generation of thromboxane by platelets in women at risk for pregnancy-induced hypertension. *N Engl J Med* 1989;321:357–62.

3. Quenby S, Mountfield S, Cartwright JE, Whitley GS, Vince G. Effects of low-molecular-weight and unfractionated heparin on trophoblast function. *Obstet Gynecol* 2004;104:354–61.

4. Han CS, Mulla MJ, Brosens JJ, Chamley LW, Paidas MJ, Lockwood CJ, Abrahams VM. Aspirin and heparin effect on basal and antiphospholipid antibody modulation of trophoblast function. *Obstet Gynecol* 2011;118:1021–8.

5. Henderson JT, Whitlock EP, O'Connor E, Senger CA, Thompson JH, Rowland MG. Low-dose aspirin for prevention of morbidity and mortality from preeclampsia: A systematic evidence review for the U.S. Preventive Services Task Force. *Ann Intern Med* 2014;160:695–703.

6. Bujold E, Roberge S, Lacasse Y, Bureau M, Audibert F, Marcoux S, Forest JC, Giguere Y. Prevention of preeclampsia and intrauterine growth restriction with aspirin started in early pregnancy: a meta-analysis. *Obstet Gynecol* 2010;116:402–14.

7. Meher S, Alfirevic Z. Aspirin for pre-eclampsia: Beware of subgroup meta-analysis. *Ultrasound Obstet Gynecol* 2013;41:479–85.

8. Duley L, Henderson-Smart DJ, Meher S, King JF. Antiplatelet agents for preventing pre-eclampsia and its complications. *Cochrane Database Syst Rev* 2007, Issue 2. Art. No.: CD004659.

9. Henderson JT, Whitlock EP, O'Conner E, Senger CA, Thompson JH, Rowland MG. Low-Dose Aspirin for the Prevention of Morbidity and Mortality From Preeclampsia: A Systematic Evidence Review for the U.S. Preventive Services Task Force. Evidence Synthesis No. 112. AHRQ Publication No. 14-05207-EF-1. Rockville, MD: Agency for Healthcare Research and Quality; 2014.

10. Askie LM, Duley L, Henderson-Smart DJ, Stewart LA, Group PC. Antiplatelet agents for prevention of pre-eclampsia: A meta-analysis of individual patient data. *Lancet* 2007;369:1791–8.

11. Roberge S, Nicolaides KH, Demers S, Villa P, Bujold E. Prevention of perinatal death and adverse perinatal outcome using low-dose aspirin: A meta-analysis. *Ultrasound Obstet Gynecol* 2013;41:491–9.

12. Ayala DE, Ucieda R, Hermida RC. Chronotherapy with low-dose aspirin for prevention of complications in pregnancy. *Chronobiol Int* 2013;30:260–79.

13. Wojtowicz A, Undas A, Huras H, Musial J, Rytlewski K, Reron A, Wilczak M, Jach R. Aspirin resistance

may be associated with adverse pregnancy outcomes. *Neuro Endocrinol Lett* 2011;32:334–9.

14. Wallenburg HC, Rotmans N. Prevention of recurrent idiopathic fetal growth retardation by low-dose aspirin and dipyridamole. *Am J Obstet Gynecol* 1987;157:1230–5.

15. CLASP: A randomised trial of low-dose aspirin for the prevention and treatment of pre-eclampsia among 9364 pregnant women. CLASP (Collaborative Low-dose Aspirin Study in Pregnancy) Collaborative Group. *Lancet* 1994;343:619–29.

16. McParland P, Pearce JM, Chamberlain GV. Doppler ultrasound and aspirin in recognition and prevention of pregnancy-induced hypertension. *Lancet* 1990;335:1552–5.

17. Viinikka L, Hartikainen-Sorri AL, Lumme R, Hiilesmaa V, Ylikorkala O. Low dose aspirin in hypertensive pregnant women: Effect on pregnancy outcome and prostacyclin-thromboxane balance in mother and newborn. *BJOG* 1993;100:809–15.

18. Caspi E, Raziel A, Sherman D, Arieli S, Bukovski I, Weinraub Z. Prevention of pregnancy-induced hypertension in twins by early administration of low-dose aspirin: A preliminary report. *Am J Reprod Immunol* 1994;31:19–24.

19. Hermida RC, Ayala DE, Iglesias M, Mojon A, Silva I, Ucieda R, Fernandez JR. Time-dependent effects of low-dose aspirin administration on blood pressure in pregnant women. *Hypertension* 1997;30:589–95.

20. Caritis S, Sibai B, Hauth J, Lindheimer MD, Klebanoff M, Thom E, Van Dorsten P, Landon M, Paul R, Miodovnik M, Meis P, Thurnau G. Low-dose aspirin to prevent preeclampsia in women at high risk. National Institute of Child Health and Human Development Network of Maternal-Fetal Medicine Units. *N Engl J Med* 1998;338:701–5.

21. Vainio M, Kujansuu E, Iso-Mustajarvi M, Maenpaa J. Low dose acetylsalicylic acid in prevention of pregnancy-induced hypertension and intrauterine growth retardation in women with bilateral uterine artery notches. *BJOG* 2002;109:161–7.

22. Yu CK, Papageorghiou AT, Parra M, Palma Dias R, Nicolaides KH, Fetal Medicine Foundation Second Trimester Screening G. Randomized controlled trial using low-dose aspirin in the prevention of pre-eclampsia in women with abnormal uterine artery Doppler at 23 weeks' gestation. *Ultrasound Obstet Gynecol* 2003;22:233–9.

23. Villa PM, Kajantie E, Raikkonen K, Pesonen AK, Hamalainen E, Vainio M, Taipale P, Laivuori H, Group PS. Aspirin in the prevention of pre-eclampsia in high-risk women: A randomised placebo-controlled

PREDO Trial and a meta-analysis of randomised trials. *BJOG* 2013;120:64–74.

24. Kingdom JC, Walker M, Proctor LK, Keating S, Shah PS, McLeod A, Keunen J, Windrim RC, Dodd JM. Unfractionated heparin for second trimester placental insufficiency: A pilot randomized trial. *J Thromb Haemost* 2011;9:1483–92.

25. Kupferminc M, Rimon E, Many A, Maslovitz S, Lessing JB, Gamzu R. Low molecular weight heparin versus no treatment in women with previous severe pregnancy complications and placental findings without thrombophilia. *Blood Coagul Fibrinolysis* 2011;22:123–6.

26. Duffett L, Rodger M. LMWH to prevent placenta-mediated pregnancy complications: An update. *Br J Haematol* 2014.

27. Greer IA, Brenner B, Gris JC. Antithrombotic treatment for pregnancy complications: Which path for the journey to precision medicine? *Br J Haematol* 2014;165:585–99.

28. Dodd JM, McLeod A, Windrim RC, Kingdom J. Antithrombotic therapy for improving maternal or infant health outcomes in women considered at risk of placental dysfunction. *Cochrane Database Sys Rev* 2013, Issue 7. Art. No.: CD006780.

29. Rodger MA, Carrier M, Le Gal G, Martinelli I, Perna A, Rey E, De Vries JI, Gris JC, Low-Molecular-Weight Heparin for Placenta-Mediated Pregnancy Complications Study G. Meta-analysis of low-molecular-weight heparin to prevent recurrent placenta-mediated pregnancy complications. *Blood* 2014;123:822–8.

30. Rodger MA, Hague WM, Kingdom J, Kahn SR, Karovitch A, Sermer M, Clement AM, Coat S, Chan WS, Said J, Rey E, Robinson S, Khurana R, Demers C, Kovacs MJ, Solymoss S, Hinshaw K, Dwyer J, Smith G, McDonald S, Newstead-Angel J, McLeod A, Khandelwal M, Silver RM, Le Gal G, Greer IA, Keely E, Rosene-Montella K, Walker M, Wells PS, Investigators T. Antepartum dalteparin versus no antepartum dalteparin for the prevention of pregnancy complications in pregnant women with

thrombophilia (TIPPS): a multinational open-label randomised trial. *Lancet* 2014;384:1673–83.

31. Mello G, Parretti E, Fatini C, Riviello C, Gensini F, Marchionni M, Scarselli GF, Gensini GF, Abbate R. Low-molecular-weight heparin lowers the recurrence rate of preeclampsia and restores the physiological vascular changes in angiotensin-converting enzyme DD women. *Hypertension* 2005;45:86–91.

32. Rey E, Garneau P, David M, Gauthier R, Leduc L, Michon N, Morin F, Demers C, Kahn SR, Magee LA, Rodger M. Dalteparin for the prevention of recurrence of placental-mediated complications of pregnancy in women without thrombophilia: A pilot randomized controlled trial. *J Thromb Haemost* 2009;7:58–64.

33. Gris JC, Chauleur C, Molinari N, Mares P, Fabbro-Peray P, Quere I, Lefrant JY, Haddad B, Dauzat M. Addition of enoxaparin to aspirin for the secondary prevention of placental vascular complications in women with severe pre-eclampsia. The pilot randomised controlled NOH-PE trial. *Thromb Haemost* 2011;106:1053–61.

34. De Vries JI, Van Pampus MG, Hague WM, Bezemer PD, Joosten JH, Investigators F. Low-molecular-weight heparin added to aspirin in the prevention of recurrent early-onset pre-eclampsia in women with inheritable thrombophilia: The FRUIT-RCT. *J Thromb Haemost* 2012;10:64–72.

35. Martinelli I, Ruggenenti P, Cetin I, Pardi G, Perna A, Vergani P, Acaia B, Facchinetti F, La Sala GB, Bozzo M, Rampello S, Marozio L, Diadei O, Gherardi G, Carminati S, Remuzzi G, Mannucci PM, Group HS. Heparin in pregnant women with previous placenta-mediated pregnancy complications: A prospective, randomized, multicenter, controlled clinical trial. *Blood* 2012;119:3269–75.

36. Greer IA, Nelson-Piercy C. Low-molecular-weight heparins for thromboprophylaxis and treatment of venous thromboembolism in pregnancy: A systematic review of safety and efficacy. *Blood* 2005;106:401–7.

37. Casele H, Haney EI, James A, Rosene-Montella K, Carson M. Bone density changes in women who receive thromboprophylaxis in pregnancy. *Am J Obstet Gynecol* 2006;195:1109–13.

Chapter

14

Prophylaxis for Fetal Growth Restriction: Nitric Oxide Donors and Sildenafil

Dietmar Schlembach

To achieve optimal fetal growth, adequate blood flow and proper uteroplacental vascular function is essential. Abnormal vasculature adaptation, resulting in aberrant uteroplacental blood flow, is a major predictor of abnormal pregnancy outcome and has been implicated as a possible cause of fetal growth restriction (FGR) [1]. The placenta generates reactive oxygen species, which may contribute to the oxidative stress seen even in normal pregnancy, but this is increased in pregnancies complicated by preeclampsia (PE) and fetal growth restriction (FGR) where oxidative stress has been clearly documented [2].

Nitric oxide (NO) plays a fundamental role in human physiology, being involved in the homeostasis of different functions, including cardiovascular reactivity and the immune response. In obstetrics NO – besides being involved in the physiology of labor and cervical ripening – possibly plays a major role in the etiology of PE and FGR. NO actively regulates embryo development, implantation, and trophoblast invasion [3,4]. The adequate morphology and function of the vascular tree of the placenta and the maternal endothelium is modulated by different environmental cues, which are related to the NO system. NO is produced by a group of enzymes called nitric oxide synthases (NOS). The vascular effects of NO are mainly generated through the endothelial nitric oxide synthase (eNOS), which is the classic "vasculoprotective" NOS isoform, but may also involve vascular expression of the neuronal (nNOS) and inducible isoforms (iNOS) of the enzyme [5]. NOS-mediated NO production requires oxygen and NADPH to convert endogenous available L-arginine into L-citrulline. NO activates soluble guanylate cyclase that catalyzes the conversion of guanosine 5'-triphosphate (GTP) to cyclic guanosine 3',5'-monophosphate (cGMP), an intracellular messenger regulating gene expression and enzyme activity. Cyclic GMP induces smooth muscle relaxation by multiple mechanisms:

- Increasing intracellular cGMP inhibits calcium entry into the cell and decreasing intracellular calcium concentrations
- Activating K+ channels, leading to hyperpolarization and relaxation
- Stimulating a cGMP-dependent protein kinase that activates myosin light chain phosphatase, the enzyme that dephosphorylates myosin light chains, which leads to smooth muscle relaxation.

Endogenous vascular NO production has been reported to be elevated in human pregnancy. A maladaptation of pregnancy, caused by inadequate implantation, may lead to an increase in oxygen-free radicals and lipid peroxides as a consequence of the vascular endothelial dysfunction, leading to a disturbed NO production. Women suffering from preeclampsia were shown to have decreased, similar, or increased levels of nitrates compared to pregnant controls [4,6]. Studying serum nitrate or nitrate levels to evaluate NO production has been found to be misleading as they are affected by many different factors, such as the patient's diet, medication regimen, and renal function. Therefore such testing has been shown to be of no clinical value [4,7]. A further possible explanation of this apparent paradox could be investigated in the dynamic evolution of placental-derived disorders such as PE or FGR: if NO production is impaired early in pregnancy, increased vascular resistance and clinical symptoms such as hypertension or FGR develop in the second part of gestation, unless a later compensatory up-regulation of NO takes place. Therefore an increase in NO metabolites can represent a compensatory response instead of the primary physiological modification of pregnancy [4].

PE and FGR are characterized by maternal endothelial dysfunction [8] and FGR is typified by increased nitric oxide production during pregnancy and after birth, which is viewed as an adaptive event to sustain placental blood flow [9]. These observations gave rise to the possibility that pharmacologic modulation of vascular endothelial function may improve uterine perfusion and fetal well-being in PE and FGR: mainly NO could play an important role in the prevention and treatment of this condition as it can improve uteroplacental circulation thereby increasing fetal blood and nutritional supply, possibly without any effect on fetal circulation. Interestingly, despite intensive research on NO and its association in pregnancy complications, there's a lack of properly designed studies on the potential value of NO donors for treatment or prevention of complications such as PE and even more isolated FGR [10].

So far, there's conflicting data on the vascular response to NO-dependent vasodilator agents in FGR and PE. Interestingly, the response to exogenous NO seems not to be altered; however, the amplitude and frequency of NO-dependent spontaneous tone oscillations are reduced in FGR chorionic arteries and can be invoked in normal vessels by inhibiting NO synthesis [3,11,12].

Because of the central role of cGMP in NO-mediated vasodilation, NO precursors (i.e., L-arginine),

NO-donors, or drugs that inhibit the breakdown of cGMP (cGMP-dependent phosphodiesterase inhibitors), such as sildenafil, may be used to enhance NO-mediated vasodilation (Figure 14.1).

Regardless of the eminent impact on pregnancy outcome and rising knowledge of the pathogenesis of FGR, besides low-dose aspirin (see Chapter 15), until now there is no effective strategy for secondary prevention.

This chapter will evaluate the current evidence on the potential benefit for prophylaxis of GR when targeting the NO system. Specifically, the mechanism and current knowledge on L-arginine (the precursor of NO), NO-donors, mainly glyceryl trinitrate (GTN) and pentaerythrityl-tetranitrate (PETN), will be highlighted. Furthermore, the effects of sildenafil citrate, a phosphodiesterase inhibitor (which enhances NO mediated smooth muscle relaxation), will be discussed.

L-arginine

The involvement of the L-arginine-NO pathway in the regulation of vascular tone suggests a possible role in the pathogenesis of FGR sustained by placental insufficiency. Arginine is an essential amino acid and the precursor for synthesis of many biologically active molecules, including nitric oxide (NO) [13]. As an effective NO donor, L-arginine has a vasodilative

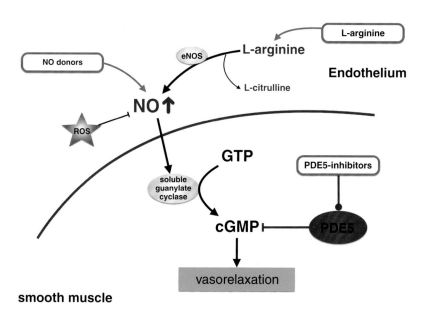

Figure 14.1 NO-biosynthesis and therapeutic strategies to upregulate vascular smooth muscle cell relaxation. NO = nitric oxide, ROS = reactive oxygen species, GTP = guanosine triphosphate, cGMP = cyclic guanylate monophosphate, PDE5 = phosphodiesterase-5.

effect. A positive influence of L-arginine on fetomaternal blood flow, based not only on the dilatation of the vessels but also on the anti-aggregative effect on the platelets, has been reported [14,15], mechanisms being synergic in improving intrauterine fetal development.

In FGR, an improvement of uteroplacental circulation has been reported in L-arginine treated FGR fetuses [14]. Subsequently, Sieroszewski and colleagues [16] published their results on long-term administration of L-arginine to pregnant women with growth-restricted fetuses: L-arginine (3 g daily orally) was found not to affect maternal plasma NO concentrations, but an improvement and acceleration of estimated fetal growth by ultrasound and an improvement of actual fetal birth weight was noted. In the treated group, the percentage of growth-restricted newborns was 29% versus 73% in the untreated group (p <0.01). Xiao and colleagues [17] evaluated the effect of L-arginine supplementation for treatment of FGR: group 1 was treated by routine therapy alone; group 2 was given L-arginine (20 g/day i.v.) in addition to routine therapy. Women with uncomplicated pregnancies were used as a control group. Mean birth weight was significantly higher in group 2 than in group 1 (p <0.05), but still lower in group 2 than in the control group (p <0.01). Unfortunately both studies were not randomized nor placebo-controlled, therefore the results have to be interpreted with care, especially as a randomized double-blinded placebo-controlled trial (verum group treated with L-arginine 14 g/day) was not able to prove the beneficial effect of L-arginine for severe FGR [18].

Nitric Oxide Donors

Drugs that can be converted by the body into nitric oxide (i.e., nitric oxide donors) are widely available, and have been used for years as therapeutic agents in cardiovascular diseases. NO donors are highly cost-effective and have beneficial effects in multiple body systems. When the body cannot generate NO via NO synthase or due to rapid turnover leading to inadequate amounts of NO available for biological homeostasis, administration of exogenous NO or prolongation of the actions of endogenous NO are practical ways to supplement NO.

In obstetric medicine, various NO donors have been investigated in complications such as preterm labor, preeclampsia, and FGR, and, so far, besides

headache, no major side effect associated with the use of nitric oxide donors in pregnancy has been reported. Nevertheless, a potential risk, associated with all vasodilators, is hypotension with subsequent reduction in the blood supply to the fetus and placenta.

Glyceryl Trinitrate (GTN)

Improvement of uterine artery flow by GTN infusion given to women with pathologic uterine artery Doppler in the absence of PE has been reported [19]. Kähler and colleagues [20] confirmed this observation in a study investigating fetal and uteroplacental blood flow after transdermal administration of GTN in pregnancies at risk for preterm delivery. A significant decrease of uterine artery resistance could be observed 24 hours following GTN application.

The clinical benefit of using NO donors as a prophylactic drug for pregnant women at risk was demonstrated for the first time by Lees and colleagues [21]: In this double-blind, randomized, placebo-controlled trial, the survival analysis of adverse events in gestation in both groups showed a 73% reduced risk of negative outcomes in the GTN group. However, this study failed to demonstrate a reduction in FGR, preterm delivery, or PE, possibly due to the small sample size. Furthermore, the use of GTN is associated with development of tachyphylaxia, i.e., nitrate tolerance, which is initiated within a few days, thus limiting the clinical effect. Interestingly, until now no further trial has been performed to further evaluate this finding. As Lees and colleagues [21] have supposed, there may be synergy of GTN and low-dose aspirin for the prophylaxis of placental pathologies, especially as it has been reported that GTN inhibits hypoxia-induced release of soluble fms-like tyrosine kinase-1 (sFlt-1), an antiangiogenic agent known to play a major role in pregnancy complications related to shallow trophoblast invasion [22].

Pentaerythrityl-Tetranitrate (PETN)

A recently published prospective randomized double-blinded trial investigated the effectiveness of the NO-donor PETN for secondary prevention of FGR, PE, and preterm birth in pregnancies at risk [23]. PETN was used, as it, in contrast to all other organic nitrates, can upregulate enzymes with a strong antioxidative capacity, thereby preventing tolerance and the development of endothelial dysfunction [24]. Women presenting with abnormal placental perfusion at mid-trimester (19–24 weeks of gestation) were randomized to either PETN (80 mg twice/day, n = 54) or placebo (n = 57). The primary endpoint of this study was FGR and/or perinatal death. PETN significantly decreased the risk for FGR and/or perinatal death (adjusted relative risk (RR) 0.410; 95% confidence interval, CI, 0.184–0.914) and for FGR (adjusted RR 0.436; 95% CI 0.196–0.970). The risk for preeclampsia was not reduced. Interestingly no placental abruption occurred in the PETN group, but five took place in the placebo group. These results suggest that secondary prophylaxis of adverse pregnancy outcome might be feasible in pregnancies exhibiting abnormal placentation using PETN. As the sample size was rather small, the authors concluded that to confirm these results further studies would be of utmost interest.

Sodium Nitroprusside (SNP)

Read and colleagues [25] examined the activity of sodium nitroprusside (SNP) in the human fetal-placental circulation in vitro in pathological and experimental conditions in which vascular function may be impaired. SNP caused a concentration-dependent reduction in fetal arterial perfusion pressure placental cotyledons. No differences were observed in the responses obtained to SNP in placentae obtained from women with normotensive pregnancies or those associated with hypertensive complications or FGR.

Using Laser Doppler fluxmetry, Koopmans and colleagues investigated the SNP-mediated vasodilation in women with FGR and could not find a difference compared to normal control pregnancies [26].

Isosorbid Mononitrate (IMN)/Isosorbide Dinitrate (IDN)

So far, no data can be found reporting the clinical use of IMN/IDN in pregnancies complicated by FGR.

Sildenafil Citrate (Viagra®)

Another group of compounds known as phosphodiesterase inhibitors (PDE5-selective inhibitors) also enhances the effects of nitric oxide. These drugs act by blocking enzymes that break down the molecule that mediates the effects of nitric oxide in the body, or cyclic guanosine monophosphate (cGMP) (Figure 14.1). Phosphodiesterase inhibitors prevent the hydrolysis of cGMP, thereby enhancing nitric oxide–mediated smooth muscle relaxation. Although no teratogenic effects have been observed in animal studies, there are currently few data on safety in human pregnancy.

Animal studies suggest that phosphodiesterase-5 (PDE5) inhibitors, such as sildenafil citrate, may improve uterine blood flow via cGMP-mediated endothelial relaxation of uterine vessels [27]. Subsequently sildenafil citrate (Viagra®) has been investigated in pregnancies complicated by PE or FGR. In 2005, Wareing and colleagues [28] reported that sildenafil citrate improves in vitro endothelial function of myometrial vessels from women whose pregnancies were complicated by FGR: increased myometrial small artery vasoconstriction and decreased endothelium-dependent vasodilatation were reported in vessels from FGR pregnancies. Sildenafil citrate significantly reduced vasoconstriction and significantly improved relaxation of FGR small arteries.

Recently, Dastjerdi and colleagues [29] reported the results of a randomized, double-blinded, and placebo-controlled trial on the effect of sildenafil citrate on fetoplacental and fetal perfusion: 41 pregnant women with growth-restricted fetuses (24–37 weeks of gestation) were evaluated for the effect of a single dose of sildenafil citrate (25–50 mg) on Doppler ultrasound parameters of the umbilical and middle cerebral arteries. Fetuses "treated" with sildenafil citrate demonstrated a significant decrease in systolic/diastolic ratios (p = 0.000) and pulsatility index (p = 0.019) for the umbilical artery and a significant increase in middle cerebral artery pulsatility index (p = 0.008). The authors conclude that treatment with sildenafil citrate may be a potential therapeutic strategy to improve uteroplacental blood flow in pregnancies with FGR, as efforts for later normalization of fetoplacental perfusion in FGR pregnancies with placental abnormalities might increase birth weight.

Nevertheless, before sildenafil may be an option for therapy or prevention of FGR, further studies are mandatory, especially as it has been reported that this drug may even have detrimental effects on uteroplacental perfusion and on the fetus [30,31]. Such a trial (STRIDER: Sildenafil Therapy In Dismal prognosis Early-onset intrauterine growth Restriction) is currently planned, and results should be available in 2020 [32].

Conclusion

Since 1992, when nitric oxide was elected "molecule of the year" by *Science* magazine, many studies have been performed in the field of perinatology. Despite a lot of good scientific evidence, the transfer from basic and preclinical experiences into clinical practice has not yet been achieved. The use of nitric oxide for prevention of preeclampsia and/or FGR appears attractive, but there is lack of evidence and properly designed randomized studies evaluating the use of NO donors in vascular complications of pregnancy, either as prophylactics or therapeutic agents. Before nitric oxide agents can be recommended for use in clinical practice, reliable evidence is required on whether they are both effective and safe.

The pathophysiology of FGR is complex, and suggests that the efficacy of L-arginine, NO donors, or sildenafil on FGR may depend, among other factors, on the degree of severity of FGR, the route and timing of the prophylactic/therapeutic drug, and the capacity to enhance arginine availability, NOS or arginase activity, or inhibit phosphodiesterase-5 activity.

In practical terms, the possible use of NO donors, L-arginine, or PDE5-inhibitors as therapeutic/prophylactic agents in the management of vascular complications of pregnancy needs further investigation, and no recommendations can be given at the present time.

Key Points

- Uteroplacental vascular function is modulated by the NO system.
- NO possibly plays a fundamental role in the etiology of preeclampsia and FGR.
- Vascular effects of NO are generated through the "vasculoprotective" endothelial nitric oxide synthase (eNOS).
- NO precursors, NO-donors, or drugs that inhibit the breakdown of cyclic GMP may be used to enhance NO-mediated vasodilation.
- Conflicting data on the vascular response to NO-dependent vasodilator agents in FGR and PE have been reported.
- Despite intensive research on NO and its association in pregnancy complications, there's a lack of properly designed studies on the potential value of NO donors for treatment or prevention of complications such as preeclampsia and even more isolated FGR.

- The possible use of NO donors, L-arginine, or PDE5-inhibitors as therapeutic/prophylactic agents in the management of vascular complications of pregnancy needs further investigation.
- Currently no definite answer for the prophylaxis of FGR via the NO system can be given.

References

1. Kaufmann P, Black S, Huppertz B. Endovascular trophoblast invasion: Implications for the pathogenesis of intrauterine growth retardation and preeclampsia. *Biol Reprod* 2003;69(1):1–7.

2. Myatt L. Review: Reactive oxygen and nitrogen species and functional adaptation of the placenta. *Placenta* 2010;31 Suppl:S66–69.

3. Krause BJ, Hanson MA, Casanello P. Role of nitric oxide in placental vascular development and function. *Placenta* 2011;32(11):797–805.

4. De Pace V, Chiossi G, Facchinetti F. Clinical use of nitric oxide donors and L-arginine in obstetrics. *J Matern Fetal Neonatal Med* 2007;20(8):569–79.

5. Govers R, Rabelink TJ. Cellular regulation of endothelial nitric oxide synthase. *Am J Physiol Renal Physiol* 2001;280(2):F193–206.

6. Lowe DT. Nitric oxide dysfunction in the pathophysiology of preeclampsia. *Nitric Oxide* 2000;4(4):441–58.

7. Bird IM, Zhang L, Magness RR. Possible mechanisms underlying pregnancy-induced changes in uterine artery endothelial function. *Am J Physiol Regul Integr Comp Physiol* 2003;284(2):R245–58.

8. Johnson MR, Anim-Nyame N, Johnson P, Sooranna SR, Steer PJ. Does endothelial cell activation occur with intrauterine growth restriction? *BJOG* 2002;109(7):836–9.

9. Pisaneschi S, Strigini FA, Sanchez AM, Begliuomini S, Casarosa E, Ripoli A, Ghirri P, Boldrini A, Fink B, Genazzani AR, Coceani F, Simoncini T. Compensatory feto-placental upregulation of the nitric oxide system during fetal growth restriction. *PLoS One* 2012;7(9):e45294.

10. Meher S, Duley L. Nitric oxide for preventing preeclampsia and its complications. *Cochrane Database Syst Rev* 2007;(2):CD006490.

11. Mills TA, Wareing M, Bugg GJ, Greenwood SL, Baker PN. Chorionic plate artery function and Doppler indices in normal pregnancy and intrauterine growth restriction. *Eur J Clin Invest* 2005;35(12):758–64.

12. Sweeney M, Wareing M, Mills TA, Baker PN, Taggart MJ. Characterisation of tone oscillations in placental and myometrial arteries from normal pregnancies and those complicated by pre-eclampsia and growth restriction. *Placenta* 2008;29(4):356–65.

13. Wu G, Bazer FW, Satterfield MC, Li X, Wang X, Johnson GA, Burghardt RC, Dai Z, Wang J, Wu Z. Impacts of arginine nutrition on embryonic and fetal development in mammals. *Amino Acids* 2013;45(2):241–56.

14. Neri I, Mazza V, Galassi MC, Volpe A, Facchinetti F. Effects of L-arginine on utero-placental circulation in growth-retarded fetuses. *Acta Obstet Gynecol Scand* 1996;75:208–12.

15. Neri I, Marietta M, Piccinini F, Volpe A, Facchinetti F. The L-arginine-nitric oxide system regulates platelet aggregation in pregnancy. *J Soc Gynecol Invest* 1998;5(4):192–6.

16. Sieroszewski P, Suzin J, Karowicz-Bilińska A. Ultrasound evaluation of intrauterine growth restriction therapy by a nitric oxide donor (L-arginine). *J Matern Fetal Neonatal Med* 2004;15(6):363–6.

17. Xiao XM, Li LP. L-arginine treatment for asymmetric fetal growth restriction. *Int J Gynaecol Obstet* 2005;88(1):15–18.

18. Winer N, Branger B, Azria E, Tsatsaris V, Philippe HJ, Rozé JC, Descamps P, Boog G, Cynober L, Darmaun D. L-arginine treatment for severe vascular fetal intrauterine growth restriction: A randomized double-bind controlled trial. *Clin Nutr* 2009;28(3):243–8.

19. Ramsay B, de Belder A, Campbell S, Moncada S, Martin JF. A nitric oxide donor improves uterine artery diastolic blood flow in normal early pregnancy and in women at high risk of pre-eclampsia. *Eur J Clin Invest* 1994;24(1):76–8.

20. Kähler C, Schleussner E, Möller A, Seewald HJ. Nitric oxide donors: Effects on fetoplacental blood flow. *Eur J Obstet Gynecol Reprod Biol* 2004;115(1):10–14.

21. Lees C, Valensise H, Black R, Harrington K, Byiers S, Romanini C, Campbell S. The efficacy and fetal-maternal cardiovascular effects of transdermal glyceryl trinitrate in the prophylaxis of pre-eclampsia and its complications: A randomized double-blind placebo-controlled trial. *Ultrasound Obstet Gynecol* 1998;12(5):334–8.

22. Barsoum IB, Renaud SJ, Graham CH. Glyceryl trinitrate inhibits hypoxia-induced release of soluble fms-like tyrosine kinase-1 and endoglin from placental tissues. *Am J Pathol* 2011;178(6):2888–96.

23. Schleussner E, Lehmann T, Kähler C, Schneider U, Schlembach D, Groten T. Impact of the nitric oxide-donor pentaerythrityl-tetranitrate on perinatal outcome in risk pregnancies: A prospective, randomized, double-blinded trial. *J Perinat Med* 2014;42(4):507–14.

24. Daiber A, Wenzel P, Oelze M, Münzel T. New insights into bioactivation of organic nitrates, nitrate tolerance and cross-tolerance. *Clin Res Cardiol* 2008;97(1):12–20.

25. Read MA, Giles WB, Leitch IM, Boura AL, Walters WA. Vascular responses to sodium nitroprusside in the human fetal-placental circulation. *Reprod Fertil Dev* 1995;7(6):1557–61.

26. Koopmans CM, Blaauw J, Van Pampus MG, Rakhorst G, Aarnoudse JG. Abnormal endothelium-dependent microvascular dilator reactivity in pregnancies complicated by normotensive intrauterine growth restriction. *Am J Obstet Gynecol* 2009;200(1):66.e1–6.

27. Zoma WD, Baker RS, Clark KE. Effects of combined use of sildenafil citrate (Viagra) and 17beta-estradiol on ovine coronary and uterine hemodynamics. *Am J Obstet Gynecol* 2004;190(5):1291–7.

28. Wareing M, Myers JE, O'Hara M, Baker PN. Sildenafil citrate (Viagra) enhances vasodilatation in fetal growth restriction. *J Clin Endocrinol Metab* 2005;90(5):2550–5.

29. Dastjerdi MV, Hosseini S, Bayani L. Sildenafil citrate and uteroplacental perfusion in fetal growth restriction. *J Res Med Sci* 2012;17(7):632–6.

30. Miller SL, Loose JM, Jenkin G, Wallace EM. The effects of sildenafil citrate (Viagra) on uterine blood flow and well being in the intrauterine growth-restricted fetus. *Am J Obstet Gynecol* 2009;200(1):102.e1–7.

31. Nassar AH, Masrouha KZ, Itani H, Nader KA, Usta IM. Effects of sildenafil in Nω-nitro-L-arginine methyl ester-induced intrauterine growth restriction in a rat model. *Am J Perinatol* 2012;29(6):429–34.

32. Ganzevoort W, Alfirevicz Z, von Dadelszen P, Kenny L, Papageorghiou A, van Wassenaer-Leemhuis A, Gluud C, Mol BW, Baker PN. STRIDER: Sildenafil Therapy In Dismal prognosis Early-onset intrauterine growth Restriction – a protocol for a systematic review with individual participant data and aggregate data meta-analysis and trial sequential analysis. *Syst Rev* 2014;3:23.

Chapter

15

Prevention and Treatment of Fetal Growth Restriction by Influencing Maternal Hemodynamics and Blood Volume

Herbert Valensise, Barbara Vasapollo, and Gian Paolo Novelli

Introduction

Fetal growth restriction (FGR) is a pregnancy disorder triggered by a defective interaction between the trophoblast and uterine tissues (suboptimal placentation) [1]. It is not clear whether the defective trophoblast development and the concomitantly arising maternal cardiovascular maladaptation are triggered by a common factor or whether abnormal trophoblast development results in poor placentation and subsequent maladaptation of the maternal cardiovascular system to pregnancy [2–4].

Both appropriate cardiovascular and uteroplacental changes appear to be important for fetal growth. In order to understand the maternal cardiovascular response during FGR, the first step is a correct understanding of the hemodynamic changes during uncomplicated pregnancies.

In the past, major interest was concentrated on the uteroplacental unit through studying the signal of the maternal uterine artery Doppler. This has led to the possibility of identification of patients at risk for pregnancy complications including FGR and was based on the supposition that the problem exclusively develops from a local dysfunction triggered by an altered placentation process. In the past two decades, clinicians widened their view in the understanding that the process that leads to the local (uteroplacental) hemodynamic alteration associated with preeclampsia and FGR might involve the whole maternal cardiovascular system and blood volume response [5–8]. The cardiovascular adaptation in uncomplicated pregnancy involves a complex physiological response by the maternal host to the presence of the conceptus. The main goal of the hemodynamic response to the pregnant state is to provide adequate uteroplacental perfusion and nutrition to facilitate fetal growth and development.

The hypothesis that the complete cardiovascular system may be involved when a complication of pregnancy develops (hypertension, preeclampsia, FGR) has allowed researchers to discover new ways to identify patients at risk through cardiac and vascular markers [9–11]. This new approach might change the way physicians look at possible interventions. Obstetricians shouldn't be only "observers" of the evolution of fetal growth, exclusively choosing the correct time to delivery, but they should try to induce improvement of fetal growth and prolongation of pregnancy. To date, the only option available to clinicians is to choose the timing of delivery of the fetus in an effort to prevent neonatal morbidity and mortality. With the knowledge and the understanding of the cardiovascular maladaptation during FGR, it might be possible to enhance the maternal cardiovascular system in order to improve the hemodynamic status of the fetus, which allows a safe prolongation of pregnancy and a gain in fetal growth, resulting in an amelioration of the neonatal outcome [12,13].

Cardiovascular and Hemodynamic Adaptation to Uncomplicated and Complicated Pregnancy

The cardiovascular adaptation to normal pregnancy involves a complex physiological response by the maternal host to the presence of the conceptus. The main goal of the hemodynamic response to the pregnant state is to provide adequate uteroplacental perfusion and nutrition for fetal development, without compromising maternal health. A series of adaptations are activated from the beginning of gestation (Table 15.1).

An understanding of cardiovascular modifications during normal pregnancy is crucial to interpret the

Table 15.1 Summary of the structural and functional cardiovascular parameters in uncomplicated and complicated pregnancy

Parameter	UP	GH	PE	FGR
→	↑	↑	↓	↓
Cardiac output	↑	↓ or ↑↑	↓↓ or ↑↑	↓
Total vascular resistance	↓	↓↓ or ↑	↓↓ or ↑↑	↑↑
Left atrial dimensions	↑	↑ or ↔		↓
Left atrial function	↑	↓	↓	↓
Left ventricular mass	↑	↑↑	↑↑	↓
Left ventricular compliance	↑	↓	↓	↓

↑: increase
↓: decrease
↔: not modified
UP, Uncomplicated Pregnancy; GH, Gestational Hypertension; PE, Preeclampsia; FGR, Fetal Growth Retardation
Source: Valensise H, Vasapollo B, Novelli GP. Maternal cardiovascular hemodynamics in normal and complicated pregnancies. *Fetal and Maternal Medicine Review* 2003; **14**:355–85.

adaptive mechanisms and to establish a reference for comparison when pregnancy becomes complicated.

During normal pregnancy, the cardiac output and plasma volume both expand by 50%, whereas the increase in red cell mass is 30%, resulting in a dilution "fall" in hemoglobin concentration. This low-resistance, high-volume, hyperdynamic, and hemodiluted pregnant state appears to be important for appropriate uteroplacental perfusion and effective fetomaternal exchange [14].

Women with growth-restricted fetuses fail to achieve these physiological cardiovascular changes and exhibit relatively non-pregnant hemodynamic features (Table 15.1).

On the other hand, mothers with *constitutional* SGA (not linked to poor placentation) fetuses show similar cardiovascular adaptations found in the mothers of appropriate-for-gestational age (AGA) fetuses [15].

Fetal Growth Restriction: Is Prevention and Treatment Possible?

Despite the many challenges in developing obstetric therapies and relative underinvestment from the pharmaceutical industry, a number of promising interventions are now emerging, many from academic–industrial partnerships.

The problem with FGR is that no therapy has been standardized so far. Some attempts have been tried and resulted in reporting general advice for the prevention of recurrent FGR (Table 15.2).

These classic interventions include the recognition of those women at risk, the reduction of risk factors, and the optimization of medical conditions. Antenatal care should include an assessment of risk factors in early pregnancy, so appropriate interventions may be instituted. Effective interventions are available for women with HIV and also for those living in malaria-endemic areas. Antiplatelet agents reduce the risk of preeclampsia and FGR in women at risk. Intrauterine treatments offer limited benefit to the baby with fetal growth restriction. Basically, the optimal management of the FGR-affected fetus, so far, has aimed to achieve the delivery of the newborn in the best possible condition, balancing the risks of prematurity against those of continued intrauterine existence [16–18].

So far, hemodynamic interventions focus on three aspects: enlargement of the amount of plasma volume during pregnancy, relaxation or distension of

Table 15.2 Effective prevention of recurrent fetal growth restriction, overview of interventions

Primary prevention (for all women)

- Reproductive plan and optimization of medical conditions (at preconception visit)
- Smoking cessation
- First-trimester ultrasound examination
- Third-trimester ultrasound examination

Secondary prevention (based on risk factor for FGR)

- Risk: women at high risk for FGR (hypertension, prior FGR, etc.)

Intervention: low-dose aspirin (start early in gestation and use dose greater than 75 mg)

- Risk: mild-to-moderate hypertension (systolic 140–169 mm Hg and/or diastolic blood pressure 90–109 mm Hg)

Intervention: avoidance of antihypertensive therapy

- Risk: women with nutritional deficiencies

Intervention: balanced energy and protein supplementation

- Risk: living in area endemic for malaria

Intervention: antimalarial prophylaxis

FGR: Fetal Growth Restriction
Source: Berghella V. Prevention of recurrent fetal growth restriction. *Obstet Gynecol* 2007; **110**:904–12.

the systemic circulation in order to increase the blood flow to the growing uterus, and, lately, efforts are made to increase selectively the uterine blood flow.

Interventions to Influence the Amount of Plasma Volume

The slower or decreased increase in whole blood volume accompanying complicated pregnancies could be stimulated by methods that increase especially the total amount of plasma volume. Several experiments have been performed on this subject. Some methods are capable of inducing small and temporary changes in plasma volume, but so far no intervention prevents or improves the complications of pregnancy.

Diuretics

Diuretics have long been used for the prevention of preeclampsia. In the 1960s, the prophylactic use was even advocated to prevent this disorder. In later years, the studies on this subject showed that preeclampsia could not be prevented [19]. Reduction of plasma volume by this intervention might theoretically even decrease birth weight [20]. Only one study looked at this aspect of the use of diuretics in pregnancy. It was concluded that birth weight was not changed; mean birth weight was non-significantly reduced with 139 grams. But this study was probably too small to draw firm conclusions; only 20 women were included [20].

Bed Rest

Bed rest has been long seen as a strategy to increase plasma volume. At least in healthy women, this is not the case. During a 13-day period of bed rest, plasma volume decreased in non-pregnant subjects by almost 10% [21]. In hypertensive pregnant women, bed rest decreased plasma volume by 14–70% [22]. This makes it unlikely that plasma volume will increase with bed rest in pregnant women with pregnancies complicated by fetal growth restriction.

Fluid Intake

Plasma volume is kept within narrow borders. Despite low or high fluid intake, plasma osmolality remains unchanged, but plasma volume may be changed by a limited percentage of about 2% by changes in fluid intake [23]. In uncomplicated pregnancies, there is a linear relationship between plasma volume and the amniotic fluid volume. Improvement of oligohydramnios by an increase in fluid intake has been proven [24]. The finding that an increase in fluid intake stimulates uterine blood flow may be a result of augmented plasma volume [25]. Since most cases of fetal growth restriction are accompanied by oligohydramnios, this intervention might be beneficial.

Administration of intravenous fluids may have the same effects as oral hydration. Use of electrolyte solutions or plasma volume expanders in the treatment of fetal growth restriction cannot be analyzed since no randomized controlled trials are available. Small case-control studies suggest improvement, especially when plasma volume expanders were used [26].

Water Immersion

Since ancient times, water immersion has been an effective method to lower maternal blood pressure. This intervention is also believed to increase plasma volume by 3–6%, depending on the gestational period of pregnancy [27]. Unless the plasma volume increases, fetal and placental circulation is not improved by this intervention [28]. A possible explanation could be that the effects of this intervention are very short lasting because water immersion cannot be done for a very long time and the effects are reversed quickly afterward.

Vasodilators

In animal experiments, administration of vasodilators like nifedipine or sodium nitrates in non-pregnant animals mimic the early pregnancy changes in hemodynamics, resulting in an increase in plasma volume [29]. The type of agent to induce these changes is obviously not important because vasodilation with both different types of medication induced the same effects. It is not clear whether treatment of pregnant women with vasodilators will lead to a chronic augmentation of plasma volume. Only one study so far examined maternal hemodynamics in pregnancy during chronic treatment with nifedipine [13]. This study did not study plasma volume changes, but the results suggest that extra measures are needed besides vasodilators to influence maternal hemodynamics. Uterine blood flow is also not influenced by chronic nifedipine use [30].

Exercise

Both in the pregnant and in the non-pregnant state, plasma volume increases as a result of physical exercise [31]. In comparison with sedentary women, in women who perform chronic exercise, plasma volume increases by 15–20% during the third trimester of pregnancy. Despite this finding, no differences were seen in birth weight or in length of gestation. Twelve weeks, postpartum these differences in plasma volume persisted.

Nitric Oxide Donors

The inadequate increase in preload shown by mothers with FGR fetuses supports the pathophysiological hypothesis of a hypovolemic state that accompanies FGR [12–14]. In the past, experimental data showed that inhibition of nitric oxide (NO) synthesis might induce maternal hypertension and growth restriction, suggesting that NO might contribute to the maintenance of low-resistance blood flow in the uteroplacental circulation during pregnancy. As a result, many investigators have administrated NO donors in such pregnancies, with controversial results. These studies, however, do not report the effects on maternal cardiac output and total peripheral resistance before and after NO administration, making it difficult to evaluate its benefits with respect to maternal hemodynamics. As stated previously, plasma volume expansion has been used in hypovolemic mothers of growth-restricted fetuses to induce a preload increase, potentially affecting stroke volume and cardiac output, with mixed results [12].

Several studies have looked at the effects of the organic nitrates glyceryl trinitrate and isosorbide dinitrate in women with preeclampsia (see Chapter 14). These have demonstrated a reduction in maternal blood pressure, uterine artery pulsatility index and resistance index, and umbilical artery resistance index with no evidence of adverse effects on fetal heart rate [32–39]. The studies so far have been small, however, looking mainly at short-term hemodynamic changes rather than outcome. Furthermore, organic nitrates are associated with tolerance, requiring nitrate-free periods. An alternative NO donor, S-nitrosoglutathione (GSNO), does not produce tolerance, reduces platelet aggregation, and increases the antioxidant glutathione [36].

In clinical practice, it appears possible to modify maternal hemodynamics with the pharmacological association of NO donors and plasma volume expansion in order to obtain a favorable effect on fetoplacental hemodynamics, although randomized controlled trials are still lacking.

Note that pregnant women with FGR fetuses usually have high TPR and therefore three simultaneous problems: (i) constriction of the resistance vessels (arteriolar compartment); (ii) low venous capacitance (venous compartment) [40]; and (iii) an underfilled vascular state. The venous compartment in the under-filled state is probably vaso-constricted in order to favor the venous return. Only by simultaneous action on these three aspects can a truly positive effect on maternal and fetoplacental hemodynamics be expected [13].

Pharmacological effects of NO donors are shown in Table 15.3. Therapy with NO donors produces a dilatation of the capacitance vessels, which increases venous pooling, acting on the problem of the low venous capacitance in these patients. If NO donors are used without the addition of fluid therapy, the overall result could be a decrease of the preload, which might already be deficient in these patients. To balance this potentially negative effect of treatment using NO donors and to increase the venous return (increasing SV and CO), an enhancement of maternal hydration could be achieved through the administration of fluids. This therapeutic strategy may allow for an improvement in positive outcomes (reduction of the afterload) while avoiding the potential threats (reduction of the preload) of therapy with NO donors. Valensise has shown that a combined pharmacological intervention with anti-hypertensives, NO donors, and hydration in hypertensive pregnancies complicated by severe fetal growth restriction has a positive effect on fetal hemodynamics and induces a prolongation of pregnancy [12]. Vasapollo used a similar therapeutic approach in hypertensive pregnant patients with high total vascular resistance. Although this study was not designed for FGR, the results showed improved neonatal outcome with higher birth weight centiles and lower rates of FGR and severe respiratory distress syndrome compared to other treatment groups [13].

Phosphodiesterase-5 (PDE5) Inhibitors

Selective treatment in order to improve the placental perfusion is one of the most recent developments in the treatment of FGR pregnancies. Uteroplacental blood flow may be improved by phosphodiesterase-5 (PDE5) inhibitors like sildenafil citrate. Evidence from *ex vivo* and animal experiments has shown

Table 15.3 Pharmacological effects of NO donors

NO Donors	Pharmacological effects	Is it positive in FGR pregnancy?
Pre-load	Decrease (dilation of the capacitance vessels, increasing venous pooling and reducing venous return to the heart)	Yes and no (venous compartment is constricted and the dilatation is a positive effect, but plasma volume is not expanded and therefore this becomes a negative effect in an already defective preload pregnancy)
Stroke volume and cardiac output	Decrease (it is an effect of the reduction of venous return)	No (already defective in FGR pregnancy)
Afterload	Decrease (dilation of the conduit vessels)	Yes (contrasts the increased afterload)
Platelet aggregation	Anti-aggregation	Yes (inhibits platelets aggregation)
Cardiac contractility	Increased	Yes (enhances cardiac function)

increases in average birth pup weight and uterine artery blood flow [41]. In human pregnancy, only one small cohort study showed a tendency toward more liveborn children who survived intact to primary discharge [42].

Conclusions

Knowledge of maternal cardiovascular function is important for the prevention and treatment of pregnancy complications like fetal growth restriction. The increase in maternal heart rate, the reduction in total vascular resistance, and the increase in cardiac output might play a role in the prophylaxis and treatment of these fetuses, since monitoring fetal heart rate and Doppler indexes serve only as predictors. The results of the ongoing research might shed new light on this problem.

Key Points

- Women undergo a variety of physiological cardiovascular adaptations including an increase in circulation volume and reduction in total vascular resistance, in order to support the development of the fetoplacental unit.

- Primary prevention of fetal growth restriction is grossly focused on smoking cessation.

- Treatment of fetal growth restriction is aimed to improve vascular filling by increasing total blood volume.

- Selective improvement of the flow through the uteroplacental unit can be achieved by therapeutic intervention.

References

1. Khong TY, De Wolf F, Robertson WB, Brosens I. Inadequate maternal vascular response to placentation in pregnancies complicated by pre-eclampsia and by small-for-gestational age infants. *BJOG* 1986;93:1049–59.

2. Roberts JM, Taylor RN, Musci TJ, Rodgers GM, Hubel CA, McLaughlin MK. Preeclampsia, an endothelial cell disorder. *Am J Obstet Gynecol* 1989;161:1200–4.

3. Taylor RN, Heilbron DC, Roberts JM. Growth factor activity in the blood of women in whom preeclampsia develops is elevated from early pregnancy. *Am J Obstet Gynecol* 1990;163:1839–44.

4. Roberts JM, Taylor RM, Goldfein A. Clinical and biochemical evidence of endothelial cell dysfunction in the pregnancy syndrome preeclampsia. *Am J Hypertens* 1991;4:700–8.

5. Duvekot JJ, Cheriex EC, Pieters FA, Peeters LH. Severely impaired fetal growth is preceded by maternal hemodynamic maladaptation in very early pregnancy. *Acta Obstet Gynecol Scand* 1995;74:693–7.

6. Duvekot JJ, Cheriex EC, Pieters FA, Menheere PP, Schouten HJ, Peeters LH. Maternal volume homeostasis in early pregnancy in relation to fetal growth restriction. *Obstet Gynecol* 1995;85:361–7.

7. Valensise H, Vasapollo B, Novelli GP, Larciprete G, Romanini ME, Arduini D, Galante A, Romanini C. Maternal diastolic function in asyptomatic pregnant women with bilateral notching of the uterine artery waveform at 24 weeks' gestation. *Ultrasound Obstet Gynecol* 2001;18:450–5.

8. Melchiorre K, Sharma R, Thilaganathan B. Cardiovascular implications in preeclampsia: An overview. *Circulation* 2014;130:703–14.

9. Valensise H, Vasapollo B, Gagliardi G, Novelli GP. Early and late preeclampsia: Two different maternal

hemodynamic states in the latent phase of the disease. *Hypertension* 2008;52:873–80.

10. Vasapollo B, Novelli GP, Valensise H. Total vascular resistance and left ventricular morphology as screening tools for complications in pregnancy. *Hypertension* 2008;51:1020–6.

11. Novelli GP, Valensise H, Vasapollo B, Larciprete G, Altomare F, Di Pierro G, Casalino B, Galante A, Arduini D. Left ventricular concentric geometry as a risk factor in gestational hypertension. *Hypertension* 2003;41:469–75.

12. Valensise H, Vasapollo B, Novelli GP, Giorgi G, Verallo P, Galante A, Arduini D. Maternal and fetal hemodynamic effects induced by nitric oxide donors and plasma volume expansion in pregnancies with gestational hypertension complicated by intrauterine growth restriction with absent end-diastolic flow in the umbilical artery. *Ultrasound Obstet Gynecol* 2008;31:55–64.

13. Vasapollo B, Novelli GP, Gagliardi G, Tiralongo GM, Pisani I, Manfellotto D, Giannini L, Valensise H. Medical treatment of early-onset mild gestational hypertension reduces total peripheral vascular resistance and influences maternal and fetal complications. *Ultrasound Obstet Gynecol* 2012;40:325–31.

14. Melchiorre K, Sutherland GR, Liberati M, Thilaganathan B. Maternal cardiovascular impairment in pregnancies complicated by severe fetal growth restriction. *Hypertension* 2012;60:437–43.

15. Vasapollo B, Valensise H, Novelli GP, Altomare F, Galante A, Arduini D. Abnormal maternal cardiac function precedes the clinical manifestation of fetal growth restriction. *Ultrasound Obstet Gynecol* 2004;24:23–9.

16. Berghella V. Prevention of recurrent fetal growth restriction. *Obstet Gynecol* 2007;110:904–12.

17. Grivell R1, Dodd J, Robinson J. The prevention and treatment of intrauterine growth restriction. *Best Pract Res Clin Obstet Gynaecol* 2009;23:795–807.

18. Sheridan C. Intrauterine growth restriction –diagnosis and management. *Aust Fam Physician* 2005;34:717–23.

19. Churchill D, Beevers GDG, Meher S, Rhodes C. Diuretics for preventing pre-eclampsia. *Cochrane Database Syst Rev* 2007, Issue 1. Art. No.: CD004451.

20. Sibai BM, Grossman RA, Grossman HG. Effects of diuretics on plasma volume in pregnancies with long-term hypertension. *Am J Obstet Gynecol* 1984;150:831–5.

21. Fortney SM, Turner C, Steinmann RN, Driscoll CNMT, Alfrey C. Blood volume responses of men and women to bed rest. *J Clin Pharmacol* 1994;34:434–9.

22. Fievet P, Pleskov L, Desailly I, Carayon A, de Fremont JF, Coevoet B, Comoy E, Demory JE, Verhoest P, Boulanger JC. Plasma renin activity, blood uric acid and plasma volume in pregnancy-induced hypertension. *Nephron* 1985;40:429–32.

23. Johnson EC, Muñoz CX, Le Bellego L, Klein A, Casa DJ, Maresh CM, Armstrong LE. Markers of the hydration process during fluid volume modification in women with habitual high or low daily fluid intakes. *Eur J Appl Physiol* 2015;115:1067–74.

24. Hofmeyr GJ, Gülmezoglu AM. Maternal hydration for increasing amniotic fluid volume in oligohydramnios and normal amniotic fluid volume. *Cochrane Database Syst Rev* 2002;(1):CD000134.

25. Flack NJ, Sepulveda W, Bower S, Fisk NM. Acute maternal hydration in third-trimester oligohydramnios: Effects on amniotic fluid volume, uteroplacental perfusion, and fetal blood flow and urine output. *Am J Obstet Gynecol* 1995;173:1186–91.

26. Heyl W, Boabang P, Faridi A, Rath W. Evaluation of the success of hemodilution therapy for fetal growth retardation by Doppler sonography. *Clin Hemorheol Microcirc* 1997;17:225–30.

27. Katz VL, McMurray R, Berry MJ, Cefalo RC. Fetal and uterine responses to immersion and exercise. *Obstet Gynecol* 1988;72:225–30.

28. Thisted DL, Nørgaard LN, Meyer HM, Aabakke AJ, Secher NJ. Water immersion and changes in the foetoplacental and uteroplacental circulation: An observational study with the case as its own control. *J Matern Fetal Neonatal Med* 2014;25:1–5.

29. Fekete A, Sasser JM, Baylis C. Chronic vasodilation produces plasma volume expansion and hemodilution in rats: Consequences of decreased effective arterial blood volume. *Am J Physiol Renal Physiol* 2011;300:F113–8.

30. Lima MM, Souza AS, Diniz C, Porto AM, Amorim MM, Moron AF. Doppler velocimetry of the uterine, umbilical and fetal middle cerebral arteries in pregnant women undergoing tocolysis with oral nifedipine. *Ultrasound Obstet Gynecol* 2009;34:311–15.

31. Pivarnik JM, Mauer ME, Ayres NA, Kirshon B, Dildy GA, Cotton DB. Effects of chronic exercise on blood volume expansion and hematologic indices during pregnancy. *Obstet Gynecol* 1994;83:264–9.

32. Krause BJ, Carrasco-Wong I, Caniuguir A, Carvajal J, Farías M, Casanello P. Endothelial eNOS/arginase imbalance contributes to vascular dysfunction in IUGR umbilical and placental vessels. *Placenta* 2013;34:20–8.

33. Schleussner E, Lehmann T, Kähler C, Schneider U, Schlembach D, Groten T. Impact of the nitric oxide-donor pentaerythrityl-tetranitrate on perinatal

outcome in risk pregnancies: A prospective, randomized, double-blinded trial. *J Perinat Med* 2014;42:507–14.

34. Di Iorio R, Marinoni E, Gazzolo D, Letizia C, Di Netta T, Cosmi EV. Maternal nitric oxide supplementation increases adrenomedullin concentrations in growth retarded fetuses. *Gynecol Endocrinol* 2002;16:187–92.

35. Lees C, Valensise H, Black R, Harrington K, Byiers S, Romanini C, Campbell S. The efficacy and fetal-maternal cardiovascular effects of transdermal glyceryl trinitrate in the prophylaxis of pre-eclampsia and its complications: A randomized double-blind placebo-controlled trial. *Ultrasound Obstet Gynecol* 1998;12:334–8.

36. Spencer RN, Carr DJ, David AL. Treatment of poor placentation and the prevention of associated adverse outcomes – what does the future hold? *Prenat Diagn* 2014;34:677–84.

37. Makino Y, Izumi H, Makino I, Shirakawa K. The effect of nitric oxide on uterine and umbilical artery flow velocity waveform in pre-eclampsia. *Eur J Obstet Gynecol Reprod Biol* 1997;73:139–43.

38. Martinez-Abundis E, Gonzalez-Ortiz M, Hernandez-Salazar F, Huerta JLMT. Sublingual isosorbide dinitrate in the acute control of hypertension in patients with severe preeclampsia. *Gynecol Obstet Invest* 2000;50:39–42.

39. Manzur-Verastegui S, Mandeville PB, Gordillo-Moscoso A, et al. Efficacy of nitroglycerine infusion versus sublingual nifedipine in severe preeclampsia: A randomized, triple-blind, controlled trial. *Clin Exp Pharmacol Physiol* 2008;35:580–5.

40. Aardenburg R, Spaanderman ME, Courtar DA, van Eijndhoven HW, de Leeuw PW, Peeters LL. A subnormal plasma volume in formerly preeclamptic women is associated with a low venous capacitance. *J Soc Gynecol Investig* 2005;12:107–11.

41. Herraiz S, Pellicer B, Serra V, Cauli O, Cortijo J, Felipo V, Pellicer A. Sildenafil citrate improves perinatal outcome in fetuses from pre-eclamptic rats. *BJOG* 2012;119:1394–402.

42. Von Dadelszen P, Dwinnell S, Magee LA, Carleton BC, Gruslin A, Lee B, Lim KI, Liston RM, Miller SP, Rurak D, Sherlock RL, Skoll MA, Wareing MM, Baker PN; Research into Advanced Fetal Diagnosis and Therapy (RAFT) Group. Sildenafil citrate therapy for severe early-onset intrauterine growth restriction. *BJOG* 2011;118:624–8.

Chapter

16

Gene Therapy in Fetal Growth Restriction

Rebecca N. Spencer, David J. Carr, and Anna L. David

Conflict of interest: ALD is an unpaid consultant and director of Magnus Growth, part of Magnus Life Science, which is aiming to take to market a novel treatment for fetal growth restriction.

Introduction

Gene therapy is the introduction of genetic material into a cell to produce a therapeutic effect. The genetic material, or transgene, is first delivered into the cell by a vector, then transcribed to produce a transgenic protein (Figure 16.1). This protein may have one of several different therapeutic actions. In monogenic disorders, such as beta-thalassemia or cystic fibrosis, the aim is to replace a protein that is faulty or absent. In other situations, the transgenic protein may supplement low levels of a naturally occurring protein or provide supra-physiological levels of an endogenous protein with beneficial effects.

When considering the potential uses of gene therapy in pregnancy, one of the most obvious and well-researched approaches is fetal gene therapy [1,2]. Here the aim is to produce transgenic protein expression within the fetus, either to cure a genetic disorder or to ameliorate its *in utero* effects. Currently, gene therapy given directly to the fetus is not considered ethically acceptable [3,4]. It also raises specific safety concerns, such as the risk of altering the fetal germ cells to produce germline transmission. In contrast, many obstetric conditions may be amenable to gene therapy delivered to the mother or possibly to the placenta. One such example is fetal growth restriction (FGR).

The term FGR is used inconsistently throughout the literature, and is often incorrectly used to describe fetuses that are constitutionally small for gestational age. In the context of this chapter, FGR refers to a fetus that has failed to meet its genetic growth potential as a result of uteroplacental insufficiency. The most common underlying problem in uteroplacental insufficiency is poor placentation, which ultimately causes a reduction in the transplacental supply of oxygen and nutrients from the mother to the fetus. While the pathophysiology will not be discussed in detail here, it is worth noting that uteroplacental insufficiency is associated with a reduction in spiral artery

remodeling, arising from the early stages of placental development [5], and a reduction in uterine artery blood volume flow [6].

This chapter considers the practicalities of how gene therapy could be used to treat FGR and will review the current evidence from *in vitro* and *in vivo* studies. It will also discuss the ethical and safety issues raised by the use of gene therapy to treat an obstetric condition and consider the practical challenges of translating such a therapy into the clinic.

Choice of Vector

As pregnancy is of finite duration, the ideal vector to deliver gene therapy for FGR would produce short-term expression in maternal tissues, at the maternal side of the placenta, or possibly within the placenta.

Gene therapy vectors may be either viral, including adenoviral vectors, retroviral vectors, and adeno-associated viral (AAV) vectors, or nonviral (Table 16.1). Adenoviral vectors efficiently transfect a wide range of cells, producing short-term protein expression, and are the most commonly used vectors in clinical trials of gene therapy [7]. One of their well-recognized side effects, however, is the potential to trigger both a B cell and a T cell mediated immune reaction [8]. This is being addressed by recent advances that are aiming to develop less immunogenic adenoviral vectors or to select serotypes to which fewer patients have preexisting immunity [9].

Adenoviral vectors enter cells through the binding of fiber proteins on their outer capsid to the coxsackie and adenovirus receptor (CAR). While this receptor is found on a wide range of cell types, it has very limited expression on the syncytiotrophoblast. This could be an advantage for a gene therapy aiming to target the maternal uteroplacental circulation without transfecting the placenta. If placental gene therapy was desired, however, a modified adenoviral vector could be used. One such example is the fiber-mutant adenovirus

Table 16.1 Gene therapy vectors commonly used in clinical trials

Vector		Expression	Advantages	Limitations	Mitigation Strategies
Viral vectors	Adenoviral vectors	Short-term	Transduce a wide range of cells Can carry a large amount of genetic information	Potential immune reaction Potential for causing abnormal liver function	Use when short-term gene transfer is required
	Retroviral and Lentiviral vectors	Long-term	Low immunogenicity	Risk of insertional mutagenesis Gamma-retroviruses can only transduce dividing cells	Self-inactivating gamma-retroviral and lentiviral constructs can reduce the probability of insertional mutagenesis by modification of the vector sequences
	Adeno-associated vectors	Long-term	Transduce a wide range of cells Less immunogenic than adenoviral vectors	Preexisting immunity to some serotypes Can only carry a limited amount of genetic information Evidence of some limited integration Cause abnormal liver function	Use serotype to which patient does not have antibodies Steroids to reduce inflammatory response
Nonviral vectors		Short-term	Potentially fewer side effects than viral vectors	Low efficiency	Apply locally in high dose

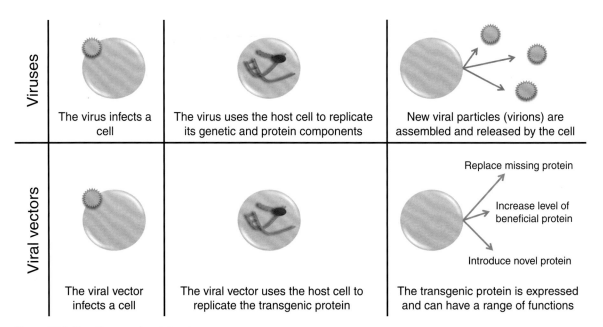

Viruses	The virus infects a cell	The virus uses the host cell to replicate its genetic and protein components	New viral particles (virions) are assembled and released by the cell
Viral vectors	The viral vector infects a cell	The viral vector uses the host cell to replicate the transgenic protein	Replace missing protein Increase level of beneficial protein Introduce novel protein The transgenic protein is expressed and can have a range of functions

Figure 16.1 Gene therapy using viral vectors.
A comparison between virus infection of a cell, and transduction of a cell with a modified viral vector.

vector carrying the Arg-Gly-Asp peptide sequence (Ad-RGD). This has modified fiber proteins, allowing it to enter cells via the integrin receptor, giving it increased tropism for placental cells [10].

Retroviral vectors, including gamma-retroviruses and lentiviruses, integrate genetic material into the host genome. While this is ideal for producing the long-term expression needed to cure a monogenic disease, it carries the risk of insertional mutagenesis, where cancer arises due to altered expression of nearby genes. Mitigation strategies such as removing parts of the vector construct to create self-inactivating vectors can reduce this risk. Long-term expression of the transgenic protein used to treat FGR may have undesirable side effects, depending on which transgenic protein is expressed. AAV vectors have a similar efficacy to adenoviral vectors, but produce less of an immune response. They generally produce short-term transgene expression, although they do have the potential for integration and can only carry a limited amount of genetic material.

Nonviral vectors generally have fewer side effects than viral vectors, but are much less efficient at introducing their transgenes into target cells [11,12]. The most commonly used nonviral vectors are liposomes, artificial lipid vesicles that bind to cell membranes to introduce the transgene that they carry. Transgenes can also be introduced by other physical and chemical means, including electrical pulses (electroporation), high-frequency ultrasound, and direct injection.

Choice of Transgenic Protein

With an increasing understanding of the molecular mechanisms underlying normal and pathological pregnancy, it is possible to identify proteins that may be suitable for treating FGR.

Vascular Endothelial Growth Factor

The growth and development of blood vessels within the placental villi is regulated by many factors. Among the key players in this process are members of the Vascular Endothelial Growth Factor (VEGF) family and their receptors [13]. So far seven VEGF proteins have been identified, of which VEGF A, B, C, and D and Placental Growth Factor (PlGF) are found in humans [14]. The formation of new blood vessels, vasculogenesis, and blood vessel growth, angiogenesis, both result from the binding of VEGF-A, or the processed forms of VEGF-C and VEGF-D, to

VEGF receptor 2 (VEGFR-2). Activation of VEGFR-2 leads to endothelial cell proliferation and migration, increased endothelial cell survival, increased vascular permeability, and activation of endothelial nitric oxide synthase (eNOS). This last effect also causes vasodilatation by increasing nitric oxide (NO) synthesis. In contrast, the soluble form of VEGFR-1, soluble fms-like tyrosine kinase 1 (sFlt-1), binds VEGF-A and PlGF, inhibiting their actions.

Uteroplacental insufficiency is associated with a shift in the normal balance of the angiogenic and anti-angiogenic factors toward an anti-angiogenic state. There is an increase in levels of sFlt-1 and a reduction in the maternal levels of bioavailable VEGF-A and PlGF [15,16]. Correcting this imbalance is therefore a potential strategy for treating FGR. However, given the angiogenic and vasodilatory actions of VEGF, it may be preferable to target increased VEGF levels to the maternal uteroplacental circulation with locally delivered gene therapy, rather than increase systemic maternal VEGF levels.

Insulin-Like Growth Factor

Insulin-like growth factors (IGFs) I and II play an important role in regulating growth, differentiation, and metabolism in almost all tissues and organs, mainly through their interaction with IGF receptor 1 (IGFR1). Their role in placental development and fetal growth makes them candidate proteins for treating FGR. During pregnancy IGF-II is produced by the mother, the placenta, and the fetus, while IGF-I expression is mainly limited to maternal and fetal tissues. IGF is predominantly bound to one of the six IGF-binding proteins (IGFBPs), which act as a reservoir and regulate IGF bioavailability. Placental factors such as pregnancy-associated plasma protein A (PAPP-A) cleave IGFBPs, increasing bioavailable levels of IGF. IGF-I helps regulate placental cell differentiation, with cord blood levels showing a positive correlation with birth weight [17,18]. IGF-II promotes trophoblast invasion through its interaction with IGFR2. Both hormones promote placental fibroblast proliferation and increase placental uptake and transfer of glucose and amino acids.

Maternal VEGF Gene Therapy for FGR

Maternal application of VEGF gene therapy has been tested in a variety of preclinical studies using adenovirus vectors.

VEGF Gene Therapy in Normal Sheep Pregnancy

The impact of Ad.VEGF on uterine blood flow (UBF) was first examined at mid-gestation in uncompromised sheep pregnancies using the VEGF-A165 isoform. UBF was quantified at baseline and at 4–7 days following direct uterine artery (UtA) injection of Ad.VEGF-A165 at laparotomy. The artery was digitally occluded during vector injection and afterward for up to 5 minutes total time to maximize transfection of the downstream endothelium [19]. By 4–7 days, volume blood flow in the UtA was increased three-fold when compared to a contralateral UtA injection of a non-vasoactive control adenoviral vector endocoding bacterial ß-galactosidase (Ad.LacZ). Ad.VEGF-A165 transduced vessels harvested at this short-term time point demonstrated an enhanced contractile response to phenylephrine and increased relaxation response to bradykinin when examined in an organ bath, as well as upregulation of endothelial nitric oxide synthase (eNOS) and VEGFR-2 [20]. Further experiments using the preprocessed short form of Ad.VEGF-D (Ad.VEGF-DΔNΔC) demonstrated similar effects on vasoreactivity, upregulation of phosphorylated eNOS, and enhanced UtA endothelial cell proliferation [20].

The effects of Ad.VEGF- A165 on UBF were next examined over a longer time period using indwelling ultrasonic flow probes. At 28 days post-injection, vessels treated with Ad.VEGF- A165 exhibited a 36.5% increase in UBF compared to just 20.1% in vessels treated with Ad.LacZ [20], which represents a virtual doubling of the normal gestational increase in UBF. A similar trend was observed long term after injection of Ad.VEGF-DΔNΔC [21]. In both studies, reduced phenylephrine-induced vasoconstriction continued to be observed, but vasorelaxation and VEGFR-2 expression no longer differed between Ad.VEGF and Ad.LacZ groups. Nevertheless at 30–45 days following treatment, there was evidence of neovascularization within the perivascular adventitia despite a complete lack of ongoing transgenic VEGF expression, which implies that the vasoactive effects of Ad.VEGF persist beyond the period of transgene expression, probably via angiogenesis mechanisms.

VEGF Gene Therapy in a Sheep Model of FGR

To determine whether Ad.VEGF-mediated changes in UBF might impact fetal growth, two separate experiments were performed using a well-established ovine model of FGR: the over-nourished adolescent ewe. Paradoxically, high nutritional intake in adolescent dams (who are themselves still growing during pregnancy) promotes maternal tissue growth at the expense of the pregnancy, leading to marked FGR (= fetal weight >2SD below the mean birth weight of genetically matched contemporaneous controls fed an optimum diet) in approximately half of cases [22–24]. The model replicates many of the key features of uteroplacental FGR in the human, including early reductions in UBF (>40%), placental weight, vascularity, secretory function and mRNA expression of VEGF and VEGFR-1, followed by asymmetrical FGR characterized by brain sparing (preserved head growth with reduced abdominal growth) and abnormal umbilical artery Doppler velocimetry [25–30].

Figure 16.2 (A/C) illustrates serial ultrasonographic measurements of the fetal abdominal circumference (AC), which is the most accurate single marker of fetal growth in humans and sheep [31,32], between mid- and late gestation. In both studies, following bilateral UtA injections of Ad.VEGF-A165 in mid-gestation, AC measurements were significantly increased by ≈20% when examined at 3 and 4 weeks following treatment compared to animals with equivalent baseline measurements receiving control treatments (Ad.LacZ or saline only) [33,34]. There was evidence of an attenuated brain-sparing effect (catch-up of abdominal to head growth). In the first cohort of pregnancies, sacrificed at 0.9 gestation (term = 145 days), significantly fewer fetuses demonstrated marked FGR (fetal weight >2SD below control mean) in Ad.VEGF-A165 compared with Ad.LacZ/saline groups (5/18 versus 17/10, respectively, p = 0.033, Figure 16.2B).

In the second cohort, culminating in spontaneous birth, lamb birth weight tended to be higher in Ad.VEGF-A165 versus saline groups (4114±230g versus 3432±303g, p = 0.081, Figure 16.2D) [34]. Thereafter Ad.VEGF-A165-treated lambs continued to grow faster in absolute terms throughout the first 12 weeks of life in the absence of any change in fractional growth velocity or markers of adiposity. Glucose tolerance testing at approximately 7 weeks of age revealed enhanced insulin secretion without any evidence of relative insulin resistance and at necropsy at 3 months of age there was evidence of increased lean tissue mass, indicative of increased

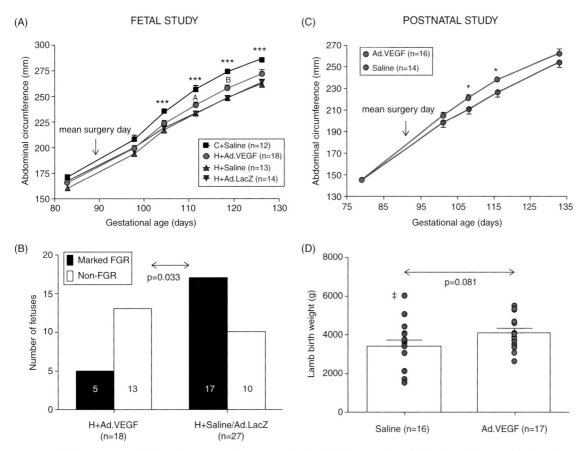

Figure 16.2 Summary of key findings from two studies of prenatal adenoviral (Ad) vascular endothelial growth factor (VEGF) gene therapy in the over-nourished adolescent model of fetal growth restriction (FGR).

In the fetal study, 57 singleton-bearing adolescent dams were offered a control-intake (C) or high-intake (H) diet to generate normal or compromised fetal growth, respectively, and received bilateral uterine artery injections of Ad.VEGF, Ad.LacZ (control vector) or saline at laparotomy in mid-gestation. The fetal abdominal circumference (AC) was measured by ultrasound at weekly intervals between 83 and 126 days' gestation. At delivery at 131 days (0.9) gestation, fetuses were categorized as marked FGR or non-FGR based on a -2SD cut-off relative to the control group mean [B]. In the postnatal study, 33 singleton-bearing over-nourished adolescent dams (all H) received either Ad.VEGF or saline and 30 underwent serial measurements of AC between 79 and 113 days' gestation [C]. Ewes were allowed to spontaneously deliver near term and lambs were weighed at birth [D]. Exact p values presented show two-group comparisons by t tests. *** p<0.001 and * p<0.05 indicate levels of significance for overall ANOVA. Post hoc comparisons are indicated by capital letters. A and B show time points at which AC measurements were significantly greater in H+Ad.VEGF versus H+Saline / H+Ad.LacZ groups (p = 0.016–0.047).

anabolic drive. DNA methylation studies found no evidence of altered epigenetic status in 10 different genes related to postnatal growth and metabolism, suggesting that these lambs were continuing to thrive rather than exhibiting signs of a "programming" effect of prenatal treatment [35]. In both studies there was evidence of increased placental efficiency (g fetus/lamb per g placenta) and in late gestation there was increased mRNA expression of VEGFR-1 and VEGFR-2 localized to the maternal placental compartment (caruncle) [36].

VEGF Gene Therapy in a Guinea Pig Model of FGR

Complementary experiments are under way to further examine the efficacy, safety, and mechanism of action of Ad.VEGF gene therapy in a second animal model of FGR induced by periconceptual nutrient deprivation of Dunkin Hartley guinea pigs. Placentation in this species more closely mimics the human, being hemochorial in nature, and shares a similar process of trophoblast cell invasion and proliferation [37,38].

In this FGR model there is a $\approx$40% reduction in fetal weight associated with uteroplacental insufficiency and brain sparing [39]. As direct injection of the UtA in the guinea pig is associated with considerable morbidity and mortality, a less invasive technique of administration has been developed using a thermosensitive Pluronic gel, which is applied externally to the uterine and radial arteries at laparotomy to achieve transduction with Ad.VEGF-A165 or Ad.LacZ at 30–34 days' gestation (term = 65) [40]. Preliminary analysis has shown that administration of Ad.VEGF-A165 in mid-gestation FGR guinea pig pregnancy results in an increase in fetal weight at term when compared to control treated animals.

Placental IGF Gene Therapy for FGR

The possibility of improving fetal growth by direct administration of IGF has been demonstrated in animal studies. However, the potential to translate this directly into clinical practice is limited by the need for a constant infusion or repeated administration of IGF. This may be surmountable with the use of gene therapy to produce IGF expression over days or weeks.

Effects of IGF Infusion in Normal Pregnancy and Animal Models of FGR

In normal guinea pig pregnancy, subcutaneous maternal administration of either IGF-I or IGF-II results in increased fetal growth. Mini osmotic pumps were fitted to pregnant IMVS colored guinea pigs on day 20 of gestation (term = 69–70), to provide a continuous infusion of IGF from day 20 to day 38. Fetal weight at day 62 was significantly higher with IGF-I or IGF-II infusion compared with infusion of a control vehicle (17% and 11%, respectively) [41]. IGF-II infusion also significantly increased the structural and functional capacity of the placenta [41] while IGF-I infusion significantly increased placental glucose uptake [42]. The increase in fetal weight was not replicated, however, in the guinea pig periconceptual nutrient restriction model of FGR [43]. This may be because the nature of the model meant that dams lacked sufficient nutrient supplies to respond to IGF treatment.

In contrast, studies in a placental embolization sheep model of FGR have shown increased fetal growth rates with IGF administration. Polystyrene microspheres were administered twice daily from day 93 to day 99, via a catheter into the maternal uterine arteries. This resulted in a significantly lower fetal weight and significantly higher brain to liver ratio at day 128 compared with non-embolized controls [44]. When embolization was followed by administration of IGF-I from day 100 to 128, either as a continuous maternal intravenous infusion (IGF-IV) or as thrice-weekly injections into the amniotic cavity (IGF-AF), the daily fetal girth increment over this period was significantly higher than after embolization alone (SAL) [44]. The fetal weights in the IGF-IV and IGF-AF groups at day 128 were intermediate between the SAL and control groups, but were not significantly different from either. A similar study, in which embolization was performed from day 103 to 109 with intra-amniotic injections on days 110, 117, and 124, also found a significantly higher fetal growth rate in animals given IGF-I injections compared with those given saline [45]. This change was accompanied by significantly higher placental mRNA expression of neutral, cationic, and branched-chain amino acid transporters in IGF versus saline groups, suggesting increasing placental amino acid transport capacity.

IGF Gene Therapy in Cell Culture

The possibility of using placental IGF gene therapy has been demonstrated *in vitro* using two different placental cell lines. Adenoviral vectors expressing IGF-I (Ad.IGF-I) and IGF-II (Ad.IGF-II) both successfully transduced human primary placental fibroblasts (PPFs) [46]. Transduced PPFs showed significantly increased proliferation and cell migration compared with non-transduced controls, as well as significantly reduced apoptosis compared with cells transduced by adenoviral vectors expressing antisense IGF-I and –II. Transduction of the BeWo choriocarcinoma cell line by Ad.IGF-I also resulted in significantly increased proliferation and significantly less apoptosis compared with the control vector Ad.LacZ [47]. Ad.IGF-I transduction also resulted in a significantly greater uptake of the amino acids 2-methylaminoisobutyric acid (MeAIB) and leucine, significantly higher mRNA expression of the sodium coupled neutral amino acid transporters (SNATs) 1 and 2 and the large neutral amino acid transporter 1 (LAT1), and significantly increased protein expression of SNAT2 compared with transfection by Ad.LacZ [47]. A similar pattern was seen in relation to glucose transport, with a significant increase in mRNA expression of glucose transporter (GLUT) 8 and protein expression of GLUT1, 3, and 8 in cells transduced by Ad.IGF-I compared with Ad.LacZ [48].

IGF Gene Therapy in a Mouse Model of FGR

The *in vivo* effects of placental IGF gene therapy have also been studied in a mouse model of uteroplacental insufficiency. At laparotomy at day 18 of gestation (term = 19–21 days), one of the two mesenteric branches of the uterine artery (MUAL) supplying a given gestational sac is selectively ligated, thereby reducing uteroplacental blood flow [49]. This insult resulted in an 11% reduction in mean pup birth weight, significantly reduced depth and volume of the placental labyrinth, and significantly reduced placental expression of IGF-I and -II compared with sham surgery. Placental protein expression of LAT1, LAT2, and GLUT8 is also significantly reduced at 20 days' gestation following MUAL compared with sham surgery [47,48]. Direct intraplacental injection of Ad.IGF-I at the time of MUAL significantly increased expression of these transporters compared to MUAL alone or MUAL combined with Ad.LacZ administration, and resulted in levels comparable to the sham surgery control group.

Taken as a whole, the research in this area suggests that increasing IGF levels has the potential to improve fetal growth and that gene therapy may be a mechanism through which this could be achieved, either through direct placental administration or potentially maternal administration. However, further work is needed to demonstrate the effects of IGF gene therapy on fetal growth.

The Ethics of Gene Therapy in Pregnancy

When considering the ethical issues around a medical intervention, one important aspect is the balance of risks and benefits [50]. As with any new therapeutic modality, the risks of maternal or placental gene therapy are not well characterized, and in most cases the efficacy is still to be determined. In 1999 the U.S. National Institute for Health (NIH) Recombinant DNA Advisory Committee laid out the minimum criteria that should be met in order for fetal gene therapy to be considered ethically acceptable; these principles could equally be applied to maternal or placental gene therapy [4]. The Committee recommended that treatment be limited to diseases with serious fetal or neonatal morbidity and mortality, which either had no effective postnatal therapy or a poor outcome despite available postnatal therapies. Furthermore, the disease should be definitively diagnosed *in utero*, have a well-defined genotype/phenotype relationship, and have an animal model for *in utero* gene transfer that recapitulates the human disease. Finally, the proposed gene therapy should correct all serious abnormalities. At that time fetal gene therapy was felt to be ethically unacceptable, in part because of concerns about fetal safety and side effects such as germline transmission. Whether a maternal or placental gene therapy is transmitted to the fetus will therefore be a key issue; this will be discussed later in this chapter.

The ethical and social acceptability of maternal gene therapy for FGR has been explored in a qualitative study, using semi-structured interviews carried out in four European countries: Germany, Spain, Sweden, and the UK [51]. Thirty-four stakeholders from professional medical bodies, patient support groups, and disability groups were interviewed, along with 24 women or couples who had experienced a previous pregnancy affected by severe early-onset FGR (Table 16.2). The idea of giving an intervention to a pregnant woman for the benefit of the fetus was felt to be acceptable, and well established in current medical practice. There was concern from stakeholders that decision-making would be challenging for women at an already psychologically stressful time. The importance of independent advice and an ongoing process of achieving informed consent were highlighted to help address this. The women, however, felt that they would have been able to make a decision about trial participation, often after discussion with their family. The fact that the proposed trial involved gene therapy was only an issue for some of the German stakeholders, who felt that this would not be acceptable to women. However, this was not borne out by any of the interviews with women in Germany. Overall the proposed trial was viewed in positive terms both by stakeholders and women.

Safety

As previously stated, in the translation of gene therapy for FGR from the laboratory to the clinic, safety to both the pregnant woman and the fetus will be of central importance.

Maternal Safety

Side effects of gene therapy may relate to the vector, for example, an immune response to an adenoviral

147

Table 16.2 Ethical issues about maternal gene therapy in pregnancy identified through qualitative stakeholder and patient interviews

Issues	Stakeholders	Patients
Who is the patient?	Broad range of attitudes: "the fetus has no legal status" "the fetus has a moral status"	For most patients the fetus was a person: "my baby"
Maternal treatment for fetal benefit	Treatment should be permissible, after careful consideration of the balance of risks and benefits.	Mother and baby's lives are intertwined. Decision to take part depends on the risk of the treatment.
Making a decision in an FGR pregnancy about trial participation	Concerned about the psychological stress put on the mother.	Most women felt able to make a decision at the time of diagnosis Discussed with family members and healthcare team. Need time to make rational decision.
Survival of fetus with disability	Not a new concept and applicable to most prenatal interventions.	Acceptable as long as disability is not due to the treatment itself.
Challenges of informed consent	Emphasized the need for independent advice for participants.	Almost all women would involve their partner.
Acceptability of gene therapy	The novelty of gene therapy was not a concern. The exception was stakeholders from Germany, where there is a negative societal view of gene therapy.	Most had a spontaneous positive reaction to a trial of a novel treatment. There were no concerns about the use of gene therapy.

vector, or to the transgenic protein, for example, the theoretical risk of malignancy or retinopathy with over-expression of VEGF. Numerous clinical trials of Ad.VEGF have been carried out in patients with peripheral vascular disease and coronary artery disease. In the 226 patients for whom short-term outcomes of Ad.VEGF have been reported, there were no serious or severe adverse events; two patients experienced a transitory rise in liver enzymes and 23 patients experienced fever. Long-term follow-up was carried out after a median of 8.1 years in 37 patients who had received intracoronary Ad.VEGF-A121 [52] and a median of 11.8 years in another 31 patients who received intramyocardial Ad.VEGF-A165 [53]. Both studies found no increase above the background incidence for mortality, new cancer diagnoses, or new diagnoses of retinopathy.

Placental Toxicity

When using gene therapy in pregnancy, particularly with intraplacental administration, the direct effects on placental tissue must also be considered. One potential side effect of using an adenoviral vector would be a local inflammatory response, manifest as an increase in placental macrophages and T cells. No such response was seen following administration of Ad.VEGF into the uterine arteries of pregnant rabbits

[54]. The findings of studies using human placentas and placental tissue have also been largely reassuring. Exposure of human placental villous explants to high-dose adenoviral vectors for 60 minutes did not produce a rise in human chorionic gonadotrophin (hCG) or lactate dehydrogenase (LDH), both of which can be released by cell damage [55]. Furthermore, *ex vivo* dual perfusion of human placentas, where the maternal cotyledon was exposed to Ad.VEGF, showed no adverse effect on placental permeability [55]. LDH levels remained significantly higher in placentas exposed to Ad.VEGF than those exposed to formulation buffer, but there was no difference in levels of hCG or alkaline phosphatase, making the clinical significance of this finding uncertain.

Placental Transfer

Significant transfer of a gene therapy across the placenta to the fetus would be undesirable, as it would carry the risk of germline transmission and may have adverse effects on fetal development. Current evidence suggests that the extent of placental transfer depends on the vector, the animal, the route of administration, and the gestation at which it is administered. Following direct intraplacental administration of adenoviral vectors, the majority of preclinical studies have found evidence of transfer to the fetus and the dam [56–60]. Maternal intravascular gene therapy using an adenoviral vector has been shown to produce transgenic protein expression in the placenta, but not the fetus, when given to pregnant sheep [19,20], mice [10], and guinea pigs [61]. In contrast, the same vector given by the same route resulted in transduction of both the placenta and the fetus when given to rabbits [54], or in multiple doses to rats [58]. Exposure of human placental villous explants to high-dose adenoviral vector showed that, where the syncytiotrophoblast was deficient, there was occasional transduction of the underlying cytotrophoblast, but no evidence of the vector crossing the basement membrane [55].

Delivery Method

In the preclinical studies of Ad.VEGF, local delivery to the uterine arteries has been achieved either by direct injection combined with proximal occlusion of the vessel or by application of a thermolabile Pluronic gel. In translation to clinical practice this could be replicated using a balloon catheter, introduced into each uterine artery in turn using x-ray-guided interventional radiology. This technique has been used for more than 30 years to treat fibroids and manage postpartum hemorrhage. It is now being used increasingly during pregnancy, with catheters and deflated balloons placed into the uterine arteries before Caesarean section when heavy bleeding is anticipated [62,63].

The preclinical studies of Ad.IGF-I have used direct intraplacental injection. This could be easily replicated in the clinical setting under ultrasound guidance, with a similar technique to chorionic villus sampling or amniocentesis. However, it is unclear whether intraplacental administration of a gene therapy would carry the same risk of miscarriage as these invasive diagnostic procedures, which is generally quoted as 1–2% [64].

Clinical Translation

Translating a novel therapeutic into the clinic requires a multidisciplinary team approach, including experts in the clinical and scientific aspects of the therapy, reproductive toxicology, regulatory affairs, and the business of experimental medicine. Early phase trials, which assess the safety of new interventions, are rare in pregnancy, in part because of underinvestment by the pharmaceutical industry in the development of new obstetric therapies [65]. This means that much

of the framework for such trials, which is well developed in other specialties like oncology, is lacking in obstetrics. Because gene therapy is an advanced therapy medicinal product (ATMP), its use is subject to specific guidelines and regulations from the European Medicines Agency (EMA) committee for advanced therapeutics (CAT), and the national competent authorities, such as the Medicines and Healthcare products Regulatory Agency (MHRA) in the UK.

Regulatory Approval

In Europe, marketing authorization for ATMPs is provided by the EMA Committee for Medicinal Products for Human Use. Such authorization requires a package of preclinical studies and clinical trials that demonstrate the safety, quality, and efficacy of the product. Early phase clinical trials, to demonstrate the safety of a product, are followed by larger trials, to demonstrate therapeutic efficacy. Within the UK all clinical trials of investigational medicinal products must receive approval from a Research Ethics Committee and from the MHRA. Similar systems are in place in other European countries, and from 2009 the Voluntary Harmonisation Procedure means that trials carried out in more than one European country can apply to the EMA for approval, rather than the national competent authorities. As yet no national ethics committee or competent authority has been asked to consider a trial of gene therapy administered to the mother or placenta as a potential treatment for FGR. A key part of any such application would be preclinical toxicology data.

Reproductive Toxicology

Before a gene therapy can be used for the first time in humans, preclinical evidence should be available on the bio-distribution and toxicity of the product [66]. These studies should use an appropriate animal model, which for obstetric diseases must include consideration of the placental structure and stages of fetal development. They should also replicate the anticipated route of administration, and use a dose that incorporates an appropriate safety margin. For clinical trials involving pregnant women, female reproductive toxicology studies must also have been completed [67]. These studies must also use a relevant animal model and dosing regimen to investigate the effects on pre- and postnatal development, including maternal function [68].

Conclusion

As research continues to uncover the physiological and pathophysiological processes that occur during pregnancy, new therapeutic possibilities become apparent. Such possibilities include the use of maternal or placental gene therapy to treat obstetric diseases. VEGF gene therapy administered into the maternal uterine arteries and either maternal or placental IGF gene therapy may provide treatment for fetal growth restriction caused by uteroplacental insufficiency. These potential therapies have yet to be translated from the laboratory into the clinic, a process that will be complicated by the lack of early phase clinical research in obstetrics. Drawing on expertise from a range of key disciplines will increase the chance of successfully developing these and other obstetric therapies, thereby providing pregnant women with new therapeutic possibilities.

Key Points

- Gene therapy can be used to produce short-term expression of a therapeutic transgenic protein.

- Maternal and placental gene therapy may be useful mechanisms for delivering treatment in a range of obstetric diseases, including fetal growth restriction.

- Adenoviral VEGF gene therapy administered via the maternal uterine arteries increases fetal growth velocity in a sheep model of FGR.

- Placental IGF gene therapy may also prove therapeutic in FGR by improving placental transfer of glucose and amino acids.

- Translating gene therapy for an obstetric disease from the laboratory to the clinic poses many challenges, and requires multidisciplinary expertise.

- The ethical and social acceptability of using gene therapy in pregnancy will be influenced by the risks to the mother and the fetus, including the potential for placental transfer.

References

1. David AL, Peebles D. Gene therapy for the fetus: Is there a future? *Best Pract Res Clin Obstet Gynaecol* 2008;22(1):203–18.

2. Mattar CN, Waddington SN, Biswas A, Davidoff AM, Choolani M, Chan JKY, et al. The case for intrauterine gene therapy. *Best Pract Res Clin Obstet Gynaecol* 2012;26(5):697–709.

3. Gene Therapy Advisory Committee. Report on the potential use of gene therapy in utero. Health Departments of the United Kingdom, November 1998. *Hum Gene Ther* 1999;10(4):689–92.

4. U. S. National Institutes of Health. Recombinant DNA Advisory Committee. Prenatal gene transfer: Scientific, medical, and ethical issues: A report of the Recombinant DNA Advisory Committee. *Hum Gene Ther* 2000;11(8):1211–29.

5. Lyall F, Robson SC, Bulmer JN. Spiral artery remodeling and trophoblast invasion in preeclampsia and fetal growth restriction: Relationship to clinical outcome. *Hypertension* 2013;62(6):1046–54.

6. Konje JC, Howarth ES, Kaufmann P, Taylor DJ. Longitudinal quantification of uterine artery blood volume flow changes during gestation in pregnancies complicated by intrauterine growth restriction. *BJOG* 2003;110(3):301–5.

7. Ginn SL, Alexander IE, Edelstein ML, Abedi MR, Wixon J. Gene therapy clinical trials worldwide to 2012 – an update. *J Gene Med* 2013;15(2):65–77.

8. Coutelle C, Waddington SN. Vector systems for prenatal gene therapy: Choosing vectors for different applications. *Methods Mol Biol* 2012;891:41–53.

9. Khare R, Chen CY, Weaver EA, Barry MA. Advances and future challenges in adenoviral vector pharmacology and targeting. *Curr Gene Ther* 2011;11(4):241–58.

10. Katayama K, Furuki R, Yokoyama H, Kaneko M, Tachibana M, Yoshida I, et al. Enhanced in vivo gene transfer into the placenta using RGD fiber-mutant adenovirus vector *Biomaterials* 2011;32(17):4185–93.

11. Al-Hendy A, Salama S. Gene therapy and uterine leiomyoma: A review. *Hum Reprod Update* 2006;12(4):385–400.

12. Stribley JM, Rehman KS, Niu H, Christman GM. Gene therapy and reproductive medicine. *Fertil Steril* 2002;77(4):645–57.

13. Ahmed A, Dunk C, Ahmad S, Khaliq A. Regulation of placental vascular endothelial growth factor (VEGF) and placenta growth factor (PlGF) and soluble Flt-1 by oxygen – a review. *Placenta* 2000;21 Suppl A:S16–24.

14. Olsson AK, Dimberg A, Kreuger J, Claesson-Welsh L. VEGF receptor signalling – in control of vascular function. *Nat Rev Mol Cell Biol* 2006;7(5):359–71.

15. Savvidou MD, Yu CK, Harland LC, Hingorani AD, Nicolaides KH. Maternal serum concentration of soluble fms-like tyrosine kinase 1 and vascular endothelial growth factor in women with abnormal uterine artery Doppler and in those with fetal growth restriction. *Am J Obstet Gynecol* 2006;195(6):1668–73.

16. Herraiz I, Droge LA, Gomez-Montes E, Henrich W, Galindo A, Verlohren S. Characterization of the soluble fms-like tyrosine kinase-1 to placental growth factor ratio in pregnancies complicated by fetal growth restriction. *Obstet Gynecol* 2014;124(2 Pt 1):265–73.

17. Roberts CT, Owens JA, Sferruzzi-Perri AN. Distinct actions of insulin-like growth factors (IGFs) on placental development and fetal growth: Lessons from mice and guinea pigs. *Placenta* 2008;29 Suppl A:S42–7.

18. Forbes K, Westwood M. The IGF axis and placental function. A mini review. *Horm Res* 2008; 69(3):129–37.

19. David AL, Torondel B, Zachary I, Wigley V, Abi-Nader K, Mehta V, et al. Local delivery of VEGF adenovirus to the uterine artery increases vasorelaxation and uterine blood flow in the pregnant sheep. *Gene Ther* 2008;15(19):1344–50.

20. Mehta V, Abi-Nader KN, Peebles DM, Benjamin E, Wigley V, Torondel B, et al. Long-term increase in uterine blood flow is achieved by local overexpression of VEGF-A(165) in the uterine arteries of pregnant sheep. *Gene Ther* 2012;19(9):925–35.

21. Mehta V, Abi-Nader KN, Shangaris P, Shaw SW, Filippi E, Benjamin E, et al. Local over-expression of VEGF-DDeltaNDeltaC in the uterine arteries of pregnant sheep results in long-term changes in uterine artery contractility and angiogenesis. *PloS One* 2014; 9(6):e100021.

22. Wallace JM, Luther JS, Milne JS, Aitken RP, Redmer DA, Reynolds LP, et al. Nutritional modulation of adolescent pregnancy outcome – a review. *Placenta* 2006;27 Suppl A:S61–8.

23. Robinson JS, Kingston EJ, Jones CT, Thorburn GD. Studies on experimental growth retardation in sheep. The effect of removal of a endometrial caruncles on fetal size and metabolism. *J Dev Physiol* 1979; 1(5):379–98.

24. Wallace JM, Aitken RP, Milne JS, Hay WW, Jr. Nutritionally mediated placental growth restriction in the growing adolescent: Consequences for the fetus. *Biol Reprod* 2004;71(4):1055–62.

25. Wallace JM, Milne JS, Matsuzaki M, Aitken RP. Serial measurement of uterine blood flow from mid to late gestation in growth restricted pregnancies induced by overnourishing adolescent sheep dams. *Placenta* 2008;29(8):718–24.

26. Wallace JM, Bourke DA, Aitken RP, Palmer RM, Da Silva P, Cruickshank MA. Relationship between nutritionally-mediated placental growth restriction and fetal growth, body composition and endocrine status during late gestation in adolescent sheep. *Placenta* 2000;21(1):100–8.

27. Carr DJ, Aitken RP, Milne JS, David AL, Wallace JM. Fetoplacental biometry and umbilical artery Doppler velocimetry in the overnourished adolescent model of fetal growth restriction. *Am J Obstet Gynecol* 2012; 207(2):141.

28. Redmer DA, Aitken RP, Milne JS, Reynolds LP, Wallace JM. Influence of maternal nutrition on messenger RNA expression of placental angiogenic factors and their receptors at midgestation in adolescent sheep. *Biol Reprod* 2005;72(4):1004–9.

29. Redmer DA, Luther JS, Milne JS, Aitken RP, Johnson ML, Borowicz PP, et al. Fetoplacental growth and vascular development in overnourished adolescent sheep at day 50, 90 and 130 of gestation. *Reproduction* 2009;137(4):749–57.

30. Lea RG, Wooding P, Stewart I, Hannah LT, Morton S, Wallace K, et al. The expression of ovine placental lactogen, StAR and progesterone-associated steroidogenic enzymes in placentae of overnourished growing adolescent ewes. *Reproduction* 2007; 133(4):785–96.

31. Carr DJ, Aitken RP, Milne JS, David AL, Wallace JM. Ultrasonographic assessment of growth and estimation of birthweight in late gestation fetal sheep. *Ultrasound Med Biol* 2011;37(10):1588–95.

32. Smith GC, Smith MF, McNay MB, Fleming JE. The relation between fetal abdominal circumference and birthweight: Findings in 3512 pregnancies. *BJOG* 1997;104(2):186–90.

33. Carr DJ, Aitken RP, Milne JS, Peebles DM, Martin JM, Zachary IC, et al. Prenatal Ad.VEGF gene therapy – a promising new treatment for fetal growth restriction. *Hum Gene Ther* 2011;22(10):A128.

34. Carr DJ, Aitken RP, Milne JS, Peebles DM, Martin JM, Zachary IC, et al. Maternal delivery of Ad.VEGF gene therapy increases fetal growth velocity in an ovine paradigm of fetal growth restriction. *Reprod Sci* 2011; 18(3 suppl):269A.

35. Carr DJ, Aitken RP, Milne JS, Peebles DM, Martin JM, Zachary IC, et al. Alterations in postnatal growth and metabolism following prenatal treatment of intrauterine growth restriction with Ad.VEGF gene therapy in the sheep. *Arch Dis Child Fetal Neonatal Ed* 2011;96:Fa7.

36. Carr DJ, Aitken RP, Milne JS, Peebles DM, Martin JF, Zachary IC, et al. Prenatal gene therapy increases fetal growth velocity and expression of VEGF receptors in

an ovine paradigm of fetal growth restriction. *Reprod Sci* 2012;19(3):78A.

37. Carter AM. Animal models of human placentation – a review. *Placenta* 2007;28 Suppl A:S41–7.

38. Mess A. The Guinea pig placenta: Model of placental growth dynamics. *Placenta* 2007;28(8–9):812–15.

39. Roberts CT, Sohlstrom A, Kind KL, Earl RA, Khong TY, Robinson JS, et al. Maternal food restriction reduces the exchange surface area and increases the barrier thickness of the placenta in the guinea-pig. *Placenta* 2001;22(2–3):177–85.

40. Mehta V, Boyd M, Martin J, Zachary I, Peebles DM, David AL. Local administration of Ad.VEGF-A165 to the uteroplacental circulation enhances fetal growth and reduces brain sparing in an FGR model of guinea pig pregnancy. *Reprod Sci* 2012;19(3):78A.

41. Sferruzzi-Perri AN, Owens JA, Pringle KG, Robinson JS, Roberts CT. Maternal insulin-like growth factors-I and -II act via different pathways to promote fetal growth. *Endocrinology* 2006;147(7):3344–55.

42. Sferruzzi-Perri AN, Owens JA, Standen P, Taylor RL, Heinemann GK, Robinson JS, et al. Early treatment of the pregnant guinea pig with IGFs promotes placental transport and nutrient partitioning near term. *Am J Physiol Endocrinol Metab* 2007;292(3):E668–76.

43. Sohlstrom A, Fernberg P, Owens JA, Owens PC. Maternal nutrition affects the ability of treatment with IGF-I and IGF-II to increase growth of the placenta and fetus, in guinea pigs. *Growth Horm IGF Res* 2001; 11(6):392–8.

44. Eremia SC, de Boo HA, Bloomfield FH, Oliver MH, Harding JE. Fetal and amniotic insulin-like growth factor-I supplements improve growth rate in intrauterine growth restriction fetal sheep. *Endocrinology* 2007;148(6):2963–72.

45. Wali JA, de Boo HA, Derraik JG, Phua HH, Oliver MH, Bloomfield FH, et al. Weekly intra-amniotic IGF-1 treatment increases growth of growth-restricted ovine fetuses and up-regulates placental amino acid transporters. *PLoS One* 2012;7(5):e37899.

46. Miller AG, Aplin JD, Westwood M. Adenovirally mediated expression of insulin-like growth factors enhances the function of first trimester placental fibroblasts. *J Clin Endocrinol Metab* 2005; 90(1):379–85.

47. Jones H, Crombleholme T, Habli M. Regulation of amino acid transporters by adenoviral-mediated human insulin-like growth factor-1 in a mouse model of placental insufficiency in vivo and the human trophoblast line BeWo in vitro. *Placenta* 2014; 35(2):132–8.

48. Jones HN, Crombleholme T, Habli M. Adenoviral-mediated placental gene transfer of IGF-1 corrects

49. Habli M, Jones H, Aronow B, Omar K, Crombleholme TM. Recapitulation of characteristics of human placental vascular insufficiency in a novel mouse model. *Placenta* 2013;34(12):1150–8.

50. David AL, Ashcroft R. Placental gene therapy. *Obstet Gynaecol Reprod Med* 2009;19(10):296–8.

51. Sheppard MK, Spencer RN, David AL, Ashcroft R. Evaluation of the ethics and social acceptability of a proposed clinical trial using maternal gene therapy to treat severe early-onset fetal growth restriction in pregnant women. *Hum Gene Ther* 2014:A98.

52. Hedman M, Muona K, Hedman A, Kivela A, Syvanne M, Eranen J, et al. Eight-year safety follow-up of coronary artery disease patients after local intracoronary VEGF gene transfer. *Gene Ther* 2009; 16(5):629–34.

53. Rosengart TK, Bishawi MM, Halbreiner MS, Fakhoury M, Finnin E, Hollmann C, et al. Long-term follow-up assessment of a phase 1 trial of angiogenic gene therapy using direct intramyocardial administration of an adenoviral vector expressing the VEGF121 cDNA for the treatment of diffuse coronary artery disease. *Hum Gene Ther* 2013;24(2):203–8.

54. Heikkila A, Hiltunen MO, Turunen MP, Keski-Nisula L, Turunen AM, Rasanen H, et al. Angiographically guided utero-placental gene transfer in rabbits with adenoviruses, plasmid/liposomes and plasmid/polyethyleneimine complexes. *Gene Ther* 2001; 8(10):784–8.

55. Brownbill P, Desforges M, Sebire N, Greenwood S, Sibley CP, David A. Human placental ex vivo studies to support an adenovirus-mediated vascular endothelial growth factor (VEGF) gene medicine for the treatment of severe early onset fetal growth restriction (FGR). *Hum Gene Ther* 2014;25(11):A60.

56. Woo YJ, Raju GP, Swain JL, Richmond ME, Gardner TJ, Balice-Gordon RJ. In utero cardiac gene transfer via intraplacental delivery of recombinant adenovirus. *Circulation* 1997;96(10):3561–9.

57. Turkay A, Saunders T, Kurachi K. Intrauterine gene transfer: Gestational stage-specific gene delivery in mice. *Gene Ther* 1999;6(10):1685–94.

58. Xing A, Boileau P, Cauzac M, Challier JC, Girard J, Hauguel-de Mouzon S. Comparative in vivo approaches for selective adenovirus-mediated gene delivery to the placenta. *Hum Gene Ther* 2000; 11(1):167–77.

59. Senoo M, Matsubara Y, Fujii K, Nagasaki Y, Hiratsuka M, Kure S, et al. Adenovirus-mediated in utero gene transfer in mice and guinea pigs: tissue distribution of recombinant adenovirus determined by quantitative

TaqMan-polymerase chain reaction assay. *Mol Genet Metab* 2000;69(4):269–76.

60. Katz AB, Keswani SG, Habli M, Lim FY, Zoltick PW, Midrio P, et al. Placental gene transfer: Transgene screening in mice for trophic effects on the placenta. *Am J Obstet Gynecol* 2009;201(5):499.e1–8.

61. Mehta V, Peebles DM, Boyd M, Zachary I, Martin J, David AL. Gene targeting to the utero-placental circulation of pregnant guinea pigs. Society for Gynaecologic Investigation 58th Annual Meeting: Reproductive Sciences; 2011. p. 332A.

62. Mok M, Heidemann B, Dundas K, Gillespie I, Clark V. Interventional radiology in women with suspected placenta accreta undergoing caesarean section. *Int J Obstet Anesth* 2008;17(3):255–61.

63. Carnevale FC, Kondo MM, de Oliveira Sousa W, Jr., Santos AB, da Motta Leal Filho JM, Moreira AM, et al. Perioperative temporary occlusion of the internal iliac arteries as prophylaxis in cesarean section at risk of hemorrhage in placenta accreta. *Cardiovasc Intervent Radiol* 2011;34(4):758–64.

64. Alfirevic Z, Sundberg K, Brigham S. Amniocentesis and chorionic villus sampling for prenatal diagnosis. *Cochrane Database Syst Rev* 2003(3):CD003252.

65. Wing DA, Powers B, Hickok D. U.S. Food and Drug Administration drug approval: Slow advances in obstetric care in the United States. *Obstet Gynecol* 2010;115(4):825–33.

66. European Medicines Agency. *Guideline on the Non-clinical Studies Required before First Clinical Use of Gene Therapy Medicinal Products (EMEA/CHMP/GTWP/125459/2006).* London: European Medicines Agency; 2008.

67. European Medicines Agency. *ICH Harmonised Tripartite Guideline E6: Note for Guidance on Good Clinical Practice (PMP/ICH/135/95).* London: European Medicines Agency; 2002.

68. European Medicines Agency. *Detection of Toxicity to Reproduction for Medicinal Products and Toxicity to Male Fertility (CPMP/ICH/386/95).* London: European Medicines Agency; 1994.

Blood Flow Volume in Umbilical Vein in Fetal Growth Restriction

Enrico Ferrazzi, Daniela Di Martino, and Tamara Stampalija

Introduction

The phrase "blood flow volume" is likely to raise concern for the reader: "flow volume" in the umbilical vein, is dangerously close to "physiology." The serendipitous results of physiological studies however have the potential to reach the bedside and impact clinical algorithms and, in the case of umbilical vein blood flow volume measurements, moving blood flow measurements further from bench to bedside. Ultrasound imaging and Doppler mode are so accurate (close to the real thing) and precise (reproducible under different conditions) that they can beat traditional methodologies adopted in animal experiments adopted for 100 years by bench physiologists. All the beauty of accuracy and precision is now packed in a 3-minute bedside measurement at any fetomaternal unit.

Controlled Burning of Carbon Chains to Get Energy for Life

To allow a living being to grow, especially at the rapidity of a developing fetus, unrestricted availability of energy is essential. The energy in eukaryotic cells is represented by adenosine tri phosphate (ATP). When for each chain of six carbon atoms (glucose, for instance) there are four molecules of oxygen (O_2x4), the molecular machines of our cells can ideally produce 36 ATPs. In reality, the efficiency of the molecular machines bring this down to 30.

A small number, just two ATPs, is produced by splitting the glucose into two pieces of three carbon atoms (pyruvate) – this is called glycolysis (step 1). This occurs in the cytoplasm. Then, if O_2 is available, the rest of the three carbon chains are moved and processed inside the mitochondria as Acetyl-CoA, in other words, pyruvate that loses a carbon with a drop (one single molecule) of O_2, and here we are with oxygen. The mitochondria are the eukaryotic cells' partners with extraordinary molecular machines that burn

short carbon chains plus O_2, to make the rest of the ATPs. This is the Krebs Cycle, or oxidative phosphorylation or citric acid cycle (step 2) (Figure 17.1). The waste products of these two steps are water and carbon dioxide (CO_2): put the water back in the plasma and breath CO_2 out.

Fatty acids are made of carbon chains as well, and are a good source of energy via oxidation to Acetyl-CoA. Carbon chains of amino acids can be also catabolized when other sources of energy are missing (an analogy is burning a table and chairs to warm up a dining room).

Energy Sources When Oxygen Is Poorly Available

In absence of O_2, as on Earth before cyanobacteria produced the huge amount of O_2 we boast in our atmosphere nowadays, carbon chains are burnt only to pyruvate to produce just two ATPs. Next, the pyruvate is reduced to lactate, a waste product of anaerobic glycolysis that can be found in various conditions: we feel it in our muscles after running too much; or it can be measured in the umbilical artery blood after a baby is delivered a bit "too late" for its energy metabolism to withstand hypoxia; or we might sample the umbilical blood in utero, in a severely growth-restricted fetus with an abnormal fetal heart rate short-term variation [1].

Which Method of Measurement of Blood Flow Volume Is the Right One?

We are fortunate that the fetus opted for a single cord instead of a network of vessels so now we can measure the blood flow volume that brings supplies for its growth. Umbilical venous blood flow volume determines the rate of fetal O_2 delivery and energy metabolism. Thus, it is among the most basic bits of information concerning the physiology of human

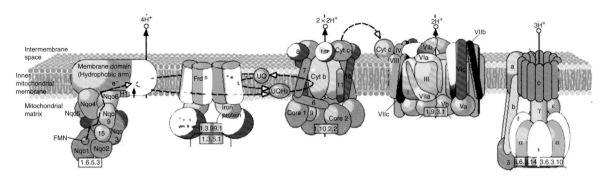

Figure 17.1 This diagram shows the beauty of the molecular machinery that eukaryotes inherited some time ago and put into our cells, the mitochondria being a free highly productive engine. The most striking machinery is on the far right, the ATP synthase, moved by hydrogen protons that at any turn produces ATP, to make 32 from each Acetyl-CoA entered into the mitochondria matrix.

intrauterine life. The delivery of O_2 substantially is parallel to that of nutrients, even though these are subject to active transfer through the placenta (i.e., amino acids and lipids) or to gradient diffusion (i.e., glucose).

Each methodology to measure umbilical venous blood flow volume so far adopted has proved to have good precision and reproducibility. However, there are major variations in absolute values. Each research group emphasizes its methodological merits, and it might be difficult to sort out which is which.

Accuracy of Measurements

The first step to approach this problem is probably to evaluate the accuracy of combining imaging, color Doppler, and Doppler velocimetry. This question has been tested independently by our group [2] and by Schmidt and coworkers [3]. Table 17.1 shows the comparison of measurements obtained by diffusion technique and combined color imaging, Doppler mode, and high-resolution imaging. The values obtained were well within the required accuracy. The accuracy of the triplex mode as described in Table 17.1 was further tested by evaluating the correlation between the vein flow volume and cotyledons' weight per vein. Fetal lambs live on two veins and fetal cotyledons are anatomically parted. Cotyledons can be counted and weighed, allowing us to observe a significant correlation between blood flow measured in each vein and the weight of perfused cotyledons ($r2 = 0.80$). The average absolute blood flow volume for the time interval of gestation of that study was 680 ml/min. Blood flow volume per unit fetal weight was 207ml/min/kg. This is in agreement with previous experimental data from the same laboratory [4] and others [5,6]. This is a magic value; it is twice the blood flow volume per kg measured in humans (approximately 120 ml/min/kg) for comparable gestational age. Fetal lambs reach their full weight (in average 3,400 grams), similar to human newborns, in 140 days, exactly half the duration of human gestation, which is 240 days; in other words, twice the flow volume to build up the same amount of tissues in half the time.

Schmidt [3] reported an overestimation of approximately 4% by Doppler technique. The sampling site chosen for the experiment was the intrahepatic portion of the umbilical vein. In his formula, Schmidt adopted the modal velocity and not the mean velocity. In slow venous flow, this can make a difference. In humans, the advantage of a single umbilical vein overturns the reasons why in most fetal lamb experiments, the best choice was the intrahepatic vein.

Umbilical Flow Volumes in the Human Fetus: Critical Methodological Issues

Work by Figueras [7] compares recent findings on umbilical venous flow volume. Figure 17.2, modified after Figueras [7], shows an apparently odd situation in which accuracy in experiments on animals (Table 17.1) reported by Galan [2] was pretty good, whereas measurement in humans appears to diverge substantially.

Figure 17.2 shows that there is recently reported data that are both close to each other (Barbera, Bellotti, and Tchirikov) and close to original data obtained in

Table 17.1 The left column shows the volume flow obtained by triplex mode in six fetal lambs between 126 and 136 days' gestation. The right column shows for each fetal lamb the values obtained by established steady state diffusion technique, a solid methodology adopted in animal experiments. The fetal lamb veins and arteries had been catheterized 5 days before as for a chronic preparation.

Sheep No.	Umbilical Vein Blood flow volume by ultrasound imaging and Doppler ml/min/kg	Umbilical Vein Blood flow volume by steady-state diffusion technique ml/min/kg
1	165.6	175.3
2	211.2	224.9
3	218.1	203.8
4	220.8	221.4
5	210.1	213.0
6	219.6	210.5
Mean ± SEM	205.5 ± 8.6	208.1 ± 7.3

the early 1980s by Gill, Eik Nes, and Van Lierde. We will call this group the "middle group." The data by Di Naro [8] are not reported in the figure because there is no equation published by this author whose mean reported value on 104 fetuses was 126/ml/min/kg. Data reported by Acharya and Kiserud on the intra-hepatic umbilical vein and by Boito on the umbilical vein lay close to each other. The upper outlier represents the data by Lees and coworkers.

Each one of these studies should require a strict methodological analysis. For instance, Acharya and Kiserud preferred as a sampling site the intrahepatic vein: the curved shape of the intrahepatic umbilical vein might cause problems to the angle of insonation of the Doppler beam. This might even be more difficult in small fetuses with little amniotic fluid. In addition to this, the umbilical insertion ring might randomly cause a turbulent flow due to differences in vein diameter between the intra-amniotic and intra-abdominal parts of the vessel, and due to the left liver lobe vein that branches at variable distance. Both Boito and Lees adopted the ellipsoid formula to measure the area of the vein on a cross-sectional plane: at 33 weeks' gestation, the authors reported areas in between $0.46cm^2$ and $0.43cm^2$. Those values are larger than the area reported by the "middle group." The mean velocity reported by Lees at 33 weeks' gestation is 10.8 cm/sec, very close to the "middle group," but alas multiplied by a large area times 60 makes probably an overfed

fetus. Opposite to this Boito decided to cut off a large part of the venous flow profile, adopting a sample volume (2–4mm) that does not interrogate the whole vessel lumen, and the reported automatically measured time-averaged velocities went down to 6.5cm/sec at 33 weeks' gestation.

Reconciliation of Physiological and Methodological Puzzles

It is very likely that this brief cross-examination makes the reader happy for the solution found in consistent data of the "middle group," but the excluded authors possibly unhappy for this short, subjective verdict. To help the verdict, a third-party support to the "middle group" derives from physiology. Oxygen concentration and partial pressure (pO_2) are well established both in human fetuses [9] and in fetal lambs [10]. Oxygen consumption is quite constant, and the theoretical difference between the mm of O_2 in the vein (approximately 6.6mm/dl) and in the arteries (4.4mm/dl, after the blood has delivered its content to the tissues) is well proved [11]. Values of umbilical vein blood flow volume reported by the "lower group" imply an arterial O_2 content (2.6 mm and 2.0 mm) and saturation (25% and 21%). Those values are found only in hypoxic fetuses.

The Simpler Methodology to Provide Accurate Measures of the Umbilical Venous Blood Flow Volume

Cross-sectional Area of the Umbilical Vein and Blood Flow Average Velocity

Figure 17.3 describes the procedure and shows the typical images to be obtained in order to measure the diameter of the vein, to visualize the same spot of the vessel by means of color imaging, to obtain a proper angle of insonation for the Doppler beam, and to obtain an adequate trace of the blood flow velocity. Present ultrasound technology allows us to optimize resolution with a procedure very similar to the one adopted for "nuchal translucency measurement."

The umbilical vein is a long vessel, and it is usually easy to find a linear segment that is at least three times as long as its diameter. This allows interrogation of a segment of the vessel with quasi-parabolic blood flow, where we can calculate the mean velocity

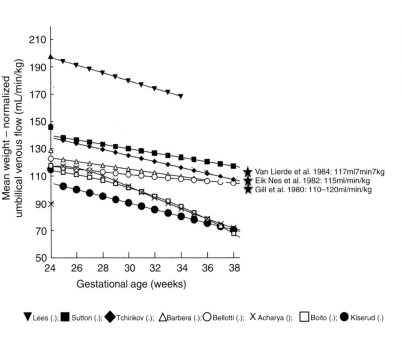

Figure 17.2 Umblical vein blood flow volume normalized per Kg of fetal weight in recent studies in human pregnancies. The text near the reported interpolating curves shows similar values obtained in the 1980s by different authors.

Van Lierde et al. 1984: 117ml7min7kg
Eik Nes et al. 1982: 115ml/min/kg
Gill et al. 1980: 110–120ml/min/kg

▼Lees (.); ■Sutton (.); ◆Tchirikov (.); △Barbera (.); ○Bellotti (.); ✕Acharya (); ☐Boito (.); ●Kiserud (.)

just by multiplying the average maximal velocity for 0.5. According to Pennati and coworkers [12], the vein flow is not exactly parabolic and the time-averaged peak velocity should be multiplied by 0.61 instead of 0.5. So far the consensus is on 0.5, and we adhere to this common value.

The Formula

The final value of umbilical vein blood flow volume is obtained by a very simple formula that includes the radius of the vessel (diameter/2 in cm), and the mean velocity (average peak velocity*0,5, in cm/sec) and time (one minute in seconds): (RxRx3,14)x(mean velocity)x60(sec).

Clinical Fallout of Physiological Background and Advanced Ultrasound Technology

Umbilical Vein Flow in FGR Fetuses with Abnormal Umbilical Pulsatility Index

Is there any use for umbilical vein blood flow in a clinical environment with a rooted efficient tradition to use Doppler waveform analysis on the arterial side of the circulation?

The good news is that all pilot studies found umbilical vein blood flow volume lower in FGR than in appropriate-for-gestational age (AGA) fetuses. These findings are independent from the methodology and possible systematic errors (precise but inaccurate methodologies). The bad news is that its value in these few severe cases is limited on clinical grounds.

Early and severe growth-restricted fetuses show well-established abnormal umbilical artery flow impedance indices. Its methodology of measure is foolproof, and its value eventually hit the guidelines and recommendations after 30 years of pilot studies and clinical and randomized trials. All this proof of principle is strongly correlated with placental impedance, usually a result of first trimester severe shallow trophoblastic invasion [13]. The key concept here is "severe."

These fetuses live in utero in a condition of relatively livable hypoxia as proved by high lactate concentration [14] due to partly aerobic but already partly anaerobic energy metabolism. This explains why meta-analysis of randomized trials proved the clinical efficacy of Doppler velocimetry [15]. In these severe cases (less than 1% of human pregnancies), the umbilical vein blood flow assessment might help on clinical grounds only to understand which fetuses might not make it in utero until a gestational age and weight with reasonable chances of extra-uterine survival [16]. We proved

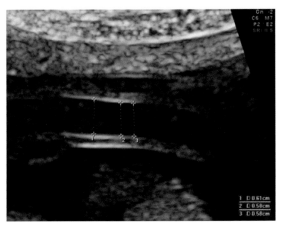 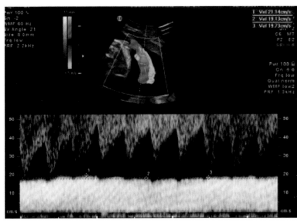

Figure 17.3 Left Panel: the area of interest (not just a digital enlargement of the whole section) is set as soon as we visualize a linear segment of the vein, three times as long as its diameter. The bright edges correspond exactly to the midsection of the vein, where the ultrasound beam is reflected and not diffracted. Three to five inner-to-inner calipers are set and averaged.

Right Panel: the color imaging is switched on at 5cm/sec, the transducer is tilted on the same spot of the vein ideally at 90°, but never less than 30°, the sample volume is set at 6 to 12 cm, depending on gestational age to include the whole lumen. The mean peak velocity is calculated.

that in extremely severe cases prior to 24 weeks' gestation, when not only the umbilical vein flow is below the norm, but also the diameter normalized for the abdominal circumference is below the norm, then the *qoad vitae* prognosis in utero is unfavorably determined.

The real clinical help of umbilical vein blood flow at the bedside is the possibility to understand fetal adaptation to progressive under-nutrition and poor oxygenation and what is happening downstream the umbilical vein. In fact, in normal pregnancies, the umbilical vein blood flow goes partly to the liver and partly directly to the right heart via ductus venosus. At mid-gestation, the percentage of flow through the ductus venosus had been estimated in between 30–40% and at 36 weeks' gestation between 15–20% [17,18].

The ductus venosus, thanks to its peculiar shape (Venturi trumpet-shaped shunt), accelerates blood from the umbilical vein straight to the median part of the right atrium. The velocity in the umbilical vein is approximately 16cm/sec; the velocity in the DV reaches 70cm/sec thanks to this hemodynamics. The ductus sucks out blood from the umbilical vein more in the first half than in the second half of pregnancy.

Under conditions of hypoxia, the inlet dilates [19] the Venturi effect is reduced in a way that velocities are decreased [20], but, since the volume flow is the squared value of the cross-section, the overall flow is increased [21,22] (Figure 17.4). This is the last compensatory mechanism that a severe FGR can deploy to protect the heart and the cerebral circulation, increasing the shunt of oxygenated placental blood. Acharya speculated that this phenomenon, when associated with the abnormal right atrial function, further reduces a-wave by the increased atrial pressure.

The paradox of this Venturi effect of the ductus venosus is that under hypoxic conditions, it sucks out blood even from the right liver lobe, and you can check it when you observe the reverse a-wave and when the pulsed Doppler sample gate is interrogating the right hepatic vein: that the flow does not go toward the lobe but from the lobe toward the hilum. Torvid and Bellotti measured the flow in the ductus venosus under these conditions, and it is higher than the umbilical vein flow. More simply, you can check the color flow of the right lobe when the ductus venosus is normal (full of angio color) and when the ductus venosus is a-wave reverse (very little angio color).

In these fetuses, glucose is burnt in an hypoxic environment at poor ATP output, lactic acid as a waste of step 1 glycolysis is increased, the fetus compensates with glicogenolysis and amino acid catabolism, and amino acidic nitrogen in the umbilical arteries might even be higher than the concentration in the vein [23]. Fetal cells are "burning the furniture to get energy to run the house"; the fetus will not grow any more, in case it might even lose lean mass, and some doctor in the ward may say that the last measurement of the fetal abdomen is wrong because it is smaller than 12 days before.

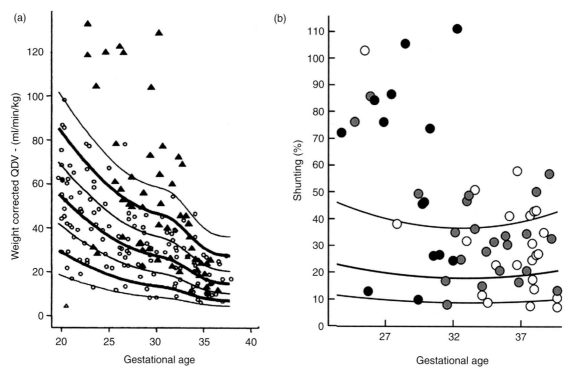

Figure 17.4 Flow volume through the ductus venosus in severe FGR versus AGA. Panel a) data from Bellotti (.) FGR fetuses with abnormal umbilical pulsatility index (black triangles) show a compensatory increase of flow in the days prior to delivery. Panel b) FGR fetuses with absent end diastolic flow (black dots) show a compensatory increase in flow prior to delivery. Both authors reported the same increase in DV inlet diameter and observed that this phenomenon occurs before 32–33 weeks' gestation and is never or very seldom observed later in gestation. The percentage of umbilical flow in a few cases is higher than 100% due to the reverse flow from the right hepatic vein into the ductus venosus. A consistent ductal dilatation was observed in studies during active uterine contractions in labor (unpublished data, MBellotti).

The Truffle randomized study proved that for short-term outcome, the measurement of the ductus venosus might compare to the computerized fetal heart rate analysis [24]. However, when long-term neurological performance at 2 years is concerned, those fetuses, recruited with an absent end diastolic flow and with an average weight of 980g, delivered because of an abnormal ductus venosus a-wave performed significantly better [25]. This might be explained by the compensatory mechanism that some fetuses activated before an ominous reduction of the short-term variability at computerize fetal heart rate analysis.

No Abnormal Umbilical Artery Doppler Means No FGR: Does It Make Sense?

From the beginning of the Doppler velocimetry era, it became clear that the placental tissue should be extensively underdeveloped due to poor trophoblastic invasion in order to be identifiable by simple Doppler velocimetry interrogation of umbilical arteries. A beautiful editorial by Brian Trudinger, published in 2007 [26], summarizes all the literature from 1982 on this topic. Figure 17.5 nicely shows the large gap of placental damage that goes undetected by umbilical artery pulsatility index.

The potential of this new, highly valuable index in detecting early and severe FGR induced some to support the idea "no abnormal umbilical artery PI, no FGR," leaving out all other small fetuses without this stigma in the uncertain realm of small-for-gestational-age (SGA) fetuses. Ambiguous sentences could be read, such as "Evaluation of placental function by umbilical artery Doppler is a clinical standard to distinguish between SGA and FGR" [27]. Constitutional small fetus became fashionable. As a matter of fact, many small fetuses with normal umbilical artery PI stubbornly continued to show abnormal metabolism in utero as regards their energetic metabolism [1], and mostly as regards their capacity to incorporate amino acids for growth [28]. In a paper that was published on top of

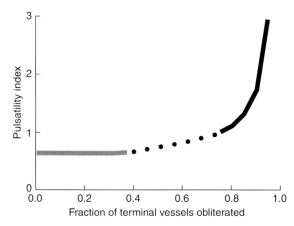

Figure 17.5 The curve reported by Trudinger in his seminal paper: "It was shown using this model that 60–70% of the small arterial channels would need to be obliterated before the umbilical artery indices of resistance became abnormal" (black line). The clinical problem is how to sort out the fetuses within the uncertain boundaries (dotted line) of placental damage.

10 years of studies in fetal lambs and in humans [29], Cetin and coworkers observed that the concentration of all nine essential and six nonessential amino acids was significantly lower in small-for-gestational-age fetuses with abnormal uterine artery Doppler and abdominal circumference <5th percentile but with normal umbilical artery PI, than in AGA fetuses for corresponding maternal concentrations. Of even higher impact was the observation that these fetuses were not different from severe FGR fetuses with abnormal umbilical PI as regards their amino acid metabolism. That is to say that, for instance, the concentration of threonine (one of the nine essential amino acids) in these fetuses was not different from that of severe FGR and was lagging below AGA of about 120 mM, for a maternal concentration in between 150–300 mM. These studies were paralleled by observations on small cohorts of FGR fetuses [30,31], showing that small fetuses (abdominal circumference <5th centile, abnormal uterine Doppler velocimetry) may exist with normal umbilical artery PI and abnormal umbilical vein blood flow.

The potential importance of this measurement is then twofold. It allows us to: a) identify a small subset of FGR fetuses with an abnormal umbilical artery PI and a normal, albeit in the lower centiles umbilical vein blood flow per unit weight; b) but mostly it allows us to identify small fetuses with normal umbilical artery PI, the otherwise undefined SGA, but with a clear reduction of umbilical vein blood flow per unit weight. The latter condition defines a case of late FGR.

Similar findings have been recently reported by Parra-Saavedra [32] on a large cohort of 193 fetuses at term with an estimated weight below the 10th percentile. According to these authors, "Multivariable analysis showed that significant contributions to prediction of emergency delivery for non-reassuring fetal status and neonatal metabolic acidosis were provided by middle cerebral artery (MCA) pulsatility index (PI) and UV blood flow normalized by fetal weight." Of interest is the finding that the value of umbilical vein blood flow of 68ml/min/kg was significantly associated with neonatal metabolic acidosis (remember anaerobic energy metabolism produces lactic acid as waste). We observed a very similar value in severe FGR in utero on the same occasion of abnormal fetal heart rate prior to iatrogenic delivery: 63ml/min/kg.

This paper that proves the clinical value of umbilical vein blood flow in term fetuses cast the background of important studies. Late FGR [33] and term FGR [34] have worse neurobiological outcomes, and have different placental energy metabolisms [35].

When, years ago, we first read about the adult consequences of being born small [36], the Barker Hypothesis, the intuitive association by resemblance, probably first stuck this concept to severe early FGR fetuses and their future outcome. Indeed, the cut-off for being considered small between 1911 and 1930 was 2,550g. In those years, and until the late 1960s, survival below 1,000g was a challenge or an exception. Understanding the physiology of late and term FGR and adopting proper diagnostic tools is probably the most important step forward that fetomaternal medicine can accomplish in the near future, and we are pretty sure that umbilical vein blood flow volume is and will be part of this future.

Key Points

- Umbilical vein flow in the human fetus in the third trimester is approximately 120ml/kg/min.

- In small fetuses, umbilical vein flow may be more sensitive than umbilical artery Doppler in identifying true growth restriction.

- At term, around 15–20% of blood returning through the umbilical vein is shunted through the ductus venosus to the right atrium.

References

1. Pardi G, Cetin I, Marconi AM, Lanfranchi A, Bozzetti P, Buscaglia M, et al. Diagnostic value of blood sampling in fetuses with growth retardation. *N Engl J Med* 1993 Oct 2;328(10):692–6.

2. Galan HL, Jozwik M, Rigano S, Regnault TR, Hobbins JC, Battaglia FC, et al. Umbilical vein blood flow determination in the ovine fetus: Comparison of Doppler ultrasonographic and steady-state diffusion techniques. *Am J Obstet Gynecol* 1999 Nov 1;181(5 Pt 1):1149–53.

3. Schmidt KG, Di Tommaso M, Silverman NH, Rudolph AM. Doppler echocardiographic assessment of fetal descending aortic and umbilical blood flows. Validation studies in fetal lambs. *Circulation* 1991 Apr 30;83(5):1731–7.

4. Meschia G, Cotter JR, Makowski EL, Burron DH. Simultaneous measurement of uterine and umbilical blood flows and oxygen uptakes. *Exp Physiol* 1967 Aug 1;52:1–18.

5. Dawes GS, Mott JC. Changes on O2 distribution and consumption in foetal lambs with variations in umbilical blood flow. *J Physiol* 1964 Jan 25;170:524–40.

6. Wallace JM, Bourke DA, Aitken RP, Leitch N, Hay WW. Blood flows and nutrient uptakes in growth-restricted pregnancies induced by overnourishing adolescent sheep. *Am J Physiol Regul Integr Comp Physiol* 2002 Feb 25;282:1027–36.

7. Figueras F, Fernández S, Hernandez-Andrade E, Gratacós E. Umbilical venous blood flow measurement: Accuracy and reproducibility. *Ultrasound Obstet Gynecol* 2008 Sep;32(4):587–91.

8. Di Naro E, Ghezzi F, Raio L, Franchi M, D'Addario V, Lanzillotti G, et al. Umbilical vein blood flow in fetuses with normal and lean umbilical cord. *Ultrasound Obstet Gynecol* 2001 Feb 28;17(3):224–8.

9. Ferrazzi E, Bellotti M, Marconi AM, Barbera AF, Pardi G. Peak velocity of the outflow of the aorta: Correlations with acid base status and oxygenation in growth retarded fetuses. 1965 Jan 4;85:663–7.

10. Meschia G, Cotter JR, Barron DH. The hemoglobin, O2, CO2, and H+ concentrations in the umbilical bloods of sheep. *Q J Exp Physiol Cogn Med Sci* 1965 Aug 4;50:185–95.

11. Battaglia FC, Meschia G. Review of studies in human pregnancies of uterine and umbilical blood flows. *Dev Period Med* 2013 Feb 7;XVIII(4):287–92.

12. Pennati G, Bellotti M, De Gasperi C, Rognoni G. Spatial velocity profile changes along the cord in normal human fetuses: Can these affect Doppler measurements of venous umbilical blood flow? *Ultrasound Obstet Gynecol* 2004 Feb 4;23(2):131–7.

13. Burton GJ, Woods AW, Jauniaux E, Kingdom JCP. Rheological and physiological consequences of conversion of the maternal spiral arteries for uteroplacental blood flow during human pregnancy. *Placenta* 2010 Nov 4;30(6):473–82.

14. Marconi AM, Cetin I, Ferrazzi E, Ferrari M, Pardi G, Battaglia FC. Lactate metabolism in normal and growth-retarded human fetuses. *Pediatr Res* 1990 Sep 28;28(6):652–6.

15. Alfirevic Z, Neilson JP. Doppler ultrasonography in high-risk pregnancies: Systematic review with meta-analysis. 1995 Jan 4;172:1379–87.

16. Rigano S, Bozzo M, Padoan A, Mustoni P, Bellotti M, Galan HL, et al. Small size-specific umbilical vein diameter in severe growth restricted fetuses that die in utero. *Prenat Diagn* 2008 Oct;28(10):908–13.

17. Bellotti M, Pennati G, De Gasperi C, Battaglia FC, Ferrazzi E. Role of ductus venosus in distribution of umbilical blood flow in human fetuses during second half of pregnancy. *Am J Physiol Heart Circ Physiol* 2000 Aug 31;279(3):H1256–63.

18. Kiserud T. Physiology of the fetal circulation. *Semin Fetal Neonatal Med* 2005 Dec;10(6):493–503.

19. Kiserud T, Ozaki T, Nishina H, Rodeck C, Hanson MA. Effect of NO, phenylephrine, and hypoxemia on ductus venosus diameter in fetal sheep. *Am J Physiol Heart Circ Physiol* 2000 Aug 31;279(3):H1166–71.

20. Bellotti M, Pennati G, Pardi G, Fumero R. Dilatation of the ductus venosus in human fetuses: Ultrasonographic evidence and mathematical modeling. *Am J Physiol Heart Circ Physiol* 1998;275(5):H1759–67.

21. Bellotti M, Pennati G, Gasperi CD, Bozzo M, Battaglia FC, Ferrazzi E. Simultaneous measurements of umbilical venous, fetal hepatic, and ductus venosus blood flow in growth-restricted human fetuses. *Am J Obstet Gynecol* 2004 May;190(5):1347–58.

22. Kiserud T, Kessler J, Ebbing C, Rasmussen S. Ductus venosus shunting in growth-restricted fetuses and the effect of umbilical circulatory compromise. *Ultrasound Obstet Gynecol* 2006;28(2):143–9.

23. Regnault TRH, Friedman JE, Wilkening RB, Anthony RV, Hay WW, Jr. Fetoplacental transport and utilization of amino acids in IUGR – a review. *Placenta* 2005 Apr;26:S52–S62.

24. Lees C, Marlow N, Arabin B, Bilardo CM, Brezinka C, Derks JB, et al. Perinatal morbidity and mortality in early-onset fetal growth restriction: Cohort outcomes of the trial of randomized umbilical and fetal flow in Europe (TRUFFLE). *Ultrasound Obstet Gynecol* 2013 Sep 23;42(4):400–8.

25. TRUFFLE *Lancet* Paper 2015.

26. Trudinger B. Doppler: More or less? *Ultrasound Obstet Gynecol* 2007;29(3):243–6.

27. Figueras F, Gardosi J. Intrauterine growth restriction: New concepts in antenatal surveillance, diagnosis, and management. *Am J Obstet Gynecol* 2011 Apr 1;204(4):288–300.

28. Cetin I, Ronzoni S, Marconi AM, Perugino G, Corbetta C, Battaglia FC, et al. Maternal concentrations and fetal-maternal concentration differences of plasma amino acids in normal and intrauterine growth-restricted pregnancies. *Am J Obstet Gynecol* 1996 May;174(5):1575–83.

29. Ronzoni S, Marconi AM, Paolini CL, Teng C, Pardi G, Battaglia FC. The effect of a maternal infusion of amino acids on umbilical uptake in pregnancies complicated by intrauterine growth restriction. *Am J Obstet Gynecol* 2002 Sep;187(3):741–6.

30. Ferrazzi E, Rigano S, Bozzo M, Bellotti M, Giovannini N, Galan H, et al. Umbilical vein blood flow in growth-restricted fetuses. *Ultrasound Obstet Gynecol* 2000 Oct 1;16(5):432–8.

31. Rigano S, Bozzo M, Ferrazzi E, Bellotti M, Battaglia FC, Galan HL. Early and persistent reduction in umbilical vein blood flow in the growth-restricted fetus: A longitudinal study. *Am J Obstet Gynecol* 2001 Oct 1;185(4):834–8.

32. Parra-Saavedra M, Crovetto F, Triunfo S, Savchev S, Parra G, Sanz M, et al. Added value of umbilical vein flow as a predictor of perinatal outcome in term small-for-gestational-age fetuses. *Ultrasound Obstet Gynecol* 2013 Jul 26;42(2):189–95.

33. Sanz-Cortés M, Figueras F, Bargalló N, Padilla N, Amat-Roldan I, Gratacós E. Abnormal brain microstructure and metabolism in small-for-gestational-age term fetuses with normal umbilical artery Doppler. *Ultrasound Obstet Gynecol* 2010 Feb 3;36(2):159–65.

34. Figueras F, Oros D, Cruz-Martinez R, Padilla N, Hernandez-Andrade E, Botet F, et al. Neurobehavior in term, small-for-gestational age infants with normal placental function. *Pediatrics* 2009 Oct 26;124(5):e934–41.

35. Mando C, De Palma C, Stampalija T, Anelli GM, Figus M, Novielli C, et al. Placental mitochondrial content and function in intrauterine growth restriction and preeclampsia. *Am J Physiol Endocrinol Metab* 2014 Feb 15;306(4):E404–13.

36. Barker JA. Fetal origins of coronary heart disease. *BMJ* 1995;311:171–4.

Chapter 18

Fetal Cardiac Function in Fetal Growth Restriction

Fàtima Crispi and Eduard Gratacós

Introduction

Normal fetal development is regulated by complex mechanisms involving various critical factors, such as the genetic profile of the embryo, maternal predispositions, placental state, fetal environment, and adequate nutrient and oxygen supply to the developing fetus. If one or more of these developmental factors is abnormal, the growth of the fetus might be impaired, resulting in low birth weight and possible remodeling of the key organs.

Accumulating evidence of a large number of epidemiological [1] and animal studies [2] performed over the past few decades confirms the existence of the direct link between the in utero environment and long-term consequences in adult life. Taken together, the data obtained suggest that the complex interaction between genetic constitution and the prenatal and early postnatal environment determines the growth and development of the fetus and defines its susceptibility to certain disorders in adult life, like hypertension, diabetes, dyslipidemia, coagulation, and neurobehavioral disorders [3]. This phenomenon is known as "fetal programming," when an insult in utero leads to structural and functional changes in key organs remaining in postnatal life and leading to a greater risk of various diseases in adulthood [2–6]. The rapid cell proliferation and differentiation during fetal growth are very sensitive to even the smallest changes damaging to the environment that can lead to permanent alterations in structural and functional constitution, which then may persist into adult life, predisposing to adult disease [3]. Numerous epidemiological studies [1,3] have demonstrated a strong association between low birth weight and cardiovascular disease and mortality in adulthood.

The main cause of low birth weight is fetal growth restriction (FGR), defined as failure of a fetus to achieve its genetic growth potential, characterized by a birth weight lower than normal with respect to the number of gestational weeks – below percentile 10 [7,8]. FGR is a major cause of perinatal morbidity and mortality and may complicate 7–10% of all pregnancies [8–10]. It is usually secondary to placental insufficiency, leading to fetal undernutrition, hypoxia, and pressure/volume overload. The heart is a critical element in the fetal adaptation to these insults. Therefore, understanding the pathophysiological cardiovascular changes that occur in FGR might be very useful in the characterization, monitoring, and prognosis of FGR.

Nowadays, recent advances in cardiovascular imaging and fetal ultrasound permit an accurate and sensitive evaluation of cardiac remodeling and dysfunction by incorporating techniques such as tissue Doppler imaging (TDI) or 2D speckle tracking [11]. These techniques have demonstrated their feasibility and validity for assessing the fetal heart [11]. The implementation of comprehensive fetal structural and functional echocardiography has allowed new pathophysiological insights into FGR [12–14]. It has also permitted us to assess the postnatal persistence of these cardiovascular changes [15] and determine its potential utility for detecting those FGR cases at higher cardiovascular risk that might benefit from early therapeutic interventions [14].

In this chapter, we will review the current evidence on the cardiovascular changes occurring in FGR prenatally and postnatally. We will also discuss the potential clinical utility of fetal cardiac function assessment in the monitoring and prognosis of FGR.

Fetal Growth Restriction

Definition of FGR

Fetal growth restriction (FGR) is defined as failure of a fetus to achieve its growth potential, characterized by a birth weight lower than expected for the gestational age – below percentile 10 [7,8]. FGR may complicate 7–10% of all pregnancies and is a major cause of perinatal and long-term morbidity and mortality [8,9,16,17].

Early- versus Late-Onset FGR

Usually FGR is displayed under two phenotypes according to the onset of the restriction [8].

Early-onset FGR (before 34 weeks' gestation) usually results from severe placental insufficiency before 34 weeks' gestation, affects less than 1% of deliveries, usually associates preeclampsia, and constitutes a main cause of perinatal mortality and morbidity [8,10]. Early-onset FGR fetuses typically present with a pattern of Doppler abnormalities that deteriorate quickly and progressively and that culminate in premature delivery of the fetus in order to preserve its life [8,10].

In contrast, **late-onset FGR** fetuses associated with a mild degree of placental insufficiency (not reflected by umbilical artery Doppler), are usually delivered near or at term, and present poorer perinatal and long-term results, including suboptimal neurobehavioral cortical development and postnatal cardiovascular outcome [8,17,18]. About two-thirds of late-onset small fetuses present severe forms of smallness, i.e., estimated fetal weight (EFW) <3rd centile, or signs of fetal-placental Doppler adaptation, defined as abnormal cerebroplacental ratio or uterine artery Doppler [8]. This group has been shown to be associated with poorer perinatal outcomes and abnormal placental histological signs [19]. The remaining third of fetuses does not present any of these features and is associated with nearly normal perinatal outcomes. By arbitrary convention, the first group is thought to represent a subset of "true FGR" within small fetuses, while the second is often defined as "constitutionally" small for gestational age (SGA) [8].

Fetal Cardiac Function

Fetal Cardiac Physiology

The primary function of the heart is to provide adequate perfusion of organs ejecting blood from the ventricle into the aorta/pulmonary artery by contracting its muscular walls [20]. To maintain normal cardiac function, both blood ejection in systole and filling of the ventricle from the atria in diastole must be adequate and occur in a synchronized manner [20,21].

The normal cardiac cycle consist of five major phases. The diastolic part of the cycle includes: (1) the *isovolumetric relaxation phase*, when after aortic/pulmonary valve closure with an isovolumetric relaxation period, no blood enters or ejects from the ventricles while the myocardium starts to relax and the intraventricular pressure drops (isovolumetric relaxation time, IRT); (2) the *early diastolic phase*, when ventricular pressure lowers the atrial pressure, the mitral/tricuspid valve opens, and blood from the atria starts to fill the ventricle in a passive manner; (3) the *atrial contraction phase*, when the atria contract and complete the filling of the ventricle (late diastole). The ejection process for the systole includes: (4) the *isovolumetric contraction phase*, when cardiomyocytes start to contract, increasing intraventricular pressure, which in turn opens the aortic/pulmonary valve (isovolumetric contraction time) without any change in volume; (5) the *ejection phase*, when due to the increased ventricular pressure, the aortic/pulmonary valves opens and the myocardium deforms, ejecting blood from the ventricle.

These main components of the cardiac cycle define the main features of cardiac blood flow movement and myocardial motion and deformation [20–22]. Myocardial *motion* is defined as the distance covered by one point over a certain period of time and is determined by displacement (distance) and velocity (distance divided by time). Accordingly, myocardial *deformation* is defined as the change in the length/thickness of a segment (two points) and is determined by strain (percentage of change) and strain rate (velocity of segment change) [22].

Fetal Cardiac Remodeling, Dysfunction, and Failure

The fetal heart will adapt to any insult with changes in its structure and function in order to keep providing blood supply to the organs. In the initial stages of an insult, the heart usually manages to adapt, undergoing a long subclinical period of **cardiac dysfunction** before the actual heart failure occurs [11,23,24]. Apart from functional changes, the heart usually undergoes changes in its shape and size in order to adapt to an insult, defining the process of **cardiac remodeling** [25].

Heart failure is defined as the inability of the heart to supply sufficient blood flow to meet the needs of the organism [26]. This is usually a late event that can be easily recognized by cardiomegaly, atrioventricular insufficiency, and fetal hydrops. It can be quantified by measuring a significant decrease in cardiac output or ejection fraction [23,26].

Determinants of Fetal Cardiac Function

Changes in cardiac function and shape are determined not only by the causal insult, but also by myocardial contractility, fiber orientation, tissue elasticity, heart geometry, segment interaction, loading conditions, electrical activation, and myocardial perfusion [22]. In the fetal heart, cardiac remodeling also depends on myocardial maturation and blood circulation [27].

Techniques for Assessing Fetal Cardiac Function

Traditionally, fetal cardiac function was assessed by measuring blood flow through conventional Doppler or cardiac morphometry in 2D or M-mode. Recently, the diagnostic evaluation has been improved by employing TDI and 2D speckle tracking imaging for the direct assessment of myocardial motion and deformation [22,28,29]. Additionally, 4D

spatiotemporal image correlation (STIC) has been proposed to evaluate more accurately cardiac dimensions and volume [30].

The most suitable parameters for assessing fetal cardiac function are mainly determined by the cause of the dysfunction [11]. Abnormal values of ejection fraction or cardiac output are usually found in the late stages of deterioration, and, therefore, more sensitive parameters have been proposed for earlier diagnosis and monitoring of fetal cardiac dysfunction. In most cases of cardiac dysfunction, diastolic parameters (such as IRT) are the first to be altered, reflecting impaired relaxation and compliance due to a stiffer or less effective heart [11]. Similarly, parameters reflecting longitudinal function (such as annular displacement or velocities) are typically affected in the early stages as compared to radial function (such as ejection fraction) (Figure 18.1) [11].

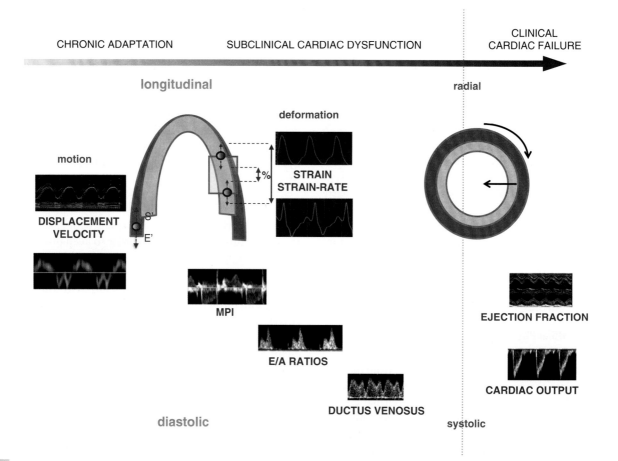

Figure 18.1 Illustration on the different stages of fetal cardiovascular adaptation, subclinical cardiac dysfunction and clinical cardiac failure, and the different fetal echocardiographic parameters that can be measured to assess systolic and diastolic function.

Conventional Doppler

Conventional Doppler allows assessing blood flow through the outflow tracts, which reflects *systolic* function and permit estimating **stroke volume** and **cardiac output** [31]. The main Doppler indices used to evaluate diastolic function are the early diastolic filling (atrial contraction), E/A ratios and precordial vein pulsatility indices, mainly **ductus venosus** (DV) [10,31–34]. In addition, Doppler can also be used to calculate time periods [31], such as isovolumetric contraction and relaxation times – time elapsed from the start of contraction/relaxation and closure/opening of the outflow valve, respectively. Time events can be evaluated individually or as a composite parameter, such as the **myocardial performance index** (MPI), which is considered a marker of global cardiac function and takes into account several systolic and diastolic time events [31,35,36].

M-mode

M-mode techniques are traditionally used in a transverse cardiac view to measure the difference in end-systolic and end-diastolic ventricular diameter and to calculate **ejection fraction**, defined as the percentage of blood ejected in each heart cycle, by applying the Teicholz formula [30,37]. M-mode can be also applied in the long axis of the heart to evaluate tricuspid and mitral annular displacement (**TAPSE** and **MAPSE**, respectively) – sensitive markers of cardiac dysfunction reflecting global longitudinal function [38,39].

Tissue Doppler Imaging (TDI)

While conventional echocardiographic techniques are based on blood flow, TDI uses frequency shifts in ultrasound waves to calculate myocardial velocity characterized by a lower velocity and higher amplitude [40]. Peak velocities evaluated at the mitral or tricuspid annulus reflect global systolic (**S'**) or diastolic (**E'** and **A'**) myocardial motion and have been demonstrated to be an early and sensitive marker of cardiac dysfunction [28,41].

TDI offline analysis can also be used to calculate myocardial **strain** and **strain-rate** [28,42].

2D Speckle Tracking

A non-Doppler technology, 2D speckle tracking, allows myocardial deformation to be quantified by using frame-by-frame tracking of bright myocardial areas (speckles) [22]. 2D speckle tracking requires post-processing and off-line analysis of 2D images and allows myocardial **strain** and **strain rate** to be measured [29,42,43].

4D Spatiotemporal Image Correlation (STIC)

4D STIC technique is based on a sweep (volume data set) of the fetal heart containing a complete reconstructed cardiac cycle and permits 3D reconstruction of the fetal heart over time, so that any target region of interest can be obtained at any stage of the cardiac cycle. 4D STIC has been proposed to measure **ventricular volumes** that allow more accurate estimation of the cardiac output and ejection fraction, and the off-line analysis also allows annulus displacement (**TAPSE** and **MAPSE**) to be assessed [30,43].

Challenges and Limitations for Assessing Fetal Cardiac Function

Fetal heart evaluation is challenging due to the smallness of the fetal heart, the high heart rate, and limited access to the fetus far from the transducer [11]. Fetal echocardiography requires specific training and expertise to acquire images and interpret the results. Several limitations should be taken into account when assessing fetal cardiac function, including fetal position and movements, small size, fetal heart rate requiring high frame rate acquisitions, maternal adiposity, impossibility to co-register electrocardiogram, changes in cardiomyocyte maturation throughout gestation, and lack of validation of some techniques for the fetal heart. These limitations are particularly important in techniques requiring offline analysis (4D-STIC, color TDI and 2D speckle tracking). Therefore any technique or parameter proposed for its assessment should follow several steps for validation before being incorporated into clinical practice [11]. The first phase is to demonstrate feasibility and reproducibility in well-designed and conducted studies. Use of the proposed parameter following strict methodological criteria is also critical to ensure proper applicability. Then, the behavior of the parameter in normal fetal conditions (physiology), as well as in each clinical disease (pathophysiology), must be described before the technique or parameter can be applied in clinical conditions.

Fetal Cardiac Remodeling and Dysfunction in FGR

The Heart as a Central Organ in Fetal Adaptive Response

The heart is a central organ in the fetal adaptive response to insults such as hypoxia, undernutrition, or pressure/volume overload during prenatal life. Consequently, assessment of fetal cardiac shape and function may be helpful in the diagnosis, monitoring, or prognosis of FGR. Actually, cardiac remodeling and dysfunction are recognized as being among the central pathophysiologic features of both early- and late-onset FGR (Figure 18.2) as fetal adaptive mechanisms to placental insufficiency [12,44]. However, cardiac dysfunction in the fetus is largely subclinical and requires sensitive methods for its identification [11].

Fetal Cardiovascular Remodeling and Dysfunction in Early-Onset FGR

Early-onset FGR usually results from severe placental insufficiency reflected by abnormal umbilical artery Doppler profile [8]. These are very severe and small cases with typically cardiomegaly, hypertrophic and globular hearts, and mild pericardial effusion [45]. The pathophysiology underlying these shape changes is complex, most probably including pressure changes and volume overload to the fetal heart, due to the chronic state of hypoxia and undernutrition and elevated placental resistances. Probably the lower availability of oxygen and nutrients has a direct effect on the myocardium, decreasing its contractility. In addition, the heart reacts to pressure overload by shifting to a more spherical shape (with a lower radius of curvature that would better tolerate pressure overload) and thickening myocardial walls (hypertrophy) (Figure 18.3). Finally, volume overload would explain the cardiomegaly and mild pericardial effusion [45].

This remodeling is usually associated with signs of cardiac dysfunction. While ejection fraction is usually preserved until very late stages of deterioration, stroke volume (volume of blood ejected in each heart beat) is usually reduced and compensated by an increase in heart rate in order to maintain cardiac output (volume of blood ejected per minute) and the adequate perfusion to organs [14]. Myocardial imaging techniques have permitted us to demonstrate a decrease in longitudinal motion such as reduced displacement (TAPSE/MAPSE) and annular systolic peak velocities [13,46]. In addition, fetuses with early FGR show signs of impaired relaxation (diastolic dysfunction) from the early stages of deterioration [12,13], as measured by increased pulsatility in precordial veins (particularly DV) [10,47], higher E/A ratios [10,12,48], increased IRT [12,49] and reduced diastolic annular peak velocities [13,46,50]. Very recently, data from 2D speckle tracking imaging have demonstrated the presence of post-systolic shortening in the basal septal part of almost half of the early-onset FGR cases [51]. This is a sign of abnormal regional myocardial deformation pointing to chronic pressure overload in these cases.

Studies evaluating cardiovascular biomarkers in cord blood of early-onset FGR support the changes measured by echocardiography, with higher fetal concentrations of B-type natriuretic peptide (BNP) [12,48], a gold standard marker of heart failure usually increased as response to hypoxia and volume overload. The most severe early-onset cases also present signs of myocardial damage as measured by increased concentrations of plasmatic troponin and heart-fatty acids finding protein [12].

Fetal Cardiovascular Remodeling and Dysfunction in Late-Onset FGR

The initial reports of cardiac function in FGR were focused on the most severe (early) cases. However, more sensitive echocardiographic techniques such as tissue Doppler have permitted demonstrating signs of cardiac dysfunction in milder cases [52]. Late-onset FGR is characterized by non-hypertrophic more globular hearts, most probably reflecting a milder degree of placental insufficiency [45]. In addition, late-onset FGR fetuses show increased values of MPI [52,53] and decreased TAPSE/MAPSE and annular peak velocities (Figure 18.3) [52,54]. These changes have been reported in late-onset FGR cases, but also in SGA fetuses without signs of severity (with EFW above 3rd centile together with normal uterine Doppler and cerebroplacental ratio) [54]. Moreover, increased cord blood levels of troponins have been detected in some late-SGA newborns [55].

Cardiac Ultrastructural Changes in FGR

Data from experimental studies suggest that FGR is not only affecting cardiac shape at the organ level, but also is associated with profound changes in the ultrastructure of the heart. Hearts from FGR cases show more prominent and dilated coronary arteries together with a decrease in longitudinal fibers compensated by

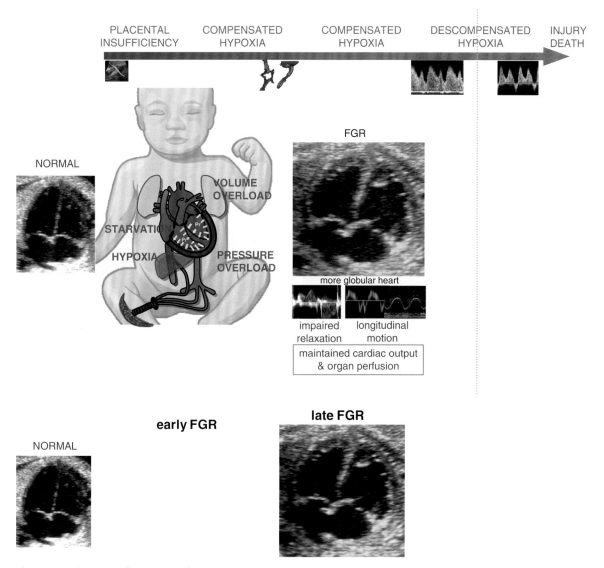

Figure 18.2 Illustration of the cascade of events in fetal growth restriction (FGR) including cardiovascular adaptation, dysfunction and failure.

a higher proportion of circumferential fibers [56]. The number of cardiomyocytes is also reduced, exhibiting more hypertrophic cells. An altered spatial arrangement of intracellular energetic units with significant increases in cytosolic space between mitochondria and myofilaments can be also observed [57]. The contractility machinery seems to also be altered with shorter sarcomere length [58] and decreased levels of sarcomeric proteins titin and myosin heavy chain [2]. Altogether, these data illustrate the profound change in the fetal heart architecture at the organ, cellular, and organelle levels.

Long-Term Cardiovascular Consequences of FGR

Persistence of Cardiac Remodeling in Children Born FGR

Recently, it has been demonstrated that cardiovascular changes in FGR persist postnatally, suggesting primary fetal cardiovascular programming [15]. In both early- and late-onset FGR children, more globular and less efficient hearts with reduced longitudinal motion and impaired relaxation were observed in a large

169

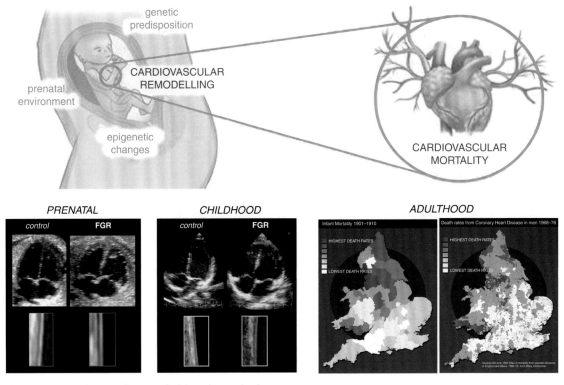

Figure 18.3 Developmental origins of adult cardiovascular disease.

cohort of 5-year-old children [15]. Late-onset FGR could compensate by increased radial function, while the more severe early-onset cases showed decreased radial function, leading to lower stroke volume and increased heart rate in order to maintain cardiac output [18]. Additionally, both groups showed signs of vascular remodeling, including increased blood pressure, as well as carotid intima-media thickness [15,18,59].

A significantly progressive increase in aortic intima-media thickness and elevated blood pressure has been described in FGR fetuses, neonates, infants, and children, suggesting predisposition to hypertension early in life and posterior increased cardiovascular risk [60,61]. Endothelial dysfunction and increased carotid stiffness have also been reported in 9-year-old children with low birth weight. Very recent data from a unique FGR cohort in Sweden also suggest the persistence of vascular dysfunction (mainly smaller dimension and higher systolic pressure wave augmentation in the aorta) in young adults who were severely growth restricted in utero [63].

Fetal Programming of Adult Cardiovascular Disease

For many years, cardiovascular diseases in adulthood were thought to be determined only by the genetic factors and the postnatal lifestyles of individuals, particularly by the amount of physical activity and quality of nutrition. However, in most cases, cardiovascular diseases seem to be triggered in early stages of life and then undergo a long subclinical phase that can last decades before the first clinical symptoms appear [64].

Already in 1989, the group of David Backer in Southampton, UK established a strong and direct correlation between low birth weight and cardiovascular disease in adulthood, including hypertension and cardiovascular mortality [1]. Accumulating evidence of a large number of epidemiological and animal studies performed over the past few decades confirms the existence of a direct link between the conditions of embryonic development and long-term consequences in adult life. Taken together, the data obtained suggest that the complex interaction between genetic constitution and prenatal and early postnatal environment determines the growth and development of the fetus and defines its susceptibility to certain disorders in adult life, like hypertension, diabetes, dyslipidemia, coagulation, and neurobehavioral disorders [3]. This phenomenon is known as "fetal programming," when an insult in utero leads to functional changes in key organs remaining in postnatal life and to a greater risk of various diseases in adulthood [3–6]. The rapid cell proliferation and differentiation during fetal growth are very sensitive to even the smallest changes damaging to the environment that can lead to permanent alterations in structural and functional constitution, which then may persist into adult life [3].

The mechanistic pathways underlying the relationship between low birth weight and cardiovascular risk are poorly understood. A number of studies support that it might be explained in part by fetal metabolic programming leading to diseases such as obesity, diabetes, or metabolic syndrome associated with cardiovascular disease. However, the cardiovascular remodeling and dysfunction described in FGR fetuses and children support the concept of primary cardiovascular programming of adult disease (Figure 18.4). Future studies are warranted to further document the dynamics of cardiovascular remodeling across the life course and to better understand the link between fetal cardiovascular dysfunction and cardiovascular disease later in life.

Implementation of Fetal Cardiac Function in a Clinical Setting

Fetal Cardiac Function for Monitoring FGR

Over the years, several cardiac parameters have been identified as the main predictors of acidemia and adverse perinatal outcome in early FGR [10,47,65]. In a recent systematic review, ductus venosus emerged as a strong predictor of mortality, with a sensitivity ranging from 40 to 60% [66] and being particularly useful between 26 and 28 weeks' gestation [67]. Although preliminary data suggested that MPI could also help to predict perinatal mortality in early FGR [68], a recent multicenter study has not confirmed these results [67]. Other fetal cardiac function parameters have shown a poor predictive value for perinatal outcomes, most probably explained by cardiac dysfunction being an inherent characteristic of growth restriction occurring in very early stages of placental insufficiency.

Prediction of Postnatal Cardiovascular Remodeling in FGR

While not useful for predicting perinatal outcomes, fetal echocardiography might help in the detection of those FGR cases with postnatal cardiovascular remodeling and higher cardiovascular risk. Actually, a recent study has demonstrated that fetal echocardiographic parameters are strongly associated with postnatal hypertension and arterial remodeling in FGR [14]. In particular, a composite score including a left ventricular sphericity index, TAPSE, IRT, and cerebroplacental ratio has demonstrated a 90% sensitivity and 70% specificity for detecting FGR cases with postnatal hypertension and increased vascular intima-media thickness, which are well-known risk factors for later cardiovascular disease [14]. If confirmed in further studies, some fetal cardiac function parameters could be incorporated as a prognostic

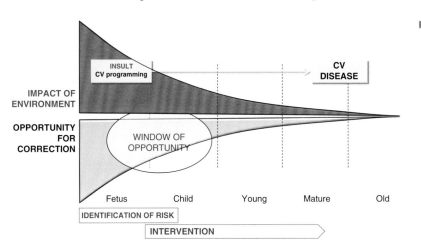

Figure 18.4

tool in FGR and help in the early detection of those cases at high cardiovascular risk that would benefit from early interventions.

Prevention of Long-Term Cardiovascular Disease in FGR

Although current clinical guidelines still do not include FGR as a cardiovascular risk factor, intensive research over the past few decades points toward the strong necessity of thorough monitoring and follow-up studies in children as well as adults who suffered FGR in fetal life. Hypertension and pre-hypertension in children has been associated with substantial long-term health risks and considered an indication for lifestyle modifications. Accordingly, it has been shown that promoting physical activity and avoiding exposure to secondary smoking or obesity together with dietary interventions significantly improve cardiovascular health in hypertensive children [69]. Particularly, high intake of dietary long-chain omega-3 fatty acids has been associated with lower blood pressure and may prevent progression of subclinical atherosclerosis in children born with low birth weight [70]. A recent randomized trial in a large cohort of children showed that inverse association of fetal growth with arterial wall thickness in childhood can be prevented by dietary omega-3 fatty acid supplementation over the first 5 years of life [71]. Breastfeeding and postnatal high intake of dietary polyunsaturated fatty acids have also demonstrated beneficial effects on cardiac and vascular remodeling in children born with FGR [72].

It is critical to adequately select the high-risk population who may benefit from these therapeutic interventions. Currently, the severity of FGR is determined mainly by the gestational age and birth centile, which are inversely related to the perinatal and neurodevelopmental outcomes [8]. For further antepartum surveillance of the FGR viable fetus, the feto-placental Doppler analysis has been proposed, thus significantly decreasing the necessity of labor induction, delivery via cesarean section, and perinatal death [8]. However, cardiovascular programming occurs not only in premature and severe FGR, but also in mild late-onset FGR cases with normal umbilical artery parameters [15,18,52]. Therefore, standard perinatal parameters such as gestational age, birth weight centile, or umbilical Doppler show poor performance for predicting long-term cardiovascular outcomes [14]. To improve diagnostic accuracy, fetal echocardiography has been

recently pointed out as a very promising tool for the early identification of those FGR cases with postnatal hypertension and arterial remodeling [14].

Considering the high prevalence of FGR and the progressing availability of intervention strategies, it is of the highest clinical relevance to detect cardiovascular risks as early as possible, to introduce timely preventive interventions, and to adapt the lifestyle, in order to improve the long-term cardiovascular health outcome of the FGR patients. While low birth weight is a recognized cardiovascular risk factor [73], FGR is still not included as a criteria for pediatric cardiovascular follow-up [74]. Given the potential benefit for the future cardiovascular health of FGR cases, such guidelines ideally should be developed and introduced into clinical practice as soon as possible.

Conclusion

The heart is a central organ in the fetal adaptive response to FGR. Placental insufficiency leads to fetal undernutrition, hypoxia, and pressure/volume overload. In order to adapt to this adverse environment, the fetal heart remodels – changes to a more globular shape – becoming less efficient [12,14]. Recent advances in fetal echocardiography have permitted us to describe that FGR present more spherical ventricles with decreased longitudinal motion (decreased annular displacement by M-mode and peak velocities by tissue Doppler) [46,52] and impaired relaxation (prolonged IRT) with maintained cardiac output [12]. These changes are more prominent in early-onset, but also present in late-onset FGR and SGA [15]. Animal studies have shown that these functional changes are associated with profound changes in the heart ultrastructure such as a shift from longitudinal to circumferential fibers, altered spatial arrangement of intracellular energetic units, and shorter sarcomere length [2,56–58]. Recent studies have also demonstrated that these cardiovascular changes in FGR persist postnatally [15], suggesting a primary fetal cardiac programming that might explain the increased cardiovascular risk later in life.

Understanding the cardiovascular changes that occur in FGR might be useful in the characterization, monitoring, and prognosis of FGR. Several cardiac parameters have been identified as main predictors of acidemia and adverse perinatal outcome in early FGR. In particular, DV has a high predictive value for perinatal mortality, particularly useful in monitoring early FGR between 26 and 28 weeks' gestation [10,67]. In addition, fetal echocardiography, including ventricular sphericity index and functional parameters such as TAPSE and IRT, shows a strong correlation with hypertension in childhood, and may be useful in the detection of those FGR cases at higher cardiovascular risk that might benefit from early therapeutic strategies [14]. Lifestyle interventions such as high intake of dietary long-chain omega-3 fatty acids, breastfeeding promotion, and avoiding obesity, may prevent the progression of subclinical cardiovascular remodeling in children born with FGR [70–72]. Considering the high prevalence of FGR and the progressing availability of intervention strategies, the implementation of cardiovascular follow-up and management could improve the future health of FGR cases, having a remarkable effect on public health. Therefore, based on the collective research data known today, the incorporation in clinical guidelines of FGR as a recognized cardiovascular risk factor for implementing a specific cardiovascular follow-up and management could benefit FGR cases by improving their future health.

Key Points

- FGR is associated with remodeled – more globular – hearts with signs of systolic and diastolic dysfunction in utero.
- Fetal cardiovascular remodeling is more severe in early-onset FGR, but also present in late-onset FGR and SGA.
- Cardiovascular remodeling secondary to FGR persists postnatally.
- FGR is associated with profound and permanent changes in the heart ultrastructure.
- Ductus venosus is useful for predicting perinatal mortality, mainly at earlygestation.
- A combination of fetal echocardiographic parameters and cerebroplacental ratio might help in the detection of FGR cases at higher postnatal cardiovascular risk.
- Postnatal lifestyle and dietary interventions may improve cardiovascular remodeling secondary to FGR.

References

1. Barker DJ, Osmond C, Golding J, Kuh D, Wadsworth ME. Growth in utero, blood pressure in childhood and adult life, and mortality from cardiovascular disease. *BMJ* 1989 Mar 4;298(6673):564–7.

2. Tintu A, Rouwet E, Verlohren S, Brinkmann J, Ahmad S, Crispi F, Van Bilsen M, Carmeliet P, Staff AC, Tjwa M, Cetin I, Gratacós E, Hernandez-Andrade E, Hofstra L, Jacobs M, Lamers WH, Morano I, Safak E, Ahmed A, le Noble F. Hypoxia induces dilated cardiomyopathy in the chick embryo: Mechanism, intervention, and long-term consequences. *PLoS One* 2009;4:e5155.

3. Gluckman PD. Developmental origins of disease paradigm: A mechanistic and evolutionary perspective. *Pediatr Res* 2004;56:311–17.

4. Palinski W, Napoli C. Impaired fetal growth, cardiovascular disease, and the need to move on. *Circulation* 2008;117:341–3.

5. Phillips D. Insulin resistance as a programmed response to fetal undernutrition. *Diabetologia* 1996;39:1119–22.

6. Gluckman PD, Hanson MA, Cooper C, Thornburg KL. Effect of in utero and early-life conditions on adult health. *N Engl J Med* 2008;359:61–73.

7. Committee on Practice Bulletins Gynecology, American College of Obstetricians and Gynecologists. Intrauterine growth restriction. Clinical management guidelines for obstetrician-gynecologists. *Int J Gynecol Obstet* 2001;72:85–96.

8. Figueras F, Gratacós E. Update on the diagnosis and classification of fetal growth restriction and proposal of a stage-based management protocol. *Fetal Diagn Ther* 2014;36:86–98.

9. Alberry M, Soothill P. Management of fetal growth restriction. *Arch Dis Child Fetal Neonatal Ed* 2007;92:62–7.

10. Baschat AA, Cosmi E, Bilardo CM, Wolf H, Berg C, Rigano S, Germer U, Moyano D, Turan S, Hartung Jm Bhide A, Muller T, Bower S, Nicolaides KH, Thilaganathan B, Gembruch U, Ferrazzi E, Hecher K, Galan H, Harman CR. Predictors of neonatal outcome in early-onset placental dysfunction. *Obstet Gynecol* 2007;109:253–61.

11. Crispi F, Gratacós E. Fetal cardiac function: Technical considerations and potential research and clinical applications. *Fetal Diagn Ther* 2012;32(1–2):47–64.

12. Crispi F, Hernandez-Andrade E, Pelsers MM, Plasencia W, Benavides-Serralde JA, Eixarch E, et al. Cardiac dysfunction and cell damage across clinical stages of severity in growth-restricted fetuses. *Am J Obstet Gynecol* 2008 Sep;199(3):254 e1–8.

13. Comas M, Crispi F, Cruz-Martinez R, Martinez JM, Figueras F, Gratacós E. Usefulness of myocardial tissue Doppler vs conventional echocardiography in the evaluation of cardiac dysfunction in early-onset intrauterine growth restriction. *Am J Obstet Gynecol* 2010;203:45.e1–45.e7.

14. Cruz-Lemini M Crispi F, Valenzuela-Alcaraz B, Figueras F, Gómez O, Sitges M, Bijnens B, Gratacós E. A fetal cardiovascular score to predict infant hypertension and arterial remodeling in intrauterine growth restriction. *Am J Obstet Gynecol 2014* Jun;210(6):552.e1–552.e22.

15. Crispi F, Bijnens B, Figueras F, Bartrons J, Eixarch E, Le Noble F, Ahmed A, Gratacós E. Fetal growth restriction results in remodeled and less efficient hearts in children. *Circulation* 2010 Jun 8;121(22):2427–36.

16. Demicheva E, Crispi F. Long-term follow-up of intrauterine growth restriction: Cardiovascular disorders. *Fetal Diagn Ther* 2014;36(2):143–53.

17. Baschat AA. Neurodevelopment following fetal growth restriction and its relationship with antepartum parameters of placental dysfunction. *Ultrasound Obstet Gynecol* 2011;37:501–14.

18. Crispi F, Figueras F, Cruz-Lemini M, Bartrons J, Bijnens B, Gratacos E. Cardiovascular programming in children born small for gestational age and relationship with prenatal signs of severity. *Am J Obstet Gynecol* 2012;207:121.e1–e9.

19. Parra-Saavedra M, Crovetto F, Triunfo S, Savchev S, Peguero A, Nadal A, Parra G, Gratacos E, Figueras F. Placental findings in late-onset SGA births without Doppler signs of placental insufficiency. *Placenta* 2013 Dec;34(12):1136–41.

20. Guyton AC. HJ. *Textbook of Medical Physiology*. 12 edn. Philadelphia, PA: Elsevier Saunder 2011.

21. Bijnens B, Cikes M, Butakoff C, Sitges M, Crispi F. Myocardial motion and deformation: What does it tell us and how does it relate to function? *Fetal Diagn Ther* 2012;32(1–2):5–16.

22. Bijnens BH, Cikes M, Claus P, Sutherland GR. Velocity and deformation imaging for the assessment of myocardial dysfunction. *Eur J Echocardiogr* 2009 Mar;10(2):216–26.

23. Huhta JC. Guidelines for the evaluation of heart failure in the fetus with or without hydrops. *Pediatr Cardiol* 2004 May–Jun;25(3):274–86.

24. Rychik J, Tian Z, Bebbington M, Xu F, McCann M, Mann S, et al. The twin-twin transfusion syndrome: Spectrum of cardiovascular abnormality and development of a cardiovascular score to assess severity of disease. *Am J Obstet Gynecol* 2007 Oct;197(4):392 e1–8.

25. Opie LH, Commerford PJ, Gersh BJ, MA. P. Controversies in ventricular remodelling. *Lancet* 2006;367:356–67.

26. Jessup M AW, Casey DE, Feldman AM, Francis GS, Ganiats TG, Konstam MA, Mancini DM, Rahko PS, Silver MA, Stevenson LW, Yancy CW. 2009 focused update: ACCF/AHA Guidelines for the Diagnosis and Management of Heart Failure in Adults: A report of the American College of Cardiology Foundation/American Heart Association Task Force on Practice Guidelines: Developed in collaboration with the International Society for Heart and Lung Transplantation. *Circulation* 2009;14(119):1977–2016.

27. Kiserud T, Acharya G. The fetal circulation. *Prenat Diagn* 2004 Dec 30;24(13):1049–59.

28. Comas M, Crispi F. Assessment of fetal cardiac function using tissue Doppler techniques. *Fetal Diagn Ther* 2012;32(1–2):30–8.

29. Germanakis I, Gardiner H. Assessment of fetal myocardial deformation using speckle tracking techniques. *Fetal Diagn Ther* 2012;32(1–2):39–46.

30. Godfrey ME, Messing B, Valsky DV, Cohen SM, Yagel S. Fetal cardiac function: M-mode and 4D spatiotemporal image correlation. *Fetal Diagn Ther* 2012;32(1–2):17–21.

31. Hernandez-Andrade E, Benavides-Serralde JA, Cruz-Martinez R, Welsh A, Mancilla-Ramirez J. Evaluation of conventional Doppler fetal cardiac function parameters: E/A ratios, outflow tracts, and myocardial performance index. *Fetal Diagn Ther* 2012;32(1–2):22–9.

32. Lee W, Allan L, Carvalho JS, Chaoui R, Copel J, Devore G, Hecher K, Munoz H, Nelson T, Paladini D, Yagel S. ISUOG consensus statement: What constitutes a fetal echocardiogram? *Ultrasound Obstet Gynecol* 2008;32:239–42.

33. Kasper DL, Braunwald E, Fauci A, et al: *Harrison's Principles of Internal Medicine*. 16 edn. New York: McGraw-Hill, 2005, p. 1346.

34. Timmerman E, Clur SA, Pajkrt E, Bilardo CM. First-trimester measurement of the ductus venosus pulsatility index and the prediction of congenital heart defects. *Ultrasound Obstet Gynecol* 2010;36:668–75.

35. Cruz-Martinez R, Figueras F, Bennasar M, Garcia-Posadas R, Crispi F, Hernandez-Andrade E, et al. Normal reference ranges from 11 to 41 weeks' gestation of fetal left modified myocardial performance index by conventional Doppler with the use of stringent criteria for delimitation of the time periods. *Fetal Diagn Ther* 2011:32(1–2):79–86.

36. Tei C, Nishimura RA, Seward JB, Tajik AJ. Noninvasive Doppler-derived myocardial performance index: Correlation with simultaneous measurements of cardiac catheterization measurements. *J Am Soc Echocardiogr* 1997;10:169–78.

37. Yagel S, Silverman NH, Gembruch U: *Fetal Cardiology: Embryology, Genetics, Physiology, Echocardiographic Evaluation, Diagnosis and Perinatal Management of Cardiac Diseases.* 2 edn. New York: Informa Healthcare USA, 2009.

38. Gardiner HM, Pasquini L, Wolfenden J, Barlow A, Li W, Kulinskaya E, et al. Myocardial tissue Doppler and long axis function in the fetal heart. *Int J Cardiol* 2006 Oct 26;113(1):39–47.

39. Carvalho JS, O'Sullivan C, Shinebourne EA, Henein MY. Right and left ventricular long-axis function in the fetus using angular M-mode. *Ultrasound Obstet Gynecol* 2001 Dec;18(6):619–22.

40. Trambaiolo P, Tonti G, Salustri A, Fedele F, Sutherland G. New insights into regional systolic and diastolic left ventricular function with tissue Doppler echocardiography: From qualitative analysis to a quantitative approach. *J Am Soc Echocardiogr* 2001 Feb;14(2):85–96.

41. Yu CM, Sanderson JE, Marwick TH, Oh JK. Tissue Doppler imaging: A new prognosticator for cardiovascular diseases. *J Am Coll Cardiol* 2007 May 15;49(19):1903–14.

42. Crispi F, Sepulveda-Swatson E, Cruz-Lemini M, Rojas-Benavente J, Garcia-Posada R, Dominguez JM, et al. Feasibility and reproducibility of a standard protocol for 2D speckle tracking and tissue Doppler-based strain and strain rate analysis of the fetal heart. *Fetal Diagn Ther* 2012;32(1–2):96–108.

43. Van Mieghem T, DeKoninck P, Steenhaut P, Deprest J. Methods for prenatal assessment of fetal cardiac function. *Prenat Diagn* 2009;29:1193–203.

44. Hecher K, Campbell S, Doyle P, Harrington K, Nicolaides K. Assessment of fetal compromise by Doppler ultrasound investigation of the fetal circulation: Arterial, intracardiac, and venous blood flow velocity studies. *Circulation* 1995;91:129–38.

45. Cruz-Lemini M, Bijnens B, Valenzuela-Alcaraz B, Sitges M, Figueras F, Crispi F, Gratacós E. Cardiac remodeling in utero in early- and late-onset intrauterine growth restriction. *Ultrasound Obstet Gynecol* 2012:40 (Issue S1):14.

46. Cruz-Lemini M, Crispi F, Valenzuela-Alcaraz B, Figueras F, Sitges M, Gomez O, et al. Value of annular M-mode displacement versus tissue Doppler velocities to assess cardiac function in intrauterine growth restriction. *Ultrasound Obstet Gynecol* 2013 Aug;42(2):175–81.

47. Bilardo CM, Wolf H, Stigter RH, Ville Y, Baez E, Visser CHA, Hecher K. Relationship between monitoring parameters and perinatal outcome in severe, early intrauterine growth restriction. *Ultrasound Obstet Gynecol* 2004;23:119–25.

48. Makikallio K, Vuolteenaho O, Jouppila P, Rasanen J. Ultrasonographic and biochemical markers of human fetal cardiac dysfunction in placental insufficiency. *Circulation* 2002;105:2058–63.

49. Niewiadomska-Jarosik K, Lipecka-Kidawska E, Kowalska-Koprek U, et al. Assessment of cardiac function in fetuses with intrauterine growth retardation using the Tei index. *Med Wieku Rozwoj* 2005;9:153–60.

50. Larsen LU, Petersen OB, Sloth E, Uldbjerg N. Color Doppler myocardial imaging demonstrates reduced diastolic tissue velocity in growth retarded fetuses with flow redistribution. *Eur J Obstet Gynecol Reprod Biol* 2011 Apr;155(2):140–5.

51. Crispi F, Bijnens B, Sepulveda-Swatson E, Cruz-Lemini M, Rojas-Benavente J, Gonzalez-Tendero A, Garcia-Posada R, Rodriguez-Lopez M, Demicheva E, Sitges M, Gratacós E. Postsystolic shortening by myocardial deformation imaging as a sign of cardiac adaptation to pressure overload in fetal growth restriction. *Circ Cardiovasc Imaging* 2014 Sep;7(5):781–7.

52. Comas M, Crispi F, Cruz-Martinez R, Figueras F, Gratacos E. Tissue Doppler echocardiographic markers of cardiac dysfunction in small-for-gestational age fetuses. *Am J Obstet Gynecol* 2011 Jul;205(1):57.e1–6.

53. Cruz-Martinez R, Figueras F, Hernandez-Andrade E, Oros D, Gratacos E. Changes in myocardial performance index and aortic isthmus and ductus venosus Doppler in term, small-for-gestational age fetuses with normal umbilical artery pulsatility index. *Ultrasound Obstet Gynecol* 2011;38(4):400–5.

54. Pérez-Cruz M, Crispi F, Fernández M, Parra J, Gómez Roig M, Gratacós E. Fetal cardiac function in late IUGR versus SGA defined by estimated fetal weight, cerebro-placental ratio and uterine artery Doppler. *Ultrasound Obstet Gynecol* 2014:44 (Issue S1): 19.

55. Chaiworapongsa T, Espinoza J, Yoshimatsu J, et al. Subclinical myocardial injury in small-for-gestational-age neonates. *J Matern Fetal Neonatal Med* 2002;11:385–90.

56. Crispi F, Gonzalez-Tendero A, Zhang C, Balicevic V, Cardenas R, Loncaric S, Bonnin A, Gratacós E, Bijnens B. Cardiac fiber orientation and coronary changes in a rabbit model of IUGR using X-ray phase-contrast synchrotron radiation-based micro-CT. *Ultrasound Obstet Gynecol* 2014; 44 (Issue S1): 133.

57. Gonzalez-Tendero A, Torre I, Garcia-Canadilla P, Crispi F, García-García F, Dopazo J, Bijnens B, Gratacós E. Intrauterine growth restriction is associated with cardiac ultrastructural and gene expression changes related to the energetic metabolism in a rabbit model. *Am J Physiol Heart Circ Physiol* 2013 Dec;305(12):H1752–60.

58. Iruretagoyena JY, Torre I, Amat-Roldan I, Psilodimitrakopoulos S, Crispi F, Garcia-Canadilla P, Gonzalez-Tendero A, Nadal A, Eixarch E, Loza-Alvarez P, Artigas D, Gratacos E. Ultrastructural analysis of myocardiocyte sarcomeric changes in relation with cardiac dysfunction in human fetuses with intrauterine growth restriction. *Am J Obstet Gynecol* 2011;204:S34.

59. Skilton MK, Evans N, Griffiths KA, Harmer JA, Celermajer D. Aortic wall thickness in newborns with intrauterine restriction. *Lancet* 2005;23:1484–6.

60. Stergiotou I, Crispi F, Valenzuela-Alcaraz B, Cruz-Lemini M, Bijnens B, Gratacos E. Aortic and carotid intima-media thickness in term small-for-gestational-age newborns and relationship with prenatal signs of severity. *Ultrasound Obstet Gynecol* 2014 Jun;43(6):625–31.

61. Cosmi E, Visentin S, Fanelli T, Mautone AJ, Zanardo V. Aortic intima media thickness in fetuses and children with intrauterine growth restriction. *Obstet Gynecol* 2009 Nov;114(5):1109–14.

62. Martin H, Hu J, Gennser G, Norman M. Impaired endothelial function and increased carotid stiffness in 9-year-old children with low birthweight. *Circulation* 2000;102:2739–44.

63. Bjarnegård N, Morsing E, Cinthio M, Länne T, Brodszki J. Cardiovascular function in adulthood following intrauterine growth restriction with abnormal fetal blood flow. *Ultrasound Obstet Gynecol* 2013 Feb;41(2):177–84.

64. Berenson GS. Childhood risk factors predict adult risk associated with subclinical cardiovascular disease. The Bogalusa Heart Study. *Am J Cardiol* 2002;90:3L–7L.

65. Girsen A, Ala-Kopsala M, Makikallio K, Vuolteenaho O, Rasanen J. Cardiovascular hemodynamics and umbilical artery N-terminal peptide of proB-type natriuretic peptide in human fetuses with growth restriction. *Ultrasound Obstet Gynecol* 2007;29:296–303.

66. Baschat AA. Ductus venosus Doppler for fetal surveillance in high-risk pregnancies. *Clin Obstet Gynecol* 2010 Dec;53(4):858–68.

67. Cruz-Lemini M, Crispi F, Van Mieghem T, Pedraza D, Cruz-Martinez R, Acosta-Rojas R, et al. Risk of perinatal death in early-onset intrauterine growth restriction according to gestational age and cardiovascular Doppler indices: A multicenter study. *Fetal Diagn Ther* 2012;32(1–2):116–22.

68. Hernandez-Andrade E, Crispi F, Benavides-Serralde JA, Plasencia W, Diesel HF, Eixarch E, Acosta-Rojas R, Figueras F, Nicolaides K, Gratacós E. Contribution of the myocardial performance index and aortic isthmus blood flow index to predicting mortality in preterm growth-restricted fetuses. *Ultrasound Obstet Gynecol* 2009 Oct;34(4):430–6.

69. Williams CL, Hayman LL, Daniels SR, Robinson TN, Steinberger J, Paridon S, Bazzarre T. Cardiovascular health in childhood: A statement for health professionals from the Committee on Atherosclerosis, Hypertension, and Obesity in the Young (AHOY) of the Council on Cardiovascular Disease in the Young, American Heart Association. *Circulation* 2002;106:143–60.

70. Skilton MR, Mikkilä V, Würtz P, Ala-Korpela M, Sim KA, Soininen P, Kangas AJ, Viikari JS, Juonala M, Laitinen T, Lehtimäki T, Taittonen L, Kähönen M, Celermajer DS, Raitakari OT. Fetal growth, omega-3 (ω-3) fatty acids, and progression of subclinical atherosclerosis: preventing fetal origins of disease? The Cardiovascular Risk in Young Finns Study. *Am J Clin Nutr* 2013;97:58–65.

71. Skilton MR, Ayer JG, Harmer JA, Webb K, Leeder SR, Marks GB, Celermajer DS. Impaired fetal growth and arterial wall thickening. A randomized trial of omega-3 supplementation. *Pediatrics* 2012;129:e698.

72. Rodriguez-Lopez M, Osorio L, Acosta R, Cruz-Lemini M, Figueras J, Figueras F, Gratacós E, Crispi F. Effect of postnatal diet on reverting cardiovascular remodelling in intrauterine growth restriction. *Ultrasound Obstet Gynecol* 2014; 44 (Issue S1): 120.

73. Mancia G, Fagard R, Narkiewicz K, Redón J, Zanchetti A, Böhm M, Christiaens T, Cifkova R, De Backer G, Dominiczak A, Galderisi M, Grobbee DE, Jaarsma T, Kirchhof P, Kjeldsen SE, Laurent S, Manolis AJ, Nilsson PM, Ruilope LM, Schmieder RE, Sirnes PA, Sleight P, Viigimaa M, Waeber B, Zannad F; Task Force Members. 2013 ESH/ESC Guidelines for the management of arterial hypertension: The Task Force for the management of arterial hypertension of the European Society of Hypertension (ESH) and of the European Society of Cardiology (ESC). *J Hypertens* 2013;31:1281–357.

74. Kavey RE, Allada V, Daniels SR, Hayman LL, McCrindle BW, Newburger JW, Parekh RS, Steinberger J. Cardiovascular risk reduction in high-risk pediatric patients: A scientific statement from

the American Heart Association Expert Panel on Population and Prevention Science; the Councils on Cardiovascular Disease in the Young, Epidemiology and Prevention, Nutrition, Physical Activity and Metabolism, High Blood Pressure Research, Cardiovascular Nursing, and the Kidney in Heart Disease; and the Interdisciplinary Working Group on Quality of Care and Outcomes Research: Endorsed by the American Academy of Pediatrics. *Circulation* 2006;114:2710–38.

Chapter

19

Heart Rate Changes and Autonomic Nervous System in Fetal Growth Restriction

Silvia M. Lobmaier, Karl-Theo M. Schneider, and Gerard H. A. Visser

Introduction

Antenatal cardiotocography (CTG) is commonly used in the surveillance of fetuses compromised by fetal growth restriction (FGR). However, interpretation of CTG patterns suffers from substantial inter- and intra-observer variability. Scoring systems have been able to reduce the inconsistency of visual assessment, but not to eliminate it. A computerized analysis known as the Oxford system has been developed by Dawes and Redman to try to solve this problem, along with short-term variation (STV) calculated from fetal heart rate (FHR) variation. Decreased FHR variation has been described to identify fetuses suffering from hypoxemia. Current assessment methods of FHR variation cannot differentiate between sympathetic and vagal influences. For this purpose, a signal processing technique derived from adult cardiology called phase-rectified signal averaging (PRSA) has been developed. PRSA can eliminate artefacts and signal perturbations of bio-signals and extract areas of interest reflecting the autonomic nervous system by the "acceleration" and "deceleration capacity." In FGR, acceleration and deceleration capacity are decreased as a result of alterations of the autonomic nervous system.

In this chapter, the autonomic nervous regulation of fetal heart rate and its variation is discussed, as are changes occurring with progressive deterioration of the fetal condition. The Dawes/Redman numerical analysis of the fetal heart rate is presented, as well as novel developments to quantify autonomic nervous system control.

Autonomic Nervous System

The Barker Hypothesis has described the inverse correlation between low birth weight and cardiovascular disease in adult life. Genetic and environmental interaction during fetal life is thought to play an important role in cardiovascular development [1]. Cardiovascular regulation depends on sympathetic and vagal autonomic control. During the development of the fetal heart, the conduction systems become enervated with autonomic nerve fibers, first sympathetic and later parasympathetic. From 18 weeks gestation onward, progressive vagal enervation of the sinoatrial and atrioventricular nodes results in a decrease of fetal heart rate. FHR variability occurs as a result of maturation of neural control [2]. During the antenatal period, FHR accelerations are almost exclusively associated with fetal movements [3].

Autonomic Nervous System and Fetal Growth Restriction

FGR will result in reduced variation in the fetal heart rate tracing [4]. Acute hypoxemia causes an immediate increase in short-term variation followed by a gradual decrease when hypoxemia becomes chronic. The initial increase in FHR variation is probably caused by the increase of fetal plasma catecholamine concentration, but STV decreases in spite of the persistent elevation in fetal plasma norepinephrine and arterial blood pressure. This might be due to a decrease in the number or sensitivity of ß-receptors in the fetal heart during chronic placental insufficiency, suggesting an alteration in the normal maturational changes of the autonomic control of fetal heart rate [5].

In small-for-gestational-age (SGA) fetuses, plasma cortisol is increased and plasma ACTH is decreased [6]. In chronic hypoxemia – a potential consequence of FGR – several hormones producing a vasoconstriction effect on the fetal circulation increase, e.g., catecholamines, arginine, vasopressin, and angiotensin II [7]. In consequence FHR rises. Activation of the sympathetic nervous system is thought to play an important role in the pathogenesis of hypertension [8]. Placental insufficiency and chronic hypoxemia might be a stimulus for catecholamine synthesis or hyper-innervation of fetal vessels by sympathetic neurons. This activation of sympathetic nervous system established in utero may be one of the mechanisms linking small size with increased blood pressure in adult life [9].

Fetal Heart Rate Patterns

With a gradual impairment in the condition of the FGR fetus there is a gradual decrease in FHR variation. On average, FHR variation falls below the normal range at the same time as decelerations occur. This condition is associated with fetal hypoxemia [10–13]. Fetal heart rate is usually slightly increased, but remains within the normal range [11]. With a further deterioration FHR variation disappears, basal fetal heart rate decreases, and late – usually shallow – decelerations occur after every Braxton Hicks contraction [14]. This condition is associated with fetal acidemia and impending intrauterine death [14,15].

The fact that the FHR pattern only becomes abnormal when fetal hypoxemia is present implies that FHR monitoring is not a useful screening tool to identify the FGR fetus. It is, however, useful to identify fetuses that have become hypoxemic. Longitudinal assessment of FHR variation may identify FGR fetuses with a consistently decreasing FHR variation, before variation has become abnormal [13].

During the preterm period, abnormal FHR patterns usually occur after blood flow velocity waveform patterns in the umbilical artery have become abnormal, but coincide with the occurrence of abnormal ductus venosus waveform patterns [17]. At term, FHR becomes abnormal before significant Doppler changes in the umbilical artery occur. This is due to the fact that abnormal flow patterns in the umbilical artery occur only when 30–50% of placental capacity is lacking; term fetuses will already be hypoxemic beforehand. Fetal movements are usually reduced in incidence only when FHR variation has become abnormal [18].

Computer Analysis of Antenatal Fetal Heart Rate Patterns

Visual assessment of FHR patterns suffers from substantial inter- and intra-observer variability [19]. Scoring systems have been found to be able to reduce the inconsistency of visual assessment, but not to eliminate it [20]. A computerized analysis known as the Oxford system has been developed by Dawes and Redman [21] to try to solve this problem, with short-term variation (STV) calculated from the basal fetal heart rate [22]. STV has been shown to be related to the fetal oxygenation [12,22,23]. The advantages of this system are:

- eliminates inter- and intra-observer variation
- quantifies fetal heart rate variation
- enables the monitoring of trends
- facilitates multicenter studies
- likely to produce more consistent clinical responses
- can be used in research
- reduces recording time (when using "Dawes/Redman criteria met" mode).

Nomograms of STV with increasing gestation have been published [23,24]. These depend on the recording length and are narrower with recordings of longer duration [25]. For longitudinal assessment of FHR variation, recording length should be about 1 hour to prevent large day-to-day fluctuations. Using such a recording length, each fetus may be used as its own control to assess changes in FHR variation with time. Generally, recording length may be considerably shorter, and the Oxford system indicates when the Dawes/Redman criteria for normality are being met.

FHR variation depends on gestational age and variation increases with increasing gestational age. It also depends on the fetal activity state and during fetal state 1F (non-REM sleep) FHR variation is lowest. At term, such episodes may last for up to 40–5 minutes. There is a negative correlation between FHR and STV, i.e., with a higher FHR, the variation will be lower. FHR variation is generally highest around midnight and lowest in the early morning [26,27]. Betamethasone, given to enhance fetal lung maturation, results in a temporary 20–30% reduction of STV 2 days after treatment has started with a normalization on day four. It also results in a 50% reduction of fetal movements and in a 90% reduction of fetal breathing movements [28,29]. Such effects are not seen after dexamethasone. This drug results in an initial increase of STV [29,30] that is less pronounced in FGR. Knowledge of these phenomena is important when assessing the fetal condition, especially in surveillance of FGR, when also fetal impairment might lead to a reduced STV.

STV has been linked to fetal oxygenation, both after caesarean section and by using data obtained at cordocentesis [31,32].

Cut-Off Values of STV When Deciding to Deliver the FGR Fetus

Ribbert and colleagues have shown that in SGA fetuses in whom STV was obtained immediately before cordocentesis, a STV <3.6 ms was always associated with severe fetal hypoxemia [12]. Conversely, Dawes and colleagues showed in a high-risk population (not all SGA!) that the risk of acidemia was low and no intrauterine deaths occurred if STV > 3 ms. If STV decreases <2.6 ms, 34% of these cases were associated with intrauterine death or metabolic acidemia [33]. Anceschi and colleagues found that a short-term variation <4.5 ms predicted acidemia with a sensitivity of 100% and a specificity of 70% [34].

The STV cut-off values used by the TRUFFLE group were:

Delivery of FGR fetuses <29 weeks gestation if STV <3.5 ms and of FGR fetuses 29–32 weeks gestation if STV <4 ms [35].

In case of steroid administration, no decision on delivery should be made on the grounds of reduced variability between 24 and 72 hours after the first intramuscular dose of steroid, unless there were spontaneous repeated persistent unprovoked decelerations on the CTG. In cases of spontaneous decelerations, delivery is generally indicated.

Advanced Techniques of Heart Rate Analysis

Newer methods on the basis of FHR variation have been developed during the past decade: linear time and frequency techniques as well as the computation of nonlinear indices may contribute to enhance the diagnostic power and reliability of fetal monitoring. The computation of different indices on FHR variability signals, either linear and nonlinear, gives helpful indications to describe pathophysiological mechanisms involved in the cardiovascular and neural system controlling the fetal heart [36,37].

Fetal magnetocardiography (fMCG) allows noninvasive, beat-to-beat analysis of fetal heart rate throughout gestation [38]. Schneider and colleagues have shown that the complexity of regulation is significantly lower in compromised FGR fetuses [39].

A quite new method derived from adult cardiology is phase-rectified signal averaging (PRSA). Artefacts, noise and non-stationarities are eliminated from a (quasi-) periodic signal. Acceleration and deceleration related time intervals are analyzed separately, giving insights to the autonomic nervous system. Autonomic nervous system impairment in FGR fetuses has been demonstrated using the PRSA method, and there is some evidence that autonomic impairment may precede reduction in STV and fetal hypoxemia [40–43].

Conclusion

CTG is useful in the antenatal surveillance of FGR since it detects fetuses that are likely to be hypoxemic. Given the large inter- and intra-observer variability of visual assessment of FHR tracings, computer analysis using the Dawes/Redman system is recommended. This holds especially for longitudinal monitoring of STV in case of FGR. The limits of normality of STV are dependent on gestational age and on the duration of the recording. Newer techniques like the PRSA method give insight in the regulation of the autonomic system and may show changes preceding the occurrence of fetal hypoxemia.

Key Points

- The fetal heart rate conduction system becomes innervated first with sympathetic and from 18 weeks gestation onward with vagal fibers.
- Chronic hypoxemia leads to decreased short-term heart rate variation, suggesting an impairment of autonomic control.
- In FGR, the fetal heart rate baseline increases, whereas with progressive deterioration of fetal condition, there is a gradual fall in heart rate variation. Reduced variation and occurrence of decelerations are associated with fetal hypoxemia.
- Computer analysis to assess FHR variation eliminates inter- and intra-observer variation. For longitudinal monitoring of FGR fetuses, recording time should be around 1 hour to assess changes occurring with time. STV increases with advancing gestational age
- Maternal betamethasone administration causes temporary decrease of STV between 24 and 72 hours after the first intramuscular dose of steroid.

- The TRUFFLE group indicated delivery of FGR fetuses <29 weeks gestation if STV <3.5 ms and of FGR fetuses 29–32 weeks gestation if STV < 4 ms.
- Newer techniques allow further insights into autonomic fetal heart rate control. This might help to identify fetuses at risk for adverse outcome, e.g., cardiovascular disease in adult life.

References

1. Barker DJ, Osmond C, Golding J, Kuh D, Wadsworth ME. Growth in utero, blood pressure in childhood and adult life, and mortality from cardiovascular disease. *BMJ* 1989;298:564–7.

2. Manning Frank A: *Fetal medicine, Principles and Practice*. Chapter 2, The fetal heart rate – genesis of fetal heart rate patterns. *Appleton & Lange Verlag, Norwalk*, CT, 1995.

3. Dawes GS, Visser GH, Goodman JD, Levine DH. Numerical analysis of the human fetal heart rate: Modulation by breathing and movement. *Am J Obstet Gynecol* 1981;140:535–44.

4. Henson GL, Dawes GS, Redman CW. Antenatal fetal heart-rate variability in relation to fetal acid-base status at caesarean section. *BJOG* 1983;90:516–21.

5. Murotsuki J, Bocking AD, Gagnon R. Fetal heart rate patterns in growth-restricted fetal sheep induced by chronic fetal placental embolization. *Am J Obstet Gynecol* 1997;176:282–90.

6. Schäffer L, Burkhardt T, Müller-Vizentini D, Rauh M, Tomaske M, Mieth RA, Bauersfeld U, Beinder E. Cardiac autonomic balance in small-for-gestational-age neonates. *Am J Physiol Heart Circ Physiol* 2008;294:H884–90.

7. Jones CT, Robinson JS. Studies on experimental growth retardation in sheep. Plasma catecholamines in fetuses with small placenta. *J Dev Physiol* 1983;5:77–87.

8. Lohmeier TE. The sympathetic nervous system and long-term blood pressure regulation. *Am J Hypertens* 2001;14:147S–154S.

9. McMillen IC, Robinson JS. Developmental origins of the metabolic syndrome: Prediction, plasticity, and programming. *Physiol Rev* 2005;85:571–633.

10. Pardi G, Cetin I, Marconi AM, Lanfranchi A, Bozzetti P, Ferrazzi E, Buscaglia M, Battaglia FC. Diagnostic value of blood sampling in fetuses with growth retardation. *N Engl J Med* 1993;328:692–6.

11. Bekedam DJ, Visser HA, Mulder EJH, Poelmann-Weesjes G. Heart rate variation and movement incidence in growth retarded fetuses: The significance

12. Ribbert LSM, Snijders RJM, Nicolaides KH, Visser GHA. Relation of fetal blood gases and data from computer assisted analysis of fetal heart rate patterns in small for gestation fetuses. *BJOG* 1991;98:820–3.

13. Snijders RJM, Ribbert LSM, Visser GHA, Mulder EJH. Numeric analysis of heart rate variation in intrauterine growth-retarded fetuses: A longitudinal study. *Am J Obstet Gynecol* 1992;166:22–7.

14. Visser GH, Redman CW, Huisjes HJ, Turnbull AC. Nonstressed antepartum heart rate monitoring: Implications of decelerations after spontaneous contractions. *Am J Obstet Gynecol* 1980;138:429–35.

15. Emmen L, Huisjes HJ, Aarnoudse JG, Visser GH, Okken A. Antepartum diagnosis of the "terminal" fetal state by cardiotocography. *BJOG* 1975;82:353–9.

16. Visser GHA, Sadovsky G, Nicolaides KH. Antepartum heart rate patterns in small-for-gestational-age third-trimester fetuses: Correlations with blood gas values obtained at cordocentesis. *Am J Obstet Gynecol* 1990;162:698–703.

17. Hecher K, Bilardo CM, Stigter RH, Ville Y, Hackelöer BJ, Kok HJ, Senat MV, Visser GH. Monitoring of fetuses with intrauterine growth restriction: A longitudinal study. *Ultrasound Obstet Gynecol* 2001;18:564–70.

18. Ribbert LS, Visser GH, Mulder EJ, Zonneveld MF, Morssink LP. Changes with time in fetal heart rate variation, movement incidences and haemodynamics in intrauterine growth retarded fetuses: A longitudinal approach to the assessment of fetal well being. *Early Hum Dev* 1993;31:195–208.

19. Figueras F, Albela S, Bonino S, Palacio M, Barrau E, Hernandez S, Casellas C, Coll O, Cararach V. Visual analysis of antepartum fetal heart rate tracings: Inter- and intra-observer agreement and impact of knowledge of neonatal outcome. *J Perinat Med* 2005;33:241–5.

20. Pardey J, Moulden M, Redman CWG. A computer system for the numerical analysis of nonstress tests. *Am J Obstet Gynecol* 2002;186:1095–103.

21. Dawes GS, Visser GHA, Goodman JDS, Redman CWG. Numerical analysis of the human fetal heart rate: The quality of ultrasound recors. *Am J Obstet Gynecol* 1981;141:43–52.

22. Street P, Dawes GS, Moulden M, Redman CWG. Short-term variation in abnormal antenatal fetal heart rate records. *Am J Obstet Gynecol* 1991;165:515–23.

23. Nijhuis IJ, Ten Hof J, Mulder EJ, Nijhuis JG, Narayan H, Taylor DJ, Visser GH. Fetal heart rate in relation to

of antenatal late heart rate decelerations. *Am J Obstet Gynecol* 1987;157:126–33.

its variation in normal and growth retarded fetuses. *Eur J Obstet Gynecol Reprod Biol* 2000;89:27–33.

24. Serra V, Bellver J, Moulden M, Redman CWG. Computerized analysis of normal fetal heart rate pattern throughout gestation. *Ultrasound Obstet Gynecol* 2009;34:74–9.

25. Nijhuis IJM, Ten Hof J, Mulder EJH, Nijhuis JG, Narayan H, Taylor DJ et al. Numerical fetal heart rate analysis: Nomograms, minimal duration of recording and intrafetal consistency. *Prenat Neonat Med* 1998;3:314–22.

26. Nijhuis IJ, Ten Hof J, Nijhuis JG, Mulder EJ, Narayan H, Taylor DJ, Visser GH. Temporal organization of fetal behavior from 24-weeks gestation onwards in normal and complicated pregnancies. *Dev Psychobiol* 1999;34:257–68.

27. Van Vliet MA, Martin CB Jr, Nijhuis JG, Prechtl HF. The relationship between fetal activity and behavioral states and fetal breathing movements in normal and growth-retarded fetuses. *Am J Obstet Gynecol* 1985;153:582–8.

28. Mushkat Y, Ascher-Landsberg J, Keidar R, Carmon E, Pauzner D, David MP. The effect of betamethasone versus dexamethasone on fetal biophysical parameters. *Eur J Obstet Gynecol Reprod Biol* 2001;97:50–2.

29. Mulder EJ, Derks JB, Visser GH. Antenatal corticosteroid therapy and fetal behaviour: A randomised study of the effects of betamethasone and dexamethasone. *BJOG* 1997;104:1239–47.

30. Dawes GS, Serra-Serra V, Moulden M, Redman CW. Dexamethasone and fetal heart rate variation. *BJOG* 1994;101:675–9.

31. Serra V, Moulden M, Bellver J, Redman CW. The value of the short-term fetal heart rate variation for timing the delivery of growth-retarded fetuses. *BJOG* 2008;115:1101–7.

32. Anceschi MM, Piazze JJ, Ruozi-Berretta A, Cosmi E, Cerekja A, Maranghi L, Cosmi EV. Validity of short term variation (STV) in detection of fetal acidemia. *J Perinat Med* 2003;31:231–6.

33. Dawes GS, Moulden M, Redman CWG. Short term fetal heart rate variation, decelerations, and umbilical flow velocity waveforms before labor. *Obstet Gynecol* 1992;80:673–8.

34. Anceschi MM, Ruozi-Berretta A, Piazze JJ, Cosmi E, Cerekja A, Meloni P, Cosmi EV. Computerized cardiotocography in the management of intrauterine growth restriction associated with Doppler velocimetry alterations. *Int J Gynaecol Obstet* 2004;86:365–70.

35. Lees CC, Marlow N, Van Wassenaer-Leemhuis A, Arabin B, Bilardo CM, Brezinka C, Calvert S, Derks JB, Diemert A, Duvekot JJ, Ferrazzi E, Frusca T, Ganzevoort W, Hecher K, Martinelli P, Ostermayer E, Papageorghiou AT, Schlembach D, Schneider KT, Thilaganathan B, Todros T, Valcamonico A, Visser GH, Wolf H; TRUFFLE study group. 2 year neurodevelopmental and intermediate perinatal outcomes in infants with very preterm fetal growth restriction (TRUFFLE): A randomised trial. *Lancet* 2015;385:2162–72.

36. Signorini MG, Fanelli A, Magenes G. Monitoring fetal heart rate during pregnancy: Contributions from advanced signal processing and wearable technology. *Comput Math Methods Med* 2014;2014:707581. doi: 10.1155/2014/707581. Epub 2014 Jan 30.

37. Gonçalves H, Rocha AP, Ayres-de-Campos D, Bernardes J. Frequency domain and entropy analysis of fetal heart rate: Appealing tools for fetal surveillance and pharmacodynamic assessment of drugs. *Cardiovasc Hematol Disord Drug Targets* 2008;8:91–8.

38. Van Leeuwen P, Lange S, Bettermann H, Grönemeyer D, Hatzmann W. Fetal heart rate variability and complexity in the course of pregnancy. *Early Hum Dev* 1999;54:259–69.

39. Schneider U, Fiedler A, Liehr M, Kähler C, Schleussner E Fetal heart rate variability in growth restricted fetuses. *Biomed Tech (Berl)* 2006;51:248–50.

40. Huhn EA, Lobmaier S, Fischer T, Schneider R, Bauer A, Schneider KT, Schmidt G: New computerized fetal heart rate analysis for surveillance of intrauterine growth restriction. *Prenat Diagn* 2011;31:509–14.

41. Lobmaier SM, Huhn EA, Pildner von Steinburg S, Müller A, Schuster T, Ortiz JU, Schmidt G, Schneider KT. Phase-rectified signal averaging as a new method for surveillance of growth restricted fetuses. *J Matern Fetal Neonatal Med* 2012;25:2523–8.

42. Graatsma EM, Mulder EJ, Vasak B, Lobmaier SM, Pildner von Steinburg S, Schneider KT, Schmidt G, Visser GH Average acceleration and deceleration capacity of fetal heart rate in normal pregnancy and in pregnancies complicated by fetal growth restriction. *J Matern Fetal Neonatal Med* 2012;25:2517–22.

43. Lobmaier SM, Mensing van Charante N, Ferrazzi E, Giussani DA, Shaw CJ, Müller A, Ortiz JU, Ostermayer E, Haller B, Prefumo F, Frusca T, Hecher K, Arabin B, Thilaganathan B, Papageorghiou AT, Bhide A, Martinelli P, Duvekot JJ, Van Eyck J, Visser GH, Schmidt G, Ganzevoort W, Lees CC, Schneider KT. Phase-rectified signal averaging method to predict perinatal outcome in infants with very preterm fetal growth restriction – a secondary analysis of TRUFFLE-trial. *Am J Obstet Gynecol* 2016. Nov;215(5):630.e1-630.e7

The Fetal Arterial and Venous Circulation in Fetal Growth Restriction

Kurt Hecher and Werner Diehl

Introduction

Fetal hemodynamic redistribution of blood flow in the presence of chronic hypoxemia due to impaired uteroplacental perfusion and subsequent placental malfunction is characterized by arterial dilatation in the brain, the suprarenal glands, and the coronary arteries. Doppler studies of the fetal circulation showing progressive changes of flow velocity waveforms (FVWs) have been used for clinical surveillance and timely delivery of affected fetuses [1–3]. A decrease in the umbilical end-diastolic flow (EDF), due to an increased placental resistance, together with a flattening of fetal growth parameters, is the earliest sonographic sign of placental dysfunction. The umbilical EDF progressively decreases, finally showing absent or reversed EDF (AREDF). Dilatation of the arterial vascular bed in the central nervous system, leading to a low-resistance flow pattern with high end diastolic velocities, is typically seen in the middle cerebral artery (MCA) and constitutes the "brain-sparing effect." Thereafter, due to progressive hypoxemia and deteriorating heart function, changes in the venous system occur. In the ductus venosus (DV), there is a decrease of velocities during atrial contraction (a-wave), which decrease to zero and finally get reversed. During the further course of fetal compromise, the presence of bi- or triphasic pulsations in the umbilical vein is an additional sign of cardiac decompensation. In severe early fetal growth restriction at gestational ages below 32 weeks, the changes in the pulsatility index (PI) of the umbilical artery and the a-wave of the DV are used clinically for timing delivery of growth-restricted fetuses in combination with other monitoring parameters such as the computer-assisted analysis of fetal heart rate (cCTG) [4]. In fetuses with a gestational age beyond 32 weeks, postponing delivery until changes in the venous circulation occur is not warranted, since the lower risks of prematurity no longer justify the risk of cardiac decompensation. This distinguishes the management of late-onset from early-onset growth-restricted fetuses. In these

cases, a decreasing resistance in the MCA leading to a low cerebroplacental ratio (CPR), in addition to deterioration of parameters such as the cCTG, may determine the optimal time for delivery.

Following the course of the fetal circulation, this chapter addresses first the redistribution of blood flow in the venous system at the level of the DV and the hepatic circulation. The DV is the first shunt of freshly oxygenated and nutrient-enriched blood returning from the placenta via the umbilical vein to the fetal heart. The second shunt, the foramen ovale, plays an important role in delivering well-oxygenated blood directly to the left ventricle. Flow patterns in the aortic isthmus (AI), MCA, and other arterial vessels contribute to the understanding of arterial redistribution in fetal growth restriction (FGR).

The Normal Venous System and Its Changes in Fetal Growth Restriction (FGR)

Oxygenated blood returning from the placenta to the fetus via the umbilical cord is partly shunted through the ductus venosus from the intrahepatic umbilical vein (UV) to the inferior vena cava and through the foramen ovale directly to the left atrium. Under normal circumstances, in the second and third trimesters, 30% and 18%, respectively, of umbilical venous blood is shunted directly to the heart [5]. Consequently, approximately 70% to 80% of blood volume of the UV is directed to the fetal liver, which shows the high priority given to this organ in fetal development. Haugen and colleagues [6] measured a DV shunting of 25% and 55% of umbilical venous flow supplying the left hepatic lobe and 20% the right hepatic lobe. At the origin of the DV, the vessel diameter is significantly smaller than that of the UV, thus resulting in an increase of flow velocities, which typically produces an aliasing effect in Doppler studies. Powered by this velocity increase, freshly oxygenated blood is thus directed to the right posterior wall of the inferior vena cava (IVC). The spatial order of the different blood streams in the inferior vena cava is depicted in Figure 20.1. The blood stream coming from the DV is located in the right posterior area, the stream of the hepatic veins draining the right lobe of the liver in the left lateral area and the stream from the lower inferior vena cava traveling anteriorly. At the level of the right atrium, owing to the arrangement of the flap of the foramen ovale and the crista dividens, the flow of the oxygenated blood stream of the right posterior area of the IVC is directed preferentially through the foramen ovale to the left heart. The blood streams entering the right atrium from the superior and distal IVC and from the hepatic veins are directed to the right ventricle through the tricuspid valve. These particular anatomic relations are crucial for effectively directing well-oxygenated blood enriched with nutrients to the left ventricle.

Partly triggered by decreasing oxygen saturation and/or suboptimal concentrations of essential nutrients owing to an impaired placental function, but also by the presence of adrenergic substances and prostaglandins, blood flow through the DV may be increased as required to meet metabolic demands of central organs [7,8]. Reduction of flow in the intrahepatic portal venous system may play an important role in venous blood flow redistribution at the level of the DV and the left portal vein system [9].

According to the degree of FGR, up to 90% of umbilical venous blood flow may be shunted through the DV [10,11], as depicted in Figure 20.2. Venous Doppler studies have even shown blood "stealing" from the left portal vein to the DV in cases of severe FGR [12,13]. Under normal circumstances, 20% of blood flow to the liver originates from portal venous flow and 80% from the umbilical vein [6]. A decrease in UV flow to the liver owing to redistribution to the DV leads to a compensatory mechanism by increasing flow through the hepatic arteries [14]. Accordingly, reduced net blood supply from the umbilical vein to the liver may be responsible for the growth restriction of the abdominal circumference and related to fetal programming [7,15]. In a study of 381 uncomplicated pregnancies, Godfrey and colleagues reported on the finding that an increased liver blood flow was associated with an increased neonatal and infant fat mass at 4 years of age [16]. In this study, pregnancies with smaller placental weight were associated with brain

sparing and increased DV shunting. Therefore, they proposed a fetal circulatory mechanism by which the allocation of nutrients and oxygen either to the brain or to the liver is prioritized according to their availability, which may depend on placentation, maternal metabolism, and diet. In an earlier observational study, fetuses of slim mothers with a balanced, healthy dietary intake in contrast to fetuses of mothers on an unbalanced diet showed an increased blood flow to the liver and a decreased shunting through the DV, thus indicating the regulation of flow distribution at the level of the DV and the left portal vein being crucial for the delivery of oxygen and nutrients from the placenta [15].

Chronic hypoxemia owing to placental insufficiency may lead to an increase in cardiac oxygen consumption due to increased cardiac afterload on the basis of high umbilico-placental resistance, and cardiac function may deteriorate. With progressive deterioration of cardiac function cardiac output decreases [17]. Increasing end-diastolic ventricular pressure and retrograde transmission of the pulse wave originating from atrial contraction (a-wave) during late ventricular diastole will cause a progressive decrease in a-wave velocities in the DV. Consequently, the pulsatility index for veins (PIV) [18,19] increases and finally, zero or reverse flow during atrial contraction may occur (Figure 20.3) [2]. Under physiological conditions, the retrograde transmission of the pulse wave of the atrial contraction is not seen in the UV, because both the change in vessel diameter and the reservoir effect of the wider UV extinguish the wave energy required to cause pulsations [20,21]. Therefore, the retrograde propagation of pulsations from the atrial contraction through the DV into the UV implies high central venous pressures and seems to be related to cardiac decompensation.

Furthermore, prolongation of diastolic time intervals, seen during the cardiac cycle and reflected FVWs of the DV, may be related to hypovolemia and consequently decreased venous return in growth-restricted fetuses [22,23]. A prolongation in ventricular filling times and/or a shortening of ejection times, in response to adrenergic stimuli, may be adaptive cardiac reactions to hypovolemia.

Highly pulsatile DV FVWs, in particular if accompanied by absent or reverse flow during the a-wave, have been investigated in clinical studies to determine the optimal time for delivery of growth-restricted fetuses at risk of cardiac decompensation [1–3].

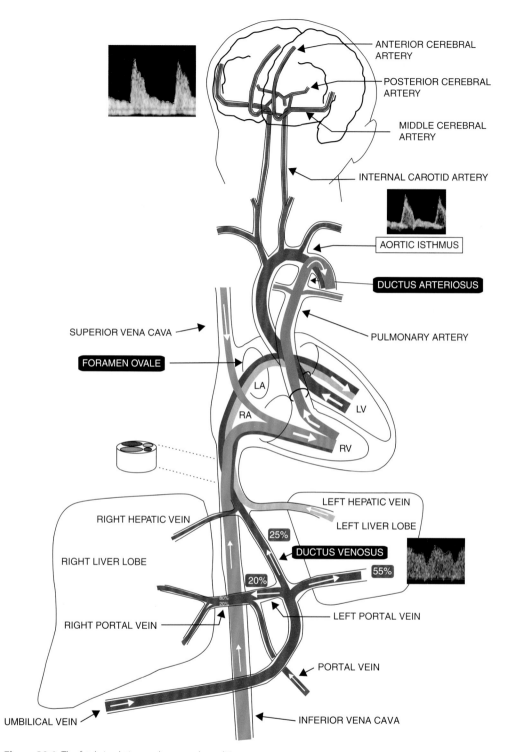

Figure 20.1 The fetal circulation under normal conditions.

The fetal circulatory system is characterized by the presence of the placenta and three shunts: ductus venosus, foramen ovale, and ductus arteriosus. Blood returning from the placenta via the umbilical vein is partly directed through the ductus venosus to the right atrium. From there, this oxygen-saturated blood crosses the foramen ovale to reach the left ventricle, where it is then directed to the aorta. From the superior and inferior vena cava, oxygen-depleted blood enters the right atrium and the right ventricle, from where it is directed to the pulmonary artery. The ductus arteriosus allows its passage to the descending aorta and the placenta. Under normal conditions, 25% of the oxygenated blood is shunted through the ductus venosus directly to the heart, while 55% supplies the left lobe of the liver.
Colors encode a scale for oxygen saturation: red, freshly oxygenated blood; blue, oxygen-depleted blood.

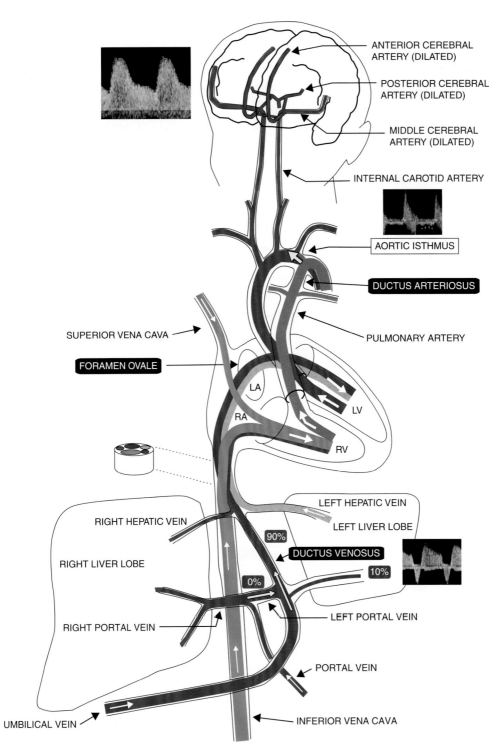

Figure 20.2 The fetal circulation in fetal growth restriction.

There is redistribution of blood flow to the brain. The amount of oxygenated blood shunted through the ductus venosus increases significantly (up to 90%) and perfusion of the liver decreases. In severe cases, reverse diastolic venous flow at the left portal vein may be seen (yellow arrow in the left portal vein). Therefore, oxygen-depleted blood may contribute to the blood flow reaching the left heart through the foramen ovale. Through the ductus arteriosus, oxygen-depleted blood travels to the descending aorta. If the umbilico-placental resistance is high and the resistance of cerebral vessels decreases due to the centralization process, an absent or reversed end-diastolic flow may be seen at the aortic isthmus (yellow arrow).

Colors encode a scale for oxygen saturation: red, freshly oxygenated blood; blue, oxygen-depleted blood.

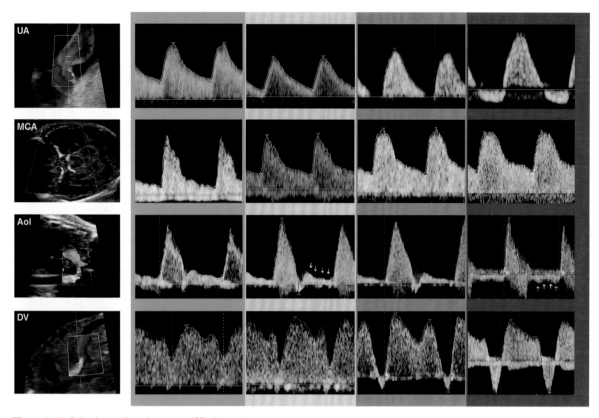

Figure 20.3 Pulsed wave Doppler curves of fetal vessels.
With progressing deterioration (encoded with background colors) significant changes in the end-diastolic phase of the velocity wave forms of the fetal vessels are recorded. In the umbilical artery (UA), increasing placental resistance causes progressively decreasing end-diastolic velocities, with zero or reverse flow in most advanced stages. In the middle cerebral artery (MCA), decreasing vascular resistance owing to dilation of cerebral vessels causes increasing end-diastolic velocities. In the aortic isthmus (AoI), the increasing downstream resistance and the decreasing cerebral resistance may lead to a reversal of end-diastolic flow. In the ductus venosus (DV), decreasing velocities of the a-wave (atrial contraction) progress to zero or reverse flow, thus indicating cardiac decompensation.
Background colors stand for progressive deterioration (green to red).

The Normal Arterial System and Its Changes in FGR

Oxygenated blood reaching the left ventricle of the heart is ejected through the aortic valve into the ascending aorta. The branches of the aortic arch supply the brain and the upper extremities with oxygenated blood, whereas after the shunting of the ductus arteriosus into the descending aorta just after the aortic isthmus (AOI), the oxygen concentration decreases due to the mixture with oxygen-depleted blood coming from the right ventricle. The descending aorta supplies the lower part of the body and the lower extremities and via the umbilical arteries blood travels to the placenta.

At the level of the aortic isthmus, which anatomically starts immediately after the origin of the left subclavian artery and ends at the aortic end of the ductus arteriosus, blood flow from the aortic arch will mix with the oxygen-depleted blood coming from the right ventricle through the main pulmonary artery and the ductus arteriosus [24]. During ventricular diastole, direction of blood flow in the AOI is influenced by the vascular resistance of the upper body, mainly determined by the brain, and the vascular resistance of the lower body, mainly determined by the placental circulation. In fetal growth restriction owing to placental insufficiency, delivery of oxygen to the fetus is impaired, leading to cerebral vasodilation, and placental resistance is increased. Both factors support retrograde blood flow during diastole in the AOI. It has been suggested that the occurrence of retrograde flow in the AOI during diastole was a sign of fetal deterioration, and some studies showed adverse neurodevelopmental outcomes in these fetuses in comparison to fetuses with antegrade diastolic flow [25]. In a cohort of growth-restricted fetuses requiring delivery before 34 weeks, Figueras and colleagues studied the sequence of changes of blood flow in the aortic isthmus and the ductus venosus, showing that flow in the umbilical artery and in the middle cerebral artery (MCA) became abnormal on average 24 and 20 days before delivery, respectively. Blood flow in the AOI and in the DV became abnormal 13 days and within the last week before delivery, respectively [26]. More recently, an isthmic systolic index has been described to express the balance of the performance of the two ventricles during pregnancy [27]. Whether the presence of diastolic reverse flow in the AOI should be clinically used in the management of FGR is still unclear.

Dilatation of the middle cerebral artery (MCA) occurs in FGR as a mechanism of blood flow redistribution to increase oxygen delivery to the brain. Nevertheless, recent data on adverse neurodevelopmental outcome in growth-restricted fetuses with normal umbilical artery Doppler and evidence of low MCA resistance [28,29] may indicate that the initially protective effect of this mechanism may get lost at some point. An increase in cerebral resistance after a phase of dilatation should not be interpreted as normalization of cerebral blood flow, but as an ominous sign [30]. Recently, other cerebral vessels have been studied confirming their participation in brain sparing, as, for instance, the posterior cerebral artery [31]. Together with the anterior cerebral artery, these vessels showed a similar vasodilatation in FGR as seen in the MCA, but with an earlier decrease of their pulsatility indices (PI) [32]. Especially for late FGR fetuses, further research is warranted to identify the ideal timing for delivery when the protective effect of brain sparing is diminished [33].

The cerebroplacental ratio (CPR), calculated as the PI of the MCA divided by the PI of the umbilical artery, offers the advantage of detecting redistribution earlier than the isolated interpretation of PI measurement of the aforementioned individual vessels [34,35]. Since in early-onset FGR the vast majority of fetuses will have abnormal umbilical and cerebral blood flow indices, the CPR is clinically not as relevant as in late-onset FGR. In a recent study, among fetuses classified as appropriate for gestational age (AGA) according to their estimated fetal weight, a subgroup with lower birth weight had significantly higher UA-PI, lower MCA-PI, and lower CPR values [36]. When using a threshold of CPR <5th centile (0.6765 MoM) derived from large-for-gestational age (LGA) fetuses as a diagnosis of failure to reach their growth potential, the percentage of fetuses with this failure increased from 1% in the 75–90th birth weight centiles to up to 6.7% in the 10–25% centiles in the AGA population. Furthermore, regardless of their expected fetal weight, a significant correlation with poor neonatal acid-base status was found in term fetuses (SGA and AGA) with low CPR in another series by the same investigators [37], thus indicating reactive late arterial cerebral dilatation and low resistance indices in late placental dysfunction.

In a series of small-for-gestational age (SGA) fetuses delivered after 34 weeks with normal umbilical artery (UA) Doppler, a recent study demonstrated the relation of histological placental signs of under perfusion with higher neonatal morbidity [38]. In this study, a standardized histologic placental classification system was used and neonatal morbidity was assessed according to a validated outcome score. In approximately two-thirds of the cases, there were histological signs of placental perfusion abnormalities, and among babies born with these placentas, there was a significantly higher rate of emergency caesarean deliveries for non-reassuring fetal status, an increased rate of neonatal metabolic acidosis and the median neonatal morbidity scores were significantly increased. The authors concluded that in late-onset FGR with normal umbilical Doppler indices, a histological substrate at the placental level correlates with adverse neonatal outcomes. In a model to predict the occurrence of emergency caesarean section or neonatal acidosis in pregnancies eligible for a trial of labor, Figueras and colleagues [39] found the presence of a low CPR (<10th centile), a mean uterine artery PI >95th centile or an expected fetal weight <3rd centile to be the best predictors. The aim of current research is to identify reliable parameters for timely delivery of fetuses at risk for neurologic sequelae, especially in late-onset FGR. Fetuses with low CPR, along with other echocardiographic predictors, have also been found to have an increased risk of cardiovascular and hypertensive disease in childhood [40], indicating fetal programming during pregnancy.

In fetal life, perfusion of the coronary arteries, with their origin just above the aortic valve annulus at the root of the ascending aorta, mainly occurs in diastole as in adult life, and diastolic peak velocities are higher than in systole when measured using Doppler velocimetry [41]. An increase of the downstream resistance, as in placental insufficiency, is related to an increased end-diastolic pressure and thus to a favorable coronary perfusion. Although the coronary arteries can be seen in normally developed fetuses at advanced gestational ages, in severe FGR with advanced levels of hypoxemia, the coronary arteries may earlier become apparent in Doppler studies and are considered an ominous sign for fetal deterioration. This so-called heart sparing effect implies an effort to optimize oxygen supply to the myocardium by a dilated coronary circulation.

Conclusion

In fetuses affected by growth restriction owing to placental dysfunction, the vascular system undergoes major adaptive changes in an effort to cope with chronic hypoxemia and suboptimal nutrient supply. These defense mechanisms are effective to prolong intrauterine life to a certain extent, but their efficacy in maintaining adequate organ development and function seems limited, especially when looking at the long-term consequences of placental dysfunction and growth restriction in later life. Understanding the underlying pathophysiology in FGR is crucial for the differentiation of fetuses coping with hypoxemia and those at risk of intrauterine demise.

The gestational age at which placental dysfunction affects fetal development plays an important role, since maturity of defense mechanisms and their respective clinical expression in terms of Doppler findings, which are used for fetal surveillance and timing of delivery, are different in early- vs. late-onset FGR. A typical differentiation limit used in clinical settings is growth restriction diagnosed before 32–34 weeks and beyond this gestational age range, with the lack of a clear line between these two groups.

In early-onset FGR, the typical sequence in which adaptive vascular changes take place seems to be constant, starting with the observation of an increased umbilical resistance and failure to achieve symmetrical growth. Thereafter, redistribution of blood flow to essential organs (brain sparing) is seen. Diastolic reverse flow in the aortic isthmus may be observed thereafter and an increase in the PI of the DV with absent or reversed flow during the a-wave as late DV pathology.

In late-onset FGR, even in fetuses in whom the estimated fetal weight shows a failure to reach its growth potential without falling below the 10th centile as defined for FGR and in the presence of a normal umbilico-placental resistance, the presence of low-resistance flow in the middle cerebral artery may lead to a low cerebroplacental ratio, which is related to adverse outcomes.

The evaluation of the fetal venous system plays a key role in distinguishing fetuses at risk for severe hypoxemia and acidemia by detecting flow patterns typical for cardiac decompensation. A DV flow pattern showing an arrested or reversed flow in the a-wave prompts for delivery in early-onset FGR. This may lead to better neurodevelopmental outcomes [42]. Since the relationship between FGR and maternal hypertensive comorbidity is high, the risk for early delivery before 29 weeks is substantially increased if preeclampsia, maternal hypertension, or HELLP-syndrome affect the pregnancy.

Fetal growth restriction is related to adaptive changes in the fetal circulation, which influence fetal programming. Structural changes in vessel architecture, with arteries showing thicker media layers and higher response to adrenergic stimuli, seem to be related to an increased propensity to hypertension, myocardial infarction, stroke, and metabolic diseases in adulthood.

Key Points

- Increased placental vascular resistance may cause early-onset fetal growth restriction and major changes in fetal circulation.

- Doppler ultrasound and measurement of pulsatility indices (PI) should be used for monitoring fetal arterial and venous blood flow.

- Decreased vascular resistance in the fetal brain leads to an increase in diastolic flow velocities and a decrease in pulsatility of cerebral arterial flow velocity waveforms (arterial redistribution affecting the middle cerebral artery and the aortic isthmus).

- Increased shunting of blood through the ductus venosus and deteriorating cardiac function lead to an increase in pulsatility of venous flow velocity waveforms (venous redistribution affecting the ductus venosus and the portal venous flow).

- A low cerebroplacental PI-ratio seems to be the most predictive diagnostic parameter in late-onset FGR.

References

1. Hecher K, Bilardo CM, Stigter RH, et al. Monitoring of fetuses with intrauterine growth restriction: A longitudinal study. *Ultrasound Obstet Gynecol* 2001;18:564–70.

2. Baschat A, Gembruch U, Harman CR. The sequence of changes in Doppler and biophysical parameters as severe fetal growth restriction worsens. *Ultrasound Obstet Gynecol* 2001;18:571–7.

3. Ferrazzi E, Bozzo M, Rigano S, et al. Temporal sequence of abnormal Doppler changes in the peripheral and central circulatory systems of the severely growth-restricted fetus. *Ultrasound Obstet Gynecol* 2002;19:140–6.

4. Bilardo CM, Wolf H, Stigter RH et al. Relationship between monitoring parameters and perinatal outcome in severe, early intrauterine growth restriction. *Ultrasound Obstet Gynecol* 2004;23:119–25.

5. Kiserud T, Rasmussen S, Skulstad SM. Blood flow and degree of shunting through the ductus venosus in the human fetus. *Am J Obstet Gynecol* 2000;182:147–53.

6. Haugen G, Kiserud T, Godfrey K, et al. Portal and umbilical venous blood supply to the liver in the human fetus near term. *Ultrasound Obstet Gynecol* 2004;24:599–605.

7. Tchirikov M, Schlabritz-Loutsevitch H, Hubbard GB, et al. Structural evidence for mechanisms to redistribute hepatic and ductus venosus blood flows in non-human primate fetuses. *Am J Obstet Gynecol* 2005;192:1146–52.

8. Haugen G, Bollerslev J, Henriksen T. Human fetoplacental and fetal liver blood flow after maternal glucose loading: A cross-sectional observational study. *Acta Obstet Gynecol Scand* 2014;93:778–85.

9. Tchirikov M, Schröder HJ, Hecher K. Ductus venosus shunting in the fetal venous circulation: Regulatory mechanisms, diagnostic methods and medical importance. *Ultrasound Obstet Gynecol* 2006;27:452–61.

10. Kessler J, Rasmussen S, Kiserud T. The fetal portal vein: Normal blood flow development during the second half of human pregnancy. *Ultrasound Obstet Gynecol* 2007;30:52–60.

11. Kiserud T, Kessler J, Ebbing C, et al. Ductus venosus shunting in growth-restricted fetuses and the effect of umbilical circulatory compromise. *Ultrasound Obstet Gynecol* 2006;28:143–9.

12. Kessler J, Rasmussen S, Kiserud T. The left portal vein as an indicator of watershed in the fetal circulation: Development during the second half of pregnancy and a suggested method of evaluation. *Ultrasound Obstet Gynecol* 2007;30:757–64.

13. Kessler J, Rasmussen S, Godfrey K, et al. Longitudinal study of umbilical and portal venous blood flow to the fetal liver: Low pregnancy weight gain is associated with preferential supply to the fetal left liver lobe. *Pediatr Res* 2008;63:315–20.

14. Ebbing C, Rasmussen S, Godfrey KM, et al. Redistribution pattern of fetal liver circulation in intrauterine growth restriction. *Acta Obstet Gynecol Scand* 2009;88:1118–23.

15. Haugen G, Hanson M, Kiserud T, et al. Fetal liver-sparing cardiovascular adaptations linked to mother's slimness and diet. *Circ Res* 2005;96:12–14.

16. Godfrey KM, Haugen G, Kiserud T, et al. Fetal liver blood flow distribution: Role in human developmental strategy to prioritize fat deposition versus brain development. *PLoS One* 2012;7:e41759.

17. Kiserud T, Ebbing C, Kessler J, Rasmussen S. Fetal cardiac output, distribution to the placenta and impact of placental compromise. *Ultrasound Obstet Gynecol* 2006;28:126–36.

18. Hecher K, Campbell S, Snijders R, et al. Reference ranges for fetal venous and atrioventricular blood flow parameters. *Ultrasound Obstet Gynecol* 1994; 4:381–90.

19. Kessler J, Rasmussen S, Hanson M, et al. Longitudinal reference ranges for ductus venosus flow velocities and waveform indices. *Ultrasound Obstet Gynecol* 2006 Dec;28:890–8.

20. Kiserud T, Kilavuz O, Hellevik LR. Venous pulsation in the fetal left portal branch: The effect of pulse and flow direction. *Ultrasound Obstet Gynecol* 2003; 21:359–64.

21. Hellevik LR, Stergiopulos N, Kiserud T, et al. A mathematical model of umbilical venous pulsation. *J Biomech* 2000;33:1123–30.

22. Wada N, Tachibana D, Kurihara Y, et al. Alterations of time-intervals of the ductus venosus and atrioventricular flow velocity waveforms in growth restricted fetuses. *Ultrasound Obstet Gynecol* 2014; doi: 10.1002/uog.14717.

23. Rigano S, Bozzo M, Ferrazzi E, et al. Early and persistent reduction in umbilical vein blood flow in the growth-restricted fetus: A longitudinal study. *Am J Obstet Gynecol* 2001;185:834–8.

24. Fouron JC. The unrecognized physiological and clinical significance of the fetal aortic isthmus. *Ultrasound Obstet Gynecol* 2003;22: 441–7.

25. Fouron JC, Gosselin J, Amiel-Tison C, et al. Correlation between prenatal velocity waveforms in the aortic isthmus and neurodevelopmental outcome between the ages of 2 and 4 years. *Am J Obstet Gynecol* 2001;184:630–6.

26. Figueras F, Benavides A, Del Rio M, et al. Monitoring of fetuses with intrauterine growth restriction: Longitudinal changes in ductus venosus and aortic isthmus flow. *Ultrasound Obstet Gynecol* 2009;33:39–43.

27. Chabaneix J, Fouron JC, Sosa-Olavarria A, et al. Profiling left and right ventricular proportional output during fetal life with a novel systolic index in the aortic isthmus. *Ultrasound Obstet Gynecol* 2014; 44:176–81.

28. Cruz-Martinez R, Figueras F, Oros D, et al. Cerebral blood perfusion and neurobehavioral performance in full-term small-for-gestational-age fetuses. *Am J Obstet Gynecol* 2009;201:474.e1–7.

29. Figueras F, Eixarch E, Meler E, et al. Small-for-gestational-age fetuses with normal umbilical artery Doppler have suboptimal perinatal and neurodevelopmental outcome. *Eur J Obstet Gynecol Reprod Biol* 2008;136:34–8.

30. Konje JC, Bell SC, Taylor DJ. Abnormal Doppler velocimetry and blood flow volume in the middle cerebral artery in very severe intrauterine growth restriction: Is the occurrence of reversal of compensatory flow too late? *BJOG* 2001;108:973–9.

31. Benavides-Serralde JA, Hernandez-Andrade E, Cruz-Martinez R, et al. Doppler evaluation of the posterior cerebral artery in normally grown and growth restricted fetuses. *Prenat Diagn* 2014;34:115–20.

32. Benavides-Serralde A, Scheier M, Cruz-Martinez R, et al. Changes in central and peripheral circulation in intrauterine growth-restricted fetuses at different stages of umbilical artery flow deterioration: New fetal cardiac and brain parameters. *Gynecol Obstet Invest* 2011;71:274–80.

33. Hernandez-Andrade E, Serralde JA, Cruz-Martinez R. Can anomalies of fetal brain circulation be useful in the management of growth restricted fetuses? *Prenat Diagn* 2012;32:103–12.

34. Baschat AA, Gembruch U. The cerebroplacental Doppler ratio revisited. *Ultrasound Obstet Gynecol* 2003;21:124–7.

35. Hecher K, Spernol R, Stettner H et al. Potential for diagnosing imminent risk to appropriate- and small-for-gestational-age fetuses by Doppler sonographic examination of umbilical and cerebral arterial blood flow. *Ultrasound Obstet Gynecol* 1992;2:266–71.

36. Morales-Roselló J, Khalil A, Morlando M, et al. Changes in fetal Doppler indices as a marker of failure to reach growth potential at term. *Ultrasound Obstet Gynecol* 2014;43:303–10.

37. Morales-Roselló J, Khalil A, Morlando M, et al. Poor neonatal acid-base status in term fetuses with low cerebroplacental ratio. *Ultrasound Obstet Gynecol* 2015;45:156–61.

38. Parra-Saavedra M, Simeone S, Triunfo S, et al. Correlation between histological signs of placental underperfusion and perinatal morbidity in late-onset small-for-gestational-age fetuses. *Ultrasound Obstet Gynecol* 2015;45:149–55.

39. Figueras F, Savchev S, Triunfo S., et al. An integrated model with classification criteria to predict small-for-gestational-age fetuses at risk of adverse perinatal outcome. *Ultrasound Obstet Gynecol* 2015;45:279–85.

40. Cruz-Lemini M, Crispi F, Valenzuela-Alcaraz B, et al. A fetal cardiovascular score to predict infant hypertension and arterial remodeling in intrauterine growth restriction. *Am J Obstet Gynecol* 2014;210:552. e1–22

41. Baschat A, Muench MV, Gembruch U. Coronary artery blood flow velocities in various fetal conditions. *Ultrasound Obstet Gynecol* 2003;21:426–9.

42. Lees C, Marlow N, van Wassenaer-Leemhuis A., et al. and the TRUFFLE Group. 2 year neurodevelopmental and intermediate perinatal outcomes in infants with very preterm fetal growth restriction (TRUFFLE): A randomised trial. *Lancet* 2015;385:2162–72.

Chapter 21

Hematological and Biochemical Findings in Fetal Growth Restriction and Relationship to Hypoxia

Irene Cetin and Chiara Mandò

Introduction

Growth of the fetus *in utero* is the result of genetic potential modulated by the availability of oxygen and nutrients and by the endocrine environment. Pregnancy is a three-compartment model, with mother, placenta, and fetus linked in a complex system that develops to ensure maintenance of fetal growth in adverse conditions.

Intrauterine growth curves based either on birth weight or on ultrasound evaluation of estimated fetal weight are widely utilized in pregnancy [1].

The clinical usefulness of the evaluation of intrauterine growth during pregnancy lies in the early identification of those pregnancies with fetuses that are growing too much or too little. The evaluation of intrauterine growth is a fundamental part of prenatal care. Indeed, normal birth weight and appropriate gestational age at delivery represent the best measure of a physiological pregnancy with normal placental function and nutrient delivery to the fetus. However, many factors can influence the process of intrauterine growth so that some fetuses do not follow their growth potential, thus altering their growth trajectory toward increased or reduced growth. This leads to adverse outcomes, both in the short term and in the long term. Some years ago, the intrauterine body composition of SGA (small for gestational age) and LGA (large for gestational age) has been compared to AGA (appropriate for gestational age) in carcasses of dead fetuses studied at delivery [2]. In these newborns, fat mass deposition was strongly increased in LGA compared to AGA in the second half of pregnancy. On the contrary, fetuses with reduced birth weights showed a significant reduction in fat mass, likely as a result of decreased nutritional supply, associated with reduced tissue deposition (Figure 21.1). A disproportionate reduction in subcutaneous fat tissue has also been reported in FGR fetuses evaluated by ultrasound

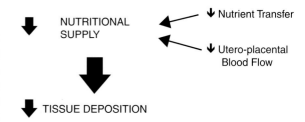

Figure 21.1 Final common mechanisms of failure of fetal growth.

[3]. Reduced tissue deposition in a fetus with a normal genetic potential can theoretically be explained by 1) reduced placental nutrient transfer to the fetus (possibly due to the mother or to the placenta) and/or 2) reduced uteroplacental blood flow.

In this chapter, we will evaluate which metabolic alterations occur in fetal growth restriction (FGR) and how they relate with the clinical severity and with the presence of hypoxia.

Relevance and Definition of FGR

Depending on definitions and on populations, FGR affects between 5–15% of pregnancies. Both prematurity and decreased weight account for the high mortality and morbidity associated with this disease [4,5]. Many studies indicate that low birth weight is associated with the development of the metabolic syndrome in adult life due to "fetal programming" and a "developmental origins of health and disease" hypothesis has been well recognized [6,7]. FGR occurs when the fetus fails to achieve its full growth potential. However, although FGR is the result of inappropriate processes likely occurring in the periconceptional phase, the clinical diagnosis of FGR is performed only in the second half of pregnancy. The recognition of a shift from the normal growth curve by ultrasound may occur independently from reductions of utero/placental/umbilical blood flows [8,9]. If we utilize a definition of growth restriction based on inappropriate intrauterine growth, then some of these fetuses may have normal levels of oxygen, while others may be, or may become, hypoxic and lactacidemic with increasing severity. Some authors prefer to define those FGR with normal placental vascularization as SGA, as this type of condition is often diagnosed only at delivery; however, although some of them may be constitutionally small, if we base our diagnosis on the intrauterine shift of growth evaluated by ultrasound, then we must consider many of them as growth restricted. Obviously, perinatal outcomes also depend on the gestational age at which these fetuses are diagnosed and delivered. Untangling the impact of growth restriction from the effects of prematurity is a difficult task for clinicians and researchers.

Does a Maternal Phenotype of FGR Exist?

A number of maternal risk factors for FGR have been described, although FGR does not present a unique maternal phenotype [10].

Indeed, maternal pre-gestational body mass index (BMI), nutritional status, diet, and exposure to environmental factors are increasingly acknowledged as potential factors affecting fetal growth both by altering nutrient availability to the fetus and by modulating fetal gene expression and placental gene expression, thus modifying placental function (Figure 21.2).

Maternal undernutrition may potentially alter fetal growth trajectory by modifying placental weight, surface, and nutrient transfer capacity, depending on the severity of the nutritional challenge and on the time of deprivation [11]. Moreover, hormone production in maternal, placental, and fetal compartments may be affected by maternal undernutrition [12]. An interesting meta-analysis reports that a balanced protein-energy supplementation is an effective intervention to reduce the risk of low birth weight and SGA births, especially in undernourished women in developing countries [13].

On the other hand, high pre-gestational BMI and maternal over-nutrition are emerging as a major health problem worldwide [14], also leading to FGR and SGA, probably through vascular alterations, metabolic derangements, altered oocytes quality [15], modifications of placental biometry [16] or altered nutrient quality. Indeed, over-nourished women are often malnourished, with macronutrient and/or micronutrient imbalances potentially affecting fetal growth [17].

Moreover, recent studies demonstrate decreased 25-hydroxyvitamin D (25-OH D) levels in fetuses of obese compared to normal-weight women (with cord blood 25-OH D levels directly correlating to neonatal percentage body fat) [18] and lower maternal serum folate concentrations, which is a rate-limiting factor for placental folate transport to the fetus, at mid- and late pregnancy [19]. Additionally, the chronic low-grade inflammation associated with obesity leads to overexpression of maternal hepcidin and C-reactive protein, negatively correlated with cord blood iron status [20].

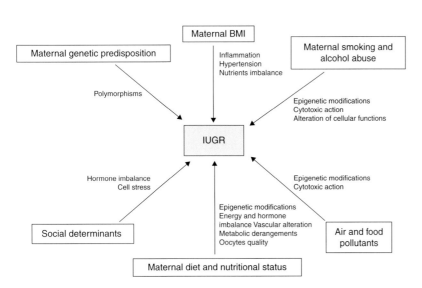

Figure 21.2 Maternal predictors of IUGR/FGR.
Source: From Cetin, I., Mandò, C., Calabrese, S. Maternal predictors of intrauterine growth restriction. *Current Opinion in Clinical Nutrition and Metabolic Care*, 2013; 16(3):310–19.

193

The role of maternal diet and of micronutrients intake seems to be of particular importance in the peri-conceptional period. In this context, folate seems to be involved not only in embryo development, but also in appropriate fetal growth. Specifically, poor adherence of the woman to the Mediterranean diet, as well as lack of folic acid pre-conceptionally, has been associated with increased risks of low birth weight and SGA in the Generation R Study conducted in the Netherlands [21].

Maternal diet also plays a central role in determining epigenetic variations, regarding DNA methylation, microRNAs, and histone modifications, that have been reported both in animal and in human placentas [22]. Indeed, macro- and micronutrients are direct regulators of DNA stability and phenotypic adaptation, by influencing the availability of methyl donors and mechanisms promoting DNA stability [23].

Placental Phenotype of FGR

Placental transport and metabolism are major players involved in fetal nutrition and metabolism since they determine the availability of oxygen and nutrients to the fetus.

For many years, it has been thought that FGR is caused by "placental insufficiency," as a result of a defective placentation process in the early phases of development. In the past decades, a specific placental phenotype has been progressively described as the results of numerous studies performed both *in vivo* and *in vitro* [24]. In particular, defects in placental metabolism and nutrient transport have been consistently reported in FGR, mainly affecting the transport of amino acids and lipids [25], but also micronutrients such as iron and folate [26,27]. However, the reason why placental development fails to be appropriate in these pregnancies is still not known.

A significant reduction in nitrogen uptake, accounting for reduced protein synthesis and fetal growth, is well recognized in FGR fetuses, independently of fetal oxygen conditions [28]. Nitrogen deposition per oxygen consumption is strongly decreased in FGR fetuses, giving rise to reduced protein utilization. Indeed, *in vivo* studies measuring amino acid transport and metabolism by stable isotope tracers, have shown decreased essential amino acid placental transport rates in intrauterine growth-restricted placentas [29,30]. In addition, decreased sodium-coupled neutral amino acid transporter 2 (SNAT2)

has been reported in human severe FGR placentas, with reduced umbilical blood flows, compared to physiological placentas [31].

Fetal growth restriction is also associated with changes in long chain-polyunsaturated fatty acids (LC-PUFA) placental handling and transfer. In normal pregnancies, the total amount of fatty acids is significantly lower in fetal than in maternal plasma, but their percentage composition is modified to favor the availability of LC-PUFA, which are needed for brain tissue accretion and membrane fluidity ("biomagnification" process). Placental supply of LC-PUFA is thus critical for the synthesis of structural lipids and for normal fetal development [32]. Decreased fetal-maternal ratios of LC-PUFA, particularly of DHA, have been reported in FGR fetuses at cordocentesis [33]. Moreover, reduced conversion ratios of LC-PUFA of the omega-3 and omega-6 series from their parent fatty acids have been demonstrated [34]. Thus, in FGR, the biomagnification process does not occur properly, and FGR fetuses are less enriched in essential fatty acids such as arachidonic acid and DHA compared to normal pregnancies [33].

Besides macronutrients, fetal growth is also importantly regulated by micronutrients' availability. Maternal iron deficiency has been associated with low birth weight and preterm delivery [35], as well as long-term neurodevelopmental outcomes [36], although there is still no sure knowledge about iron levels in mothers and fetuses with FGR. Interestingly, decreased gene and protein expression of placental Transferrin Receptor 1 (TfR1), responsible for iron transfer from the mother to the fetus, has been shown in FGR [26]. Altered macro- and micronutrient placental transport is thus recognized in growth-restricted pregnancies.

However, regulation of these pathways still needs to be fully understood. A placental regulation of iron transfer and levels might occur, due by the increased expression of proteins derived from the inflammation state characterizing FGR, such as hepcidin [37]. Moreover, amino acid restriction, that has been consistently shown in FGR, can alter the uptake of both iron and copper [35]. Finally, human placental mesenchymal stromal cells have recently been investigated, showing an impaired angiogenic potential as well as increased capacity for adipocyte differentiation [38].

Role of Oxygen

Many alterations occurring in FGR placentas can be explained by changes in oxygen (O_2) concentrations.

Indeed, while in normal pregnancies, the placenta acts as a venous equilibrator, with pO_2 in the umbilical vein lower and proportional to values in the uterine vein, in FGR, both uterine venous pO_2 and uterine-umbilical venous gradients are increased, leading to decreased coefficients of uterine oxygen extraction and thus to reduced oxygen delivery to the FGR fetus [39,40]. This may be the result of decreased placental permeability and/or increased placental oxygen utilization.

Oxygen is used in mitochondria to produce ATP by oxidative phosphorylation. Mitochondria have also a critical function in mediating apoptosis signals and multiple cellular signaling pathways, as well as in the production of reactive oxygen species (ROS), that can generate oxidative stress, protein and lipid oxidation and DNA damage, if not properly inactivated by endogenous enzymes. FGR is highly associated with increased oxidative stress, which is a powerful inducer of both apoptotic and necrotic changes [41,42]. Mitochondrial DNA (mtDNA) levels, accounting for the number of mitochondria in the cell, are significantly increased in placental tissue of growth-restricted compared to physiological pregnancies [43]. Interestingly, in the analyzed population, there was a significant negative correlation between mtDNA levels and umbilical vein pO_2 (Figure 21.3), suggesting a compensatory mechanism, leading to mitochondrial biogenesis up-regulation with FGR increasing in severity. When oxygen becomes a limiting factor, the modulation of mitochondrial function plays an important role in overall biologic adaptation. Different mitochondrial responses seem to depend on the degree of hypoxia, on the age at exposure to hypoxia, and on the duration of exposure [44].

Mitochondrial DNA levels increase significantly in maternal blood during gestation [45], possibly due to placental syncytial fragments released in maternal circulation. Indeed, increased mtDNA levels have also been shown in maternal blood of FGR pregnancies in the third trimester of gestation, compared to physiological pregnancies of the same gestational age. So it has been hypothesized that the increase of mtDNA content in FGR pregnancies could represent a compensatory mechanism to hypoxia [45].

Mitochondrial content and function were also measured in cytotrophoblast cells, an important cell type for placental function. Although higher mtDNA

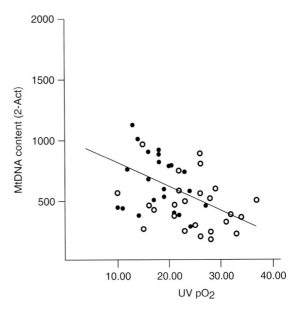

Figure 21.3 Relationship between placental mtDNA and umbilical venous pO_2 in fetuses with appropriate for gestational age weights (white circles) and FGR (black circles) (y=-20.344x + 1014.8; r^2=0.228; p=0.001).
Source: From Lattuada D, Colleoni F, Martinelli A, Garretto A, Magni R, Radaelli T, Cetin I. Higher mitochondrial DNA content in human IUGR placenta. *Placenta*. 2008;29(12):1029-33.

content was confirmed in FGR placental whole tissue, in cytotrophoblast cells significantly lower levels of both mtDNA levels and the gene and protein expression of the mitochondrial-biogenesis activator NRF1 (Nuclear Respiratory Factor 1) were reported in FGR compared to normal pregnancies. However, functionality of these mitochondria, measured by cell oxygen consumption, was higher in FGR cytotrophoblast cells compared to normal cells, particularly in more severe FGR, presenting altered umbilical cord pulsatility index and more severe hypoxic conditions [46]. Altered mitochondrial content and function have also been reported in FGR human placental mesenchymal stromal cells, possibly indicating a shift from anaerobic to aerobic metabolism, with the loss of metabolic characteristics that are typical of undifferentiated multipotent cells [38].

Reduced energy substrate may also lead to placental mitochondria dysfunction. Indeed, "malnourished" placentas during rat pregnancy present increased mitochondria dependent apoptosis [47]. A number of proteins sensitive to nutritional changes and involved in mitochondria replication and energy production are also involved in epigenetic processes such as histone deacetylation and DNA methylation

195

[48]. These mechanisms may therefore be pivotal in the development of the placental phenotype of FGR and in the responses occurring with increased severity.

Fetal Phenotype of FGR

An abnormal placental phenotype has thus been demonstrated in FGR pregnancies. How do these placental changes regulate fetal metabolism (and growth) in FGR?

FGR fetuses are undergoing a number of progressive adaptations. At first, decreased nutrient delivery occurs, particularly for amino acids, likely because they utilize complex and energy-dependent active transport systems. Reduced amino acid concentrations have been consistently reported in umbilical venous blood of FGR compared to AGA fetuses sampled both at cordocentesis and at cesarean section [49–51]. Nitrogen uptake is thus reduced and as a consequence protein tissue deposition is reduced. At the same time, essential lipids such as DHA become less available, affecting the composition and fluidity of membranes, particularly in the brain [52]. On the other hand, glucose availability does not seem to be affected in normoxemic FGR fetuses, and no evidence of glucogenesis has been demonstrated in FGR fetuses in an elegant stable isotope study performed by maternal steady state ^{13}C-UL-glucose infusion prior to cordocentesis [53].

A low metabolic status clearly occurs in FGR fetuses. Fetal oxygen uptake, measured as the venous-arterial difference in O_2 content times the umbilical vein flow (according to the Fick principle), is significantly lower in FGR, even on a per-kg basis [25]. Metabolic changes are related to the severity of FGR, evaluated by umbilical arterial Doppler pulsatility index (PI_{ua}) together with fetal heart rate (FHR) evaluation (Table 21.1). Recently, increased mtDNA levels have been reported in the cord blood of FGR, and mtDNA epigenetic modifications have been proposed to possibly be responsible for these changes [54].

In particular, type 1 FGR fetuses, characterized by normal PI_{ua} and normal FHR, have normal umbilical vein oxygen and lactate levels; type 2 FGR, with abnormal PI_{ua} and normal FHR show a slight, although not significant decrease; type 3 FGR, characterized by abnormal PI_{ua}, together with abnormal FHR, have significantly lower oxygen and higher lactate levels [8]. These findings occur independently of gestational age.

For glucose, changes in the fetal-maternal gradient also seem to occur when fetuses become hypoxic, likely as a consequence of decreased fetal utilization [55]. However, average hemoglobin levels are significantly higher in all types of FGR fetuses [8], and this may suggest that even FGR with normal umbilical arterial PI may be characterized by moderate degrees of relatively mild and likely intermittent episodes of hypoxia.

A progressive reduction of O_2 supply leading to subsequent systemic metabolic acidosis has been utilized as a sheep model of FGR in order to investigate acute changes in fetal brain metabolism [56]. This *in vivo* study was able to provide data by quantitative proton magnetic resonance spectroscopy showing changes in cerebral metabolite concentrations, particularly increases in lactate production by the fetal lamb brain, as the consequence of both decreased fetal arterial oxygen saturation and the subsequent systemic metabolic acidosis.

In humans, the presence of a lactate peak has been reported in the brain of a 28-week severely affected FGR fetus (type 3), presenting abnormal umbilical artery Doppler and fetal heart rate tracings (Figure 21.4). These measures were correlated with the low oxygen content and high lactic acid concentration observed in umbilical blood obtained at delivery [57]. In the same study, FGR fetuses of type 1 and type 2 did not show cerebral lactate peaks, suggesting that lactate brain production is a severe feature characterizing significant metabolic changes occurring in the fetal brain of the most severe FGR.

Table 21.1 Fetal metabolic changes related to the severity of FGR at cordocentesis

	Gestational age (weeks)	O2 content (mM)	Lactate (mM)
Normal-growth fetuses	27.8±6.9	6.0±0.9	0.8±0.2
FGR fetuses			
TYPE 1	33.3±2.3	6.0±0.8	0.9±0.2
TYPE 2	32.2±2.5	5.4±1.0	1.1±0.4
TYPE 3	29.2±2.8	4.0±1.2*	2.5±1.0*

TYPE 1 FGR: normal umbilical arterial Doppler pulsatility index (PI_{ua}) and normal fetal heart rate (FHR). TYPE 2 FGR: abnormal PI_{ua} and normal FHR. TYPE 3 FGR: abnormal PI_{ua} and abnormal FHR.
*p <0.05 vs normal-growth fetuses.

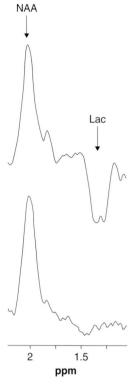

Figure 21.4 Fetal brain lactate detection by magnetic resonance spectroscopy. The region of the spectra between 1.00 and 2.25 ppm is represented. A, In the most severe FGR case (FGR type 3), lactate is clearly detectable, because the typical inverted doublet is centered at 1.33 ppm. B, Conversely, no lactate peak is detected in a case of similar gestational age but with a less severe FGR (FGR type 2). Spectra A and B are normalized to the NAA peak. Lac, lactate; NAA, N-acetylaspartate.

Source: From Cetin I, Barberis B, Brusati V, Brighina E, Mandia L, Arighi A, Radaelli T, Biondetti P, Bresolin N, Pardi G, Rango M. Lactate detection in the brain of growth-restricted fetuses with magnetic resonance spectroscopy. *Am J Obstet Gynecol*. 2011;205(4):350.e1–7.

In FGR, studies performed to evaluate cerebral outcomes are always potentially biased by the difficulty of separating the burden of prematurity from the impact of growth restriction. To overcome this problem, changes occurring in the brain of FGR fetuses have been studied by magnetic resonance imaging performed at term-corrected age, and compared to a group of premature babies with no FGR [58]. While results were similar in the two groups taken as a whole, significantly reduced cerebral myelination was reported in those FGR neonates with abnormal middle cerebral artery Doppler indexes. The occurrence of the so-called brain sparing (cerebral artery vasodilation) has long been thought of as an attempt by the fetus to maintain cerebral substrate supply. However, these findings suggest that vasodilation of the middle cerebral artery does not always guarantee a full protection for brain development and may indeed be already detrimental. The idea that cerebral vasodilation is an adaptive and benign process has now been challenged also by studies showing adverse neurodevelopmental outcome in FGR fetuses with cerebral blood redistribution [59,60], particularly to the frontal regions of the brain [61,62].

There is a need to better comprehend the "natural history" of fetal growth restriction. Uncertainty occurs as to whether clinical differences in FGR represent different degrees of severity or different pathologies. Indeed, we do not completely understand whether and why some FGR have a very rapid evolution to hypoxia and fetal distress, while others seem to have an adaptation to the decrease in growth, and may evolve slowly *in utero*. Although the decrease in growth rate has an epigenetic "cost," the burden of prematurity has to be carefully weighted in clinical terms. Moreover, maternal preeclampsia may be associated with FGR, thus making the picture more complex. In this context, inflammation and oxygen reduction may also occur on the maternal side and this may have significant and additive effects on fetal well-being.

Conclusion

Fetal growth restriction is a complex disease characterized by differences related to severity of placental compromise. In less severe late-gestation FGR presenting normal umbilical blood flows and normal fetal heart rate, oxygen, lactate, and glucose concentrations are not modified in fetal blood. However, fetal availability of amino acids and lipids are already altered compared to normal pregnancies, suggesting that changes in complex placental nutrient transport systems precede FGR, also affecting intrauterine programming. Differently, when umbilical blood flows are impaired, fetal oxygen uptake becomes insufficient and metabolic acidosis occurs, together with altered mitochondrial content and function, leading to a severe picture of the pathology, in which delivery should be carefully planned, also in relation to gestational age.

Mild fetal brain damage may occur already in relation to early vascular brain redistribution, and this may become severe as oxygen delivery is significantly reduced, leading to significant lactate production within the fetal brain.

This evidence highlights that placental phenotype of FGR changes in relation to severity, from adaptation to failure.

The picture of hematological findings in FGR derives from studies with single fetal sampling, performed either at cordocentesis or at delivery. Therefore, we still lack direct and clear evidence about the *in utero* metabolic changes related to the evolution from normal to abnormal growth. However, as clinicians, we must know that FGR is accompanied by severe metabolic costs; as researchers, we need to better understand how to develop potential therapeutic tools to prevent premature deliveries and adverse outcomes.

Key Points

- Many risk factors in the mother can contribute to develop FGR [10].

- Maternal pre-gestational BMI, nutritional status, diet, and exposure to environmental factors are potential factors affecting fetal growth both by altering nutrient availability to the fetus and by modulating placental gene expression, thus modifying placental function. Indeed, maternal diet also plays a central role in determining epigenetic variations, regarding DNA methylation, microRNAs, and histone modifications.

- A specific placental phenotype called "placental insufficiency" associated with defects in placental metabolism and nutrient transport has been found in FGR, mainly affecting the transport of amino acids and lipids [25], but also micronutrients such as iron and folate [26,27].

- Many alterations in FGR can be explained by changes in oxygen concentration. Indeed, in FGR both uterine venous pO2 and uterine-umbilical venous gradients are increased, leading to decreased coefficient of uterine extraction and thus to reduced oxygen delivery to the FGR fetus (24.37). This may be the result of decreased placental permeability and/or increased placental oxygen utilization.

- Oxygen alteration within the placenta may be responsible for impaired mitochondria biogenesis and function. This may lead to defects in cell production of energy, as well as excessive ROS production leading to oxidative stress, DNA damage, defects in the regulation of cell apoptosis, and many cell dysfunctions.

References

1. Cetin I, Boito S, Radaelli T. Evaluation of fetal growth and fetal well-being. *Seminars in Ultrasound CT and MRI* 2008;29:136–46.

2. Sparks JW. *Semin Perinatol* 1984;8:74–93.

3. Padoan A, Rigano S, Ferrazzi E, et al. Differences in fat and lean mass proportions in normal and growth-restricted fetuses. *Am J Obstet Gynecol* 2004;191(4):1459–64.

4. Baschat AA. Fetal responses to placental insufficiency: an update. *BJOG* 2004;111:1031–41.

5. Alexander GR, Kogan M, Bader D, et al. US birth weight/gestational age-specific neonatal mortality: 1995–1997 rates for whites, Hispanics, and blacks. *Pediatrics* 2003;111:e61–6.

6. De Rooij SR, Painter RC, Holleman F, et al. The metabolic syndrome in adults prenatally exposed to the Dutch famine. *Am J Clin Nutr* 2007;86:1219–24.

7. Painter RC, Osmond C, Gluckman P, et al. Transgenerational effect of prenatal exposure to the Dutch famine on neonatal adiposity and health in later life. *BJOG* 2008;115:1243–9.

8. Pardi G, Cetin I, Marconi AM, et al. Diagnostic value of blood sampling in fetuses with growth retardation. *N Engl J Med* 1993;328:692–6.

9. Unterscheider J, Daly S, Geary MP, et al. Optimizing the definition of intrauterine growth restriction: The multicenter prospective PORTO Study. *Am J Obstet Gynecol* 2013;208(4):290.e1–6.

10. Cetin, I., Mandò, C., Calabrese, S. Maternal predictors of intrauterine growth restriction. *Curr Opin Clin Nutr Metab Care* 2013;16(3):310–19.

11. Vaughan OR, Sferruzzi-Perri AN, Coan PM, et al. Environmental regulation of placental phenotype: Implications for fetal growth. *Reprod Fertil Dev* 2012;24:80–96.

12. Igwebuike UM. Impact of maternal nutrition on ovine foetoplacental development: A review of the role of insulin-like growth factors. *Anim Reprod Sci* 2010; 121:189–96.

13. Imdad A, Bhutta ZA. Maternal nutrition and birth outcomes: Effect of balanced protein-energy supplementation. *Paediatr Perinat Epidemiol* 2012; 26 (Suppl 1):178–90.

14. McKnight JR, Satterfield MC, Li X, et al. Obesity in pregnancy: Problems and potential solutions. *Front Biosci* (Elite Ed) 2011; 3:442–52; Review.

15. Luzzo KM, Wang Q, Purcell SH, et al. High fat diet induced developmental defects in the mouse: Oocyte meiotic aneuploidy and fetal growth retardation/brain defects. *PLoS One* 2012;7:e49217.

16. Mandò C, Calabrese S, Mazzocco MI, Novielli C, Anelli GM, Antonazzo P, Cetin I. Sex specific adaptations in placental biometry of overweight and obese women. *Placenta* 2016;38:1–7.

17. Moran LJ, Sui Z, Cramp CS, Dodd JM. A decrease in diet quality occurs during pregnancy in overweight and obese women which is maintained postpartum. *Int J Obes* (Lond) 2013;37(5):704–11.

18. Josefson JL, Feinglass J, Rademaker AW, et al. Maternal obesity and vitamin D sufficiency are associated with cord blood vitamin D insufficiency. *J Clin Endocrinol Metab* 2013;98:114–19.

19. Kim H, Hwang JY, Kim KN, et al. Relationship between body-mass index and serum folate concentrations in pregnant women. *Eur J Clin Nutr* 2012;66:136–38.

20. Dao MC, Sen S, Iyer C, et al. Obesity during pregnancy and fetal iron status: Is Hepcidin the link? *J Perinatol* 2013;33(3):177–81.

21. Timmermans S, Jaddoe VW, Hofman A, et al. Periconception folic acid supplementation, fetal growth and the risks of low birth weight and preterm birth: The Generation R Study. *Br J Nutr* 2009;102(5):777–85.

22. Novakovic B, Saffery R. The ever growing complexity of placental epigenetics – Role in adverse pregnancy outcomes and fetal programming. *Placenta* 2012; 33:959–70.

23. Sebert S, Sharkey D, Budge H, et al. The early programming of metabolic health: Is epigenetic setting the missing link? *Am J Clin Nutr* 2011;94 (Suppl):1953S–1958S.

24. Sibley CP, Turner MA, Cetin I, et al. Placental phenotypes of intrauterine growth. *Pediatr Res* 2005;58(5):827–32.

25. Cetin I, Alvino G. Intrauterine growth restriction: Implications for placental metabolism and transport. A review. *Placenta* 2009;30 (Suppl A):S77–S82.

26. Mandò C, Tabano S, Colapietro P, et al. Transferrin receptor gene and protein expression and localization in human IUGR and normal term placentas. *Placenta* 2011;32:44–50.

27. Furness D, Fenech M, Dekker G, et al. Vitamin B12, Vitamin B6 and homocysteine: Impact on pregnancy outcome. *Matern Child Nutr* 2013;9(2):155–66.

28. Cetin I, Ronzoni S, Marconi AM, et al. Maternal concentrations and fetal-maternal concentration differences of plasma amino acids in normal and intrauterine growth-restricted pregnancies. *Am J Obstet Gynecol* 1996;174(5):1575–83.

29. Marconi AM1, Paolini CL, Stramare L, et al. Steady state maternal-fetal leucine enrichments in normal and intrauterine growth-restricted pregnancies. *Pediatr Res* 1999;46(1):114–19.

30. Paolini CL, Marconi AM, Ronzoni S, et al. Placental transport of leucine, phenylalanine, glycine, and proline in intrauterine growth-restricted pregnancies. *J Clin Endocrinol Metab* 2001;86(11):5427–32.

31. Mandò C, Tabano S, Pileri P, et al. SNAT2 expression and regulation in human growth-restricted placentas. *Pediatr Res* 2013;74(2):104–10.

32. Haggarty P. Placental regulation of fatty acid delivery and its effect on fetal growth – a review. *Placenta* 2002;23(Suppl. A):S28–38.

33. Cetin I, Giovannini N, Alvino G, et al. Intrauterine growth restriction is associated with changes in polyunsaturated fatty acid fetal-maternal relationships. *Pediatr Res* 2002;52(5):750–5.

34. Cetin I, Koletzko B. Long-chain u-3 fatty acid supply in pregnancy and lactation. *Curr Opin Clin Nutr Metab Care* 2008;11:297–302.

35. McArdle HJ, Andersen HS, Jones H, et al. Copper and iron transport across the placenta: regulation and interactions. *J Neuroendocrinol* 2008;20(4):427e31. Review.

36. Zimmerman MB, Hurrel RF. Nutritional iron deficiency. *Lancet* 2007;370: 511e20.

37. Nicolas G, Chauvet C, Viatte L, Danan JL, Bigard X, Devaux I, Beaumont C, Kahn A, Vaulont S. The gene encoding the iron regulatory peptide hepcidin is regulated by anemia, hypoxia, and inflammation. *J Clin Invest* 2002;110:1037–44.

38. Mandò C, Razini P, Novielli C, Anelli GM, Belicchi M, Erratico S, Banfi S, Meregalli M, Tavelli A, Baccarin M, Rolfo A, Motta S, Torrente Y, Cetin I. Impaired angiogenic potential of human placental mesenchymal stromal cells in intrauterine growth restriction. *Stem Cells Transl Med* 2016;5(4):451–63.

39. Pardi G, Cetin I, Marconi AM, et al. Venous drainage of the human uterus: Respiratory gas studies in normal and fetal growth-retarded pregnancies. *Am J Obstet Gynecol* 1992;166(2):699–706.

40. Sibley Cp, Pardi G, Cetin I, et al. Workshop Report: Pathogenesis of intrauterine growth restriction (IUGR) – conclusions derived from a European Union Biomed 2 Concerted Action Project "Importance of Oxygen Supply in Intrauterine Growth Restricted Pregnancies." *Trophoblast Research* 2002;23:S75–S79.

41. Tjoa ML, Cindrova-Davies T, Spasic-Boskovic O, et al. Trophoblastic oxidative stress and the release of cell-free feto-placental DNA. *Am J Pathol* 2006;169:400–4.

42. Yung HW, Calabrese S, Hynx D, et al. Evidence of placental translation inhibition and endoplasmic reticulum stress in the etiology of human intrauterine growth restriction. *Am J Pathol* 2008;173:451–62.

43. Lattuada D, Colleoni F, Martinelli A, et al. Higher mitochondrial DNA content in human IUGR placenta. *Placenta* 2008;29(12):1029–33.

44. Lynn EG, Lu Z, Minerbi D, et al. The regulation, control, and consequences of mitochondrial oxygen utilization and disposition in the heart and skeletal muscle during hypoxia. *Antioxid Redox Signal* 2007;9:1353–61.

45. Colleoni F, Lattuada D, Garretto A, et al. Maternal blood mitochondrial DNA content during normal and intrauterine growth restricted (IUGR) pregnancy. *Am J Obstet Gynecol* 2010;203(4):365.e1–6.

46. Mandò C, De Palma C, Stampalija T, et al. Placental mitochondrial content and function in intrauterine growth restriction and preeclampsia. *Am J Physiol Endocrinol Metab* 2014;306(4):E404–13.

47. Belkacemi L, Jelks A, Chen CH, et al. Altered placental development in undernourished rats: Role of maternal glucocorticoids. *Reprod Biol Endocrinol* 2011;9:105.

48. Sebert S, Sharkey D, Budge H, et al. The early programming of metabolic health: is epigenetic setting the missing link? *Am J Clin Nutr* 2011; 94(Suppl):1953S–8S.

49. Cetin I, Marconi AM, Bozzetti P, et al. Umbilical amino acid concentrations in appropriate and small for gestational age infants: a biochemical difference present in utero. *Am J Obstet Gynecol* 1988;158(1):120–6.

50. Cetin I, Corbetta C, Sereni LP, et al. Umbilical amino acid concentrations in normal and growth-retarded fetuses sampled in utero by cordocentesis. *Am J Obstet Gynecol* 1990;162(1):253–61.

51. Cetin I, Ronzoni S, Marconi AM, et al. Maternal concentrations and fetal-maternal concentration differences of plasma amino acids in normal and intrauterine growth-restricted pregnancies. *Am J Obstet Gynecol* 1996;174(5):1575–83.

52. Cetin I, Giovannini N, Alvino G, et al. Intrauterine growth restriction is associated with changes in polyunsaturated fatty acid fetal–maternal relationships. *Pediatr Res* 2002;52:750–5.

53. Marconi Am, Cetin I, Davoli E, et al. An evaluation of fetal glucogenesis in intrauterine growth retarded pregnancies by a comparison of steady state fetal and maternal enrichments of plasma glucose at cordocentesis. *Metabolism* 1993;42:860–4.

54. Novielli C, Mandò C, Tabano SM, Anelli GM, Fontana L, Antonazzo P, Miozzo M, Cetin I. Mitochondrial DNA content and methylation in fetal blood of pregnancies with placental insufficiency. *Placenta* 2017;55:63–70.

55. Marconi AM, Paolini C, Buscaglia M, et al. The impact of gestational age and fetal growth on the maternal-fetal glucose concentration difference. *Obstet Gynecol* 1996;87(6):937–42.

56. Van Cappellen AM, Heerschap A, Nijhuis JG, et al. Hypoxia, the subsequent systemic metabolic acidosis, and their relationship with cerebral metabolite concentrations: An in vivo study in fetal lambs with proton magnetic resonance spectroscopy. *Am J Obstet Gynecol* 1999;181(6):1537–45.

57. Cetin I, Barberis B, Brusati V, et al. Lactate detection in the brain of growth-restricted fetuses with magnetic resonance spectroscopy. *Am J Obstet Gynecol* 2011;205(4):350.e1–7.

58. Ramenghi LA, Martinelli A, De Carli A, et al. Cerebral maturation in IUGR and appropriate for gestational age preterm babies. *Reprod Sci* 2011;18(5):469–75.

59. Scherjon S, Briet J, Oosting H, et al. The discrepancy between maturation of visual-evoked potentials and cognitive outcome at five years in very preterm infants with and without hemodynamic sign of fetal brain sparing. *Pediatrics* 2000;105:385–91.

60. Flood K, Unterscheider J, Daly S, et al. The role of brain sparing in the prediction of adverse outcomes in intrauterine growth restriction: Results of the multicenter PORTO Study. *Am J Obstet Gynecol* 2014;211(3):288.e1–5.

61. Cruz-Martinez R, Figueras F, Oros D, et al. Cerebral blood perfusion and neurobehavioral performance in full-term small-for-gestational-age fetuses. *Am J Obstet Gynecol* 2009;201(5):474.e1–7.

62. Eixarch E, Meler E, Iraola A, et al. Neurodevelopmental outcome in 2-years-old infants who were small-for-gestational age term fetus with cerebral blood flow redistribution. *Ultrasound Obstet Gynecol* 2008;32:849–99.

Chapter

22

Management of Early-Onset Fetal Growth Restriction (Less than 34 Weeks)

Tullia Todros and Giovanna Oggé

Introduction

Early-onset intrauterine fetal growth restriction (FGR) (less than 34 weeks' gestation) is a major issue for modern obstetrics: indeed, perinatal mortality associated with early-onset FGR has been reported to be as high as 41%, depending on definition, study population, and gestational age (GA) [1]. Moreover, early-onset FGR is strongly associated with severe neonatal morbidity (such as central nervous system, respiratory, and gastroenteric complications) [2,3], infant neurodevelopmental impairment [4,5], and cardiovascular and metabolic disease in adulthood in agreement with the "Barker hypothesis" of fetal programming of adult disease [5,6].

To date, the main known determinants of short- and long-term prognosis are: fetal cardiovascular status, birthweight, and GA at birth [7–9].

Fetal cardiovascular condition, as indicated by Doppler velocimetry of arterial and venous vessels and by fetal heart rate (FHR) tracings, is strictly related to the fetal acid-base status: hence serial testing with Doppler ultrasound and cardiotocography allows us to follow the transition from fetal normal oxygenation to hypoxemia, hypoxia, and acidemia, which in turn appears to be the nearest fetal antecedent of perinatal mortality and infant neurodevelopmental delay [10].

Birth weight is the expression of both GA at birth and the severity of fetal malnutrition and correlates with major neonatal morbidity [7] and abnormal neurodevelopment in infancy and childhood [8,9] independently of Doppler parameters in early-onset FGR.

On the other hand, prematurity (as a result of iatrogenic preterm delivery of fetuses considered at high risk of intrauterine acidemia and demise) is an independent predictor of neonatal mortality and severe neonatal complications associated with abnormal neurodevelopmental outcomes in FGR fetuses [7–11]. A multicenter cohort trial conducted between 2000 and 2006 in 12 centers of perinatal medicine in the United States and Europe reports neonatal outcomes of 604 singleton live born with FGR delivered between 24 and 32 weeks + 6 days. Mortality within 28 days of life was 20%, while the incidence of severe neonatal morbidity was 36%; however, the rate of neonatal death decreased by 2% per each day of pregnancy prolongation between 24 and 27 weeks of GA. In contrast, after this threshold, Doppler velocimetry of the venous circulation and arterial pH were the only independent variables predictive of neonatal mortality, while GA at delivery was not a determinant of neonatal survival. Similarly, GA was the main predictor of severe neonatal morbidity until 29 weeks, but it was replaced by venous Doppler velocimetry between 29 and 33 weeks [7].

More favorable data on neonatal mortality and morbidity are reported by the Trial of Randomized and Fetal Flow in Europe (TRUFFLE). This is a randomized clinical trial (RCT) conducted between 2005 and 2010 in 20 European centers, in which 503 fetuses with early-onset FGR (diagnosed between 26 weeks and 31 weeks + 6 days of GA) were randomly allocated to be delivered according to one of three criteria (cardiotocographic criteria, early abnormalities in the venous Doppler velocimetry, or late abnormalities in the venous Doppler velocimetry as discussed extensively later). When the short-term outcomes of the whole cohort, regardless of the arm of randomization, were analyzed, neonatal mortality before discharge from hospital was 5.5% of all live born, and severe morbidity was 24%. Besides GA and birth weight, the major determinant of poor outcome was the occurrence of maternal hypertensive disease, which shortened the interval between diagnosis of FGR and delivery [12].

Based on these data, the aim of clinical management of early-onset FGR fetuses is currently focused on optimizing the timing of delivery in order to balance the risks of prolonged intrauterine hypoxia versus the complications associated with preterm birth.

As standardized protocols are not available, the main target of clinical research is to identify the most efficient tool (or combination of tools) for monitoring the deterioration of the fetal condition and selection of those fetuses that will benefit from timely delivery and those that will take advantage from further intrauterine maturation. Furthermore, as early-onset FGR is frequently associated with hypertensive disorders of pregnancy [13], the decision to deliver will necessarily take into account a strict follow-up of maternal conditions as well.

This chapter will cover available evidence about methods of fetal monitoring and intrapartum care and suggest a flow-chart for obstetrical management of pregnancies complicated by early-onset FGR.

Fetal Monitoring

Doppler Velocimetry

Doppler velocimetry of different fetal vessels allows us to follow hemodynamic deterioration, which typically involves progression from increased resistance in feto-placental circulation, to redistribution of fetal blood flow, to cardiac compromise, although variability occurs in the exact sequence of vessels changes and in the length of intervals between them.

Technique and information obtained by Doppler evaluation of single fetal vessels are discussed in detail in Chapter 20.

Fetal Heart Rate Tracing and Biophysical Profile Score

Cardiotocography

The visual analysis of fetal heart rate through antepartum cardiotocography (CTG) has been the first noninvasive test introduced in obstetric practice to detect fetal hypoxemia and acidemia in FGR fetuses, as well as in other conditions. The single parameters that are most strongly associated with hypoxemia/acidemia are late decelerations and reduced heart rate variability [19,20].

CTG is characterized by high sensitivity, but is limited by disappointing specificity and positive predictive value and low inter-observer reproducibility [21]. The problem of reduced reproducibility of traditional CTG has been overcome by the development of computerized heart rate analysis, which provides quantitative parameters. The most appropriate parameter for the monitoring of fetuses at risk for intrauterine hypoxemia appears to be short-term variation (STV). STV is determined by a computerized system (Sonicaid System 8002, Huntleigh) on a minimum of 40 minutes of FHR recording. This software fits a FHR baseline and calculates short term FHR variation as the difference in beat-to-beat intervals between successive epochs of 3.75 seconds [22].

STV is determined by the balance between the two branches of the autonomous nervous system input, with the sympathetic system contributing to accelerations and the parasympathetic system contributing to decelerations [23]. A persistent reduction in fetal heart variability is a sign of central nervous system depression secondary to chronic hypoxemia [24]. There is a clear correlation between reduced STV and both fetal acidemia [25] and intrauterine death [26] in FGR fetuses. In a large, retrospective cohort of SGA fetuses (birth weight below the 3rd percentile) delivered between 26 and 42 weeks, STV <3 msec predicted metabolic acidosis at birth with sensitivity of 52.5%, specificity of 91.4%, positive predictive value of 64.6%, and negative predictive value of 86.6% [27]. Reduction of STV is a late event that tends to occur very close to changes in the ductus venosus (DV) Doppler velocimetry. However the order of presentation of the two signs is variable, as some fetuses present the reduction of STV first, while in other cases increased PI of the DV occurs earlier [27,28].

When compared with changes in DV pulsatility index (PI), STV alone has a lower predictive value for adverse neonatal outcome [29].

Biophysical Profile Score

An alternative approach to improve the predictive value of traditional CTG is to incorporate it in a composite test that also includes other variables of the fetal status.

In the biophysical profile, fetal breathing, body movements, muscular tone, the amount of amniotic fluid, and fetal reactivity (on CTG) are assessed synoptically as a score, instead of evaluating the individual criteria.

Fetal biophysical profile score correlates with antepartum umbilical vein pH [30] and in the majority of cases, a decline in the biophysical profile is preceded by arterial and venous Doppler velocities deterioration [31].

The biophysical profile is less accurate than umbilical arteries (UA) and venous Doppler velocimetry in the prediction of fetal acidemia [32,33]. Interestingly, the performance of biophysical profile in the prediction of low pH at birth improves when traditional evaluation of CTG is replaced by computerized STV [32].

Currently there is no evidence that the integration of the different components of the biophysical profile in a single score provides any advantage over the separate evaluation of FHR and multi-vessel Doppler velocimetry on outcomes of FGR fetuses.

The TRUFFLE Study

The TRUFFLE study is, to date, the only RCT comparing the effects of different strategies of fetal monitoring on infant neurologic and neurodevelopmental outcomes in early-onset FGR [34]. Five hundred and three singleton fetuses with FGR were recruited between 26 $^{+0}$ and 31 $^{+6}$ weeks of gestation in 20 European centers and were randomly allocated to be delivered according to one of the following criteria:

1) reduced short term variability (STV) in a 60-minute FHR tracing, defined as <3.5 msec at 26 $^{+0}$ – 28 $^{+6}$ weeks and <4 msec at 29 $^{+0}$ – 32 $^{+0}$ weeks;

2) early changes in the DV waveform, defined as PI >95th percentile for GA;

3) late changes in the DV waveform, defined as absent or reversed flow during the a wave.

Regardless of the group of randomization, delivery was mandatory whenever one of the following "safety criteria" was met: very low STV (<2.6 msec at 26 $^{+0}$ – 28 $^{+6}$ weeks, <3 msec at 29 $^{+0}$ – 32 $^{+0}$ weeks); spontaneous repeated decelerations at CTG; absent end-diastolic flow in the UA after 32 weeks of gestation and reversed end-diastolic flow in the UA after 30 weeks of GA. After 32 weeks the decision to deliver was based on local criteria.

Among survivors, normal neurodevelopmental outcome at 2 years was significantly more frequent in the group randomized to delivery following late changes in the DV compared to the group randomized to delivery following reduced STV (95% vs. 85%, p = 0.005), although this was associated with a nonsignificant increase in overall mortality (10% in the DV late changes group, 7% in the DV early changes group, 8% in the STV group). Mortality was significantly higher for babies entered before 29 weeks than later (14% vs. 4%), but the incidence of abnormal neurodevelopment was comparable (8% vs. 9%).

Noteworthy, however, a considerable proportion of fetuses was not delivered according to the randomization

arm: 24% because they met "safety net" criteria, 11% because of fetal indications out of the study protocol (as suspected abruptio placentae or visual assessment of CTG), 11% because of maternal indications, and 29% were delivered after 32 weeks according to local criteria.

Thus the study suggests that in case of FGR before 32 weeks of GA, delaying delivery until late changes in the DV flow occur is associated with the best neurodevelopmental outcomeat 2 years of age unless other well-standardized signs of severe deterioration in the FHR and/or umbilical artery occur (TRUFFLE safety net criteria).

Patterns of Cardiovascular Deterioration

The sequence of fetal hemodynamic changes associated with chronic hypoxemia due to placental dysfunction is presently well established, from increased impedance in the placental circulation (increased PI in the UA up to reversed end-diastolic velocities), to the redistribution of arterial flow with brain sparing (reduced PI in the middle cerebral artery), to cardiac impairment with venous flow abnormalities (elevated PI in the DV up to reversal of a wave), to FHR abnormalities and abnormal biophysical profile score, to death [28,29,31,35–38]. However, the speed of the progression and the time interval between each stage is variable, due to gestational age, severity of placental damage, concomitant maternal disease, individual susceptibility to hypoxemia, and probably other factors [31,39]. Thus when a specific Doppler abnormality is documented in a growth-restricted fetus, it is not possible to predict how long it will take until it will reach most severe deterioration prompting delivery to avoid fetal death.

In a longitudinal observational study including 668 Doppler examinations on 104 fetuses with FGR, Turan and colleagues identified three different patterns of cardiovascular velocities deterioration:

1) severe early-onset placental dysfunction: abnormal UA velocities present early in gestation (median 26 weeks) and progress rapidly, resulting in very preterm delivery (median 30 weeks);

2) progressive placental dysfunction: abnormal UA Doppler velocities appear slightly later (median 29 weeks) and progress steadily but less rapidly than in the previous case, allowing us to delay delivery to a safer gestational age (median 33 weeks);

3) mild placental dysfunction: UA Doppler abnormalities are milder and do not progress beyond flow redistribution, i.e., they do not evolve into cardiac dysfunction; this pattern is more typical of late-onset FGR (median GA at first Doppler abnormality 31 weeks, median GA at delivery 35 weeks) [39].

Maternal Monitoring

As FGR is basically a "placental disease," it is often associated with maternal preeclampsia of placental origin [13]. In the TRUFFLE study, the number of women with any hypertensive complication of pregnancy increased from 60% at study entry to 73% at delivery [34]. On the other hand, the presence of hypertensive disease of pregnancy increases the risk of FGR by three- to four-fold [38,40–42]. Moreover, maternal hypertension has a negative impact on fetal prognosis, by reducing the interval from diagnosis of FGR to delivery [34].

It is therefore important, once the diagnosis of FGR is made, to assess uterine artery Doppler velocimetry that is highly predictive of the development of severe preeclampsia [43] and to strictly monitor maternal conditions: blood pressure, urine output, renal function, neurological symptoms, cardiopulmonary impairment, signs of HELLP syndrome (Hemolysis, Elevated Liver enzymes, Low Platelet count) [44,45].

Flow Chart

As previously mentioned, the purpose of clinical management of early-onset FGR is to establish the timing of delivery in order to minimize both the risk of death or short- and long-term morbidity derived from preterm birth and the risk of fetal death and irreversible neurological damage due to intrauterine hypoxemia and acidemia. Unfortunately, neither an adequate single test nor a widely agreed protocol is to date available to this aim.

Based on the review of the best available evidence, monitoring and delivery of early-onset FGR should be based on the following principles:

1) early-onset FGR should be referred to highly specialized centers, with high-quality equipment, with experienced operators in the performance and interpretation of prenatal tests, in monitoring maternal and fetal conditions and in counseling these patients, and with availability of a neonatal intensive care unit;

2) fetal monitoring needs to be based on the integration of multiple tests, including multi-vessel Doppler velocimetry and FHR analysis;

3) in the assessment of early-onset FGR fetuses, the evaluation of FHR should preferably be based on computerized analysis of STV;

4) the cut-off of fetal deterioration that indicates delivery needs to vary according to gestational age, as the latter is the main determinant of perinatal mortality and intact survival;

5) in very preterm FGR (<32 weeks), based on the only available RCT, the most adequate test to provide optimal infant neurological outcome appears to be the occurrence of either late changes in the DV (absent or reversed a wave) or severe alterations in FHR (very low STV);

6) after 32 weeks, the decision to deliver should also be based on abnormalities in the umbilical artery waveforms, namely absence of end-diastolic velocities at umbilical Doppler.

Figure 22.1 illustrates a flow chart for clinical management of early-onset FGR stratified by GA and severity of umbilical artery abnormality. UA Doppler velocimetry is used to prompt delivery when absent end-diastolic velocities are seen at or beyond 32 weeks or reversed end-diastolic velocities are found at or beyond 30 weeks, even if the other biophysical tests are normal. Before this GA, the severity of UA velocities abnormalities is useful to dictate the frequency and type of fetal surveillance, but not to take action about delivery. If UA Doppler velocities are abnormal, but end-diastolic velocities are present, CTG, Doppler velocimetry of DV, evaluation of amniotic fluid index, and ultrasonographic fetal biometry should be performed every 1 to 2 weeks, depending on the severity of FGR. It must be underscored that fetal growth can be assessed only taking into account measurements obtained at least 2 weeks apart. If the fetus is growing and the biophysical variables remain normal, pregnancy may continue beyond 34 weeks. Intensification of fetal surveillance or delivery are needed when the results of one or more biophysical variables become abnormal. In cases of AED before 32 weeks or RED before 30 weeks, intensive fetal surveillance is needed, with computerized CTG performed at least daily and Doppler velocimetry and amniotic fluid index every 2/3 days. Delivery is indicated when late changes in the DV (absent or reversed a wave) or severe alterations in FHR (very low STV and persistent decelerations) occur.

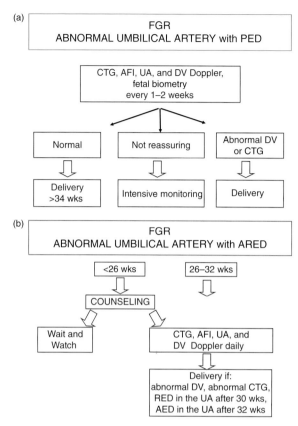

Figure 22.1 Flow chart of fetal monitoring and timing of delivery in early-onset FGR with present end-diastolic flow in the umbilical artery (a), and with absent or reversed end-diastolic flow in the umbilical artery (b). FGR: fetal growth restriction; PED: positive end-diastolic flow velocities; CTG: cardiotocography; AFI: amniotic fluid index; UA: umbilical artery; DV: ductus venosus; ARED: absent or reversed end-diastolic flow velocities; AED absent end-diastolic flow velocities; RED: reversed end-diastolic flow velocities.

Cesarean section is the mode of delivery in the vast majority of cases [7,9,12,46] and fetal hypoxia/acidosis is usually the indication. Corticosteroids for lung maturity might be administered [47,48], although the actual effect of steroid treatment on morbidity and mortality of FGR fetuses is still debated [49]. Noteworthy, FHR variability can be reduced in the 24–72 hours following the first dose: therefore no decision on delivery should be made based only on reduced FHR variation.

Conclusions

The management of early onset FGR remains one of the main challenges of maternal-fetal medicine. In the absence of pharmacologic therapy, the only treatment is timed delivery, balancing the risk of prematurity and the risk of too long an exposure to hypoxia and undernutrition *in utero*. Recent data show that results in terms of survival and intact survival of these fetuses are improving, and overall good. Both survival and intact survival rates, at least at 2 years of age, dramatically increase with GA at delivery between 26 and 32–34 weeks. Therefore, the aim of management is to prolong pregnancy as long as possible, at the same time avoiding fetal death or irreversible damage. Unfortunately, there is no single test indicating the break point, in spite of the many tests reflecting fetal conditions and their deterioration that have been developed in the past decades: UA and DV Doppler velocimetry, computerized CTG, ultrasound for assessment of fetal growth, and amniotic fluid index. At the moment the best management is based on the integration of the results of the different tests, also taking into account GA and possible complicating conditions such as maternal preeclampsia.

Key Points

- Early-onset FGR must be managed in specialized centers where both maternal-fetal medicine and neonatal intensive care units are present.

- Pregnancy should be prolonged as long as possible between 25–26 and 32–34 weeks, while avoiding intrauterine death or irreversible damage.

- Timing of delivery is based on integration of results of biophysical tests: umbilical artery Doppler, ductus venosus Doppler, computerized CTG.

References

1. Mari G, Hanif F, Treadwell MC, Kruger M. Gestational age at delivery and Doppler waveforms in very preterm intrauterine growth-restricted fetuses as predictors of perinatal mortality. *J Ultrasound Med* 2007 May;26:555–9.

2. Garite TJ, Clark R, Thorp JA. Intrauterine growth restriction increases morbidity and mortality among premature neonates. *Am J Obstet Gynecol* 2004; 191:481–7.

3. Aucott SW, Donohue PK, Northington FJ. Increased morbidity in severe early intrauterine growth restriction. *J Perinatol* 2004;24:435–40.

4. Morsing E, Asard M, Ley D, Stjernqvist K, Marsál K. Cognitive function after intrauterine growth

restriction and very preterm birth. *Pediatrics* 2011;127:e874–82.

5. Guellec I, Lapillonne A, Renolleau S, Charlaluk ML, Roze JC, Marret S, Vieux R, Monique K, Ancel PY; EPIPAGE Study Group. Neurologic outcomes at school age in very preterm infants born with severe or mild growth restriction. *Pediatrics* 2011;127:e883–91.

6. Barker DJ, Osmond C. Infant mortality, childhood nutrition, and ischaemic heart disease in England and Wales. *Lancet* 1986; 1: 1077–81Kanaka-Gantenbein C. Fetal origins of adult diabetes. *Ann N Y Acad Sci* 2010;1205:99–105.

7. Baschat AA, Cosmi E, Bilardo CM, Wolf H, Berg C, Rigano S, Germer U, Moyano D, Turan S, Hartung J, Bhide A, Müller T, Bower S, Nicolaides KH, Thilaganathan B, Gembruch U, Ferrazzi E, Hecher K, Galan HL, Harman CR. Predictors of neonatal outcome in early-onset placental dysfunction. *Obstet Gynecol* 2007;109:253–61.

8. Baschat AA, Viscardi RM, Hussey-Gardner B, Hashmi N, Harman C. Infant neurodevelopment following fetal growth restriction: Relationship with antepartum surveillance parameters. *Ultrasound Obstet Gynecol* 2009;33:44–50.

9. Torrance HL, Bloemen MC, Mulder EJ, Nikkels PG, Derks JB, de Vries LS, Visser GH. Predictors of outcome at 2 years of age after early intrauterine growth restriction. *Ultrasound Obstet Gynecol* 2010; 36:171–7.

10. Soothill PW, Ajayi RA, Campbell S, Ross EM, Candy DC, Snijders RM, Nicolaides KH. Relationship between fetal acidemia at cordocentesis and subsequent neurodevelopment. *Ultrasound Obstet Gynecol* 1992;2:80–3.

11. Bernstein IM, Horbar JD, Badger GJ, Ohlsson A, Golan A. Morbidity and mortality among very-low-birth-weight neonates with intrauterine growth restriction. The Vermont Oxford Network. *Am J Obstet Gynecol* 2000;182:198–206.

12. Lees C, Marlow N, Arabin B, Bilardo CM, Brezinka C, Derks JB, Duvekot J,Frusca T, Diemert A, Ferrazzi E, Ganzevoort W, Hecher K, Martinelli P, Ostermayer E, Papageorghiou AT, Schlembach D, Schneider KT, Thilaganathan B, Todros T, Van Wassenaer-Leemhuis A, Valcamonico A, Visser GH, Wolf H; TRUFFLE Group. Perinatal morbidity and mortality in early-onset fetal growth restriction: Cohort outcomes of the trial of randomized umbilical and fetal flow in Europe (TRUFFLE). *Ultrasound Obstet Gynecol* 2013; 42:400–8.

13. Groom KM, North RA, Poppe KK, Sadler L, McCowan LM. The association between customised small for gestational age infants and pre-eclampsia or gestational hypertension varies with gestation at delivery. *BJOG* 2007;114:478–84.

14. Hofstaetter C, Dubiel M, Gudmundsson S. Two types of umbilical venous pulsations and outcome of high-risk pregnancy. *Early Hum Dev* 2001;61:111–17.

15. Baschat AA, Gembruch U, Weiner CP, Harman CR. Qualitative venous Doppler waveform analysis improves prediction of critical perinatal outcomes in premature growth-restricted fetuses. *Ultrasound Obstet Gynecol* 2003;22:240–5.

16. Baschat AA, Gembruch U, Gortner L, Reiss I, Weiner CP, Harman CR. Coronary artery blood flow visualization signifies hemodynamic deterioration in growth-restricted fetuses. *Ultrasound Obstet Gynecol* 2000;16:425–31.

17. Chaoui R. Coronary arteries in fetal life: Physiology, malformations and the "heart-sparing effect." *Acta Paediatr Suppl* 2004;93:6–12.

18. Rizzo G, Capponi A, Pietrolucci ME, Boccia C, Arduini D. The significance of visualising coronary blood flow in early onset severe growth restricted fetuses with reverse flow in the ductus venosus. *J Matern Fetal Neonatal Med* 2009;22:547–51.

19. Flynn AM, Kelly J, O'Conor M. Unstressed antepartum cardiotocography in the management of the fetus suspected of growth retardation. *BJOG* 1979;86:106–10.

20. Visser GH, Redman CW, Huisjes HJ, Turnbull AC. Nonstressed antepartum heart rate monitoring: Implications of decelerations after spontaneous contractions. *Am J Obstet Gynecol* 1980; 138:429–35.

21. Ayres-de-Campos D, Bernardes J, Costa-Pereira A, Pereira-Leite L. Inconsistencies in classification by experts of cardiotocograms and subsequent clinical decision. *BJOG* 1999;106:1307–10.

22. Dawes GS, Lobb M, Moulden M, Redman CW, Wheeler T. Antenatal cardiotocogram quality and interpretation using computers. *BJOG* 1992;99:791–7.

23. Van Ravenswaaij-Arts CM, Kollée LA, Hopman JC, Stoelinga GB, Van Geijn HP. Heart rate variability. *Ann Intern Med* 1993;118:436–47.

24. Visser GH, Bekedam DJ, Ribbert LS. Changes in antepartum heart rate patterns with progressive deterioration of the fetal condition. *Int J Biomed Comput* 1990;25:239–46.

25. Guzman ER, Vintzileos AM, Martins M, Benito C, Houlihan C, Hanley M. The efficacy of individual computer heart rate indices in detecting acidemia at birth in growth-restricted fetuses. *Obstet Gynecol* 1996;87:969–74.

26. Street P, Dawes GS, Moulden M, Redman CW. Short-term variation in abnormal antenatal fetal heart rate records. *Am J Obstet Gynecol* 1991;165:515–23.

27. Serra V, Moulden M, Bellver J, Redman CW. The value of the short-term fetal heart rate variation for timing the delivery of growth-retarded fetuses. *BJOG* 2008; 115:1101–7.

28. Hecher K, Bilardo CM, Stigter RH, Ville Y, Hackelöer BJ, Kok HJ, Senat MV, Visser GH. Monitoring of fetuses with intrauterine growth restriction: A longitudinal study. *Ultrasound Obstet Gynecol* 2001; 18:564–70.

29. Bilardo CM, Wolf H, Stigter RH, Ville Y, Baez E, Visser GH, Hecher K. Relationship between monitoring parameters and perinatal outcome in severe, early intrauterine growth restriction. *Ultrasound Obstet Gynecol* 2004;23:119–25.

30. Walkinshaw S, Cameron H, MacPhail S, Robson S. The prediction of fetal compromise and acidosis by biophysical profile scoring in the small for gestational age fetus. *J Perinat Med* 1992;20:227–32.

31. Baschat AA, Gembruch U, Harman CR. The sequence of changes in Doppler and biophysical parameters as severe fetal growth restriction worsens. *Ultrasound Obstet Gynecol* 2001;18:571–7.

32. Turan S, Turan OM, Berg C, Moyano D, Bhide A, Bower S, Thilaganathan B, Gembruch U, Nicolaides K, Harman C, Baschat AA. Computerized fetal heart rate analysis, Doppler ultrasound and biophysical profile score in the prediction of acid-base status of growth-restricted fetuses. *Ultrasound Obstet Gynecol* 2007; 30:750–6.

33. Yoon BH, Romero R, Roh CR, Kim SH, Ager JW, Syn HC, Cotton D, Kim SW. Relationship between the fetal biophysical profile score, umbilical artery Doppler velocimetry, and fetal blood acid-base status determined by cordocentesis. *Am J Obstet Gynecol* 1993;169:1586–94.

34. Ferrazzi E, Bozzo M, Rigano S, Bellotti M, Morabito A, Pardi G, Battaglia FC, Galan HL. Temporal sequence of abnormal Doppler changes in the peripheral and central circulatory systems of the severely growth-restricted fetus. *Ultrasound Obstet Gynecol* 2002;19:140–6.

35. Lees C; Marlow N, Van Wassenaer-Leemhuis A, Arabin B, Bilardo CM, Brezinka C, Calvert S, Derks JB, Diemert A, Duvekot JJ, Ferrazzi E, Frusca T, Ganzevoort W, Hecher K, Martinelli P, Ostermayer E, Papageorghiou AT, Schlembach D, Schneider KTM, Thilaganathan B, Todros T, Valcamonico A, Visser GHA, Wolf H on behalf of the TRUFFLE Group. The Trial of Randomized Umbilical and Fetal Flow in Europe (TRUFFLE) study: Two year neurodevelopmental and intermediate perinatal outcomes. *Lancet* 2015;385:2162–72.

36. Figueras F, Benavides A, Del Rio M, Crispi F, Eixarch E, Martinez JM, Hernandez-Andrade E, Gratacós E. Monitoring of fetuses with intrauterine growth restriction: Longitudinal changes in ductus venosus and aortic isthmus flow. *Ultrasound Obstet Gynecol* 2009;33:39–43.

37. Arduini D, Rizzo G, Romanini C. Changes of pulsatility index from fetal vessels preceding the onset of late decelerations in growth-retarded fetuses. *Obstet Gynecol* 1992;79:605–10.

38. Baschat AA. Neurodevelopment following fetal growth restriction and its relationship with antepartum parameters of placental dysfunction. *Ultrasound Obstet Gynecol* 2011;37:501–14

39. Turan OM, Turan S, Gungor S, Berg C, Moyano D, Gembruch U, Nicolaides KH, Harman CR, Baschat AA. Progression of Doppler abnormalities in intrauterine growth restriction. *Ultrasound Obstet Gynecol* 2008;32:160–7.

40. Odegård RA, Vatten LJ, Nilsen ST, Salvesen KA, Austgulen R. Preeclampsia and fetal growth. *Obstet Gynecol* 2000;96:950–5.

41. Rasmussen S, Irgens LM. Fetal growth and body proportion in preeclampsia. *Obstet Gynecol* 2003; 101:575–83.

42. Allen VM, Joseph K, Murphy KE, Magee LA, Ohlsson A. The effect of hypertensive disorders in pregnancy on small for gestational age and stillbirth: A population based study. *BMC Pregnancy Childbirth* 2004;4:17.

43. Khalil A, Garcia-Mandujano R, Maiz N, Elkhaouli M, Nicolaides KH. Longitudinal changes in uterine artery Doppler and blood pressure and risk of pre-eclampsia. *Ultrasound Obstet Gynecol* 2014;43:541–7.

44. Royal College of Obstetricians and Gynaecologists. Hypertension in pregnancy: The management of hypertensive disorders during pregnancy. www.nice.org.uk/guidance/cg107 (accessed January 18, 2015).

45. American College of Obstetricians and Gynecologists. Task Force on Hypertension in Pregnancy. Hypertension in Pregnancy. www.acog.org/Womens-Health/Preeclampsia-and-Hypertension-in-Pregnancy (accessed January 18, 2015).

46. Brodszki J, Morsing E, Malcus P, Thuring A, Ley D, Marsál K. Early intervention in management of very preterm growth-restricted fetuses: 2-year outcome of infants delivered on fetal indication before 30 gestational weeks. *Ultrasound Obstet Gynecol* 2009; 34:288–96.

47. Royal College of Obstetricians and Gynaecologists. The Investigation and Management of the Small-for-Gestational-Age Fetus. Green-top Guideline No. 31. 2nd Edition. February 2013. Minor revisions January 2014. www.rcog.org.uk/globalassets/documents/guidelines/gtg_31.pdf (accessed January 18, 2015).

48. American College of Obstetricians and Gynecologists. ACOG Practice bulletin no. 134: Fetal growth restriction. *Obstet Gynecol* 2013;121:1122–33.

49. Torrance HL, Derks JB, Scherjon SA, Wijnberger LD, Visser GH. Is antenatal steroid treatment effective in preterm IUGR fetuses? *Acta Obstet Gynecol Scand* 2009;88:1068–73.

Chapter

23

Late-Onset Fetal Growth Restriction

C. M. Bilardo and Francesc Figueras

Identification Issues

Antenatal detection of babies with defective growth often falls short, missing up to 75% of babies at risk of being small for gestational age (SGA) before delivery [1].

This is due to the fact that ultrasound growth assessment has intrinsic limitations and the quest for effective early prediction methods for the later growth impairment is still ongoing [2,3].

In low-risk pregnancies, prenatal detection of defective growth is worse (~15%) [4]. Such poor performance takes a toll, given that undetected SGA status significantly raises the risks of adverse perinatal outcomes and stillbirth [5,6]; and many instances of avoidable stillbirth are linked to failure in antenatal SGA detection [7].

By combining first- or second-trimester uterine Doppler findings with baseline maternal characteristics, detection of early-onset (needing delivery at <34 weeks) growth restriction (GR) nears acceptable levels [8]. Furthermore, up to 60% of early-onset GR cases are marked by preeclampsia [9]. Unfortunately, growth restriction in late pregnancy is still largely overlooked [10,11], while accounting for the largest fraction of adverse perinatal outcomes and stillbirths [12,13]. Within this subset, the chief correlate in stillbirth, perinatal complications, and abnormal neurodevelopment is severe growth restriction (generally birth weight <3rd percentile) [14–16]. Detecting late-onset growth restriction, especially severe states, is thus central to third-trimester screening.

Current third-trimester strategies to monitor growth involve symphysis-fundal height determination. However, only 16% of SGA infants are detected this way in low-risk populations [10]. Consequently, most SGA births are full-term [17]. Third-trimester ultrasound (US) monitoring of fetal growth is done routinely in some countries, boosting detection rates to 40–80% [5,11,18]. However, the impact on perinatal outcomes remains unclear. A systematic review of randomized trials fails to demonstrate any real benefit from routine third-trimester scanning [19]. However, it may be argued that the older pooled data hold limited contemporary validity [20]. The most recent study [21] (as part of this meta-analysis) claimed a 30% reduction in fetal growth restriction (FGR) when third-trimester US was performed. Furthermore, many of the studies involved no change in management if a diagnosis of FGR was made, which does not reflect current modes of practice. And finally, just three of the included trials [21–23] (contributing only 12% of subjects overall) routinely performed US studies after 34 weeks, which is when FGR due to placental insufficiency is more likely to be phenotypically apparent and thus more readily detected by ultrasound. A recent randomized study shows that in low-risk women, detection at 37 weeks is more effective than at 34 weeks [24]. Including maternal characteristics in addition to ultrasound data in the prediction model may also boost detection rates [25].

Detecting SGA in advance of delivery has several potential benefits. Detection prompts further investigations, such as umbilical artery Doppler study, which has been shown to reduce stillbirth and increase preterm delivery without increasing neonatal mortality [26]. Detection also alerts clinicians and mothers to the increased risk involved, enabling institution of appropriate monitoring intervals, awareness of fetal movements patterns by the mother, and deliberations on the optimal timing of delivery. Depending on severity of FGR, the risk of stillbirth may be increased by 5- to 10-fold [27]. A population-based study in the United States reported a significantly increased risk of stillbirth in pregnancies complicated by SGA when delivered after the 37th week [28]; and another [6] in the UK, where 92,218 normally formed singletons (including 389 stillbirths) were analyzed, found a reduced stillbirth rate (per 1,000 births) of 9.7 with antenatal FGR detection, compared with 19.8 when growth restriction remained undetected. The impact of timely recognition and delivery of SGA babies is also underscored by the fact that in this study, gestational age in instances of detected vs. non-detected SGA differed by only 10 days (270 vs. 280 days), but resulted in a 50% lower incidence of stillbirths. Similarly, another large single-center retrospective study by Lindqvist and colleagues [5] found that fetuses with severe FGR (i.e., weight deviation ≤−22% or approximately <3rd percentile) that went undetected before delivery showed a fourfold increase in risk of adverse fetal outcome.

The Distinction between Late FGR and SGA

SGA represents a heterogeneous population that comprises several phenotypes: (i) fetuses with congenital malformations (including chromosomopathies) or infections are a marginal proportion; (ii) fetuses that do not achieve their endowed growth potential mainly due to placental insufficiency. Thus, they could be considered true cases of FGR; (iii) finally, the largest fraction of the small babies are constitutionally small (i.e., they have a low growth potential). By convention, these last two groups are normally referred to as FGR versus SGA.

From a clinical point of view, the distinction between late FGR and SGA is relevant because of the correlation with perinatal outcome. Whereas FGR represents a pathological condition associated with adverse perinatal outcome, SGA merely is the end of the spectrum of healthy babies. While conceptually FGR and SGA are clearly distinct conditions, from a clinical point of view, their differentiation is rather challenging.

Recent literature on optimal fetal growth [29,30] challenges the concept of constitutionally determined growth potential [31]. In fact, fetuses from eight different countries and ethnicities show a homogeneous growth with a narrow band of variation, provided maternal nutrition and health care are adequate and similar [29].

A challenging group is represented by fetuses that have failed to reach their maximum growth potential, but with biometry still falling within the range of normality. These cases may be identified by a deflecting growth pattern, i.e., a growth trajectory that falls in a lower centile with advancing gestation, rather than following the same percentile line [33].

Umbilical artery has proven a good screening method for early placental insufficiency, but unfortunately does not capture late-onset placental insufficiency.

A sizable body of evidence shows that the umbilical artery does not reliably reflect placental insufficiency and does not predict adverse outcome in late-onset FGR [33,34]. It is intriguing that while most cases of late-onset SGA present signs of placental underperfusion [35,36], this is not reflected in the umbilical artery Doppler. One could speculate that the degree of the extension accounts for this finding. Indeed, animal [37] and mathematical [38] experimental models of placental vessel obliteration have suggested that umbilical artery Doppler become abnormal only if an extensive part of the placenta is involved.

Improving the Definition of FGR by Incorporating Predictors of Adverse Outcome

The current evidence suggests that there is not a single marker to differentiate FGR and SGA phenotypes.

The use of middle cerebral artery (MCA) Doppler in this setting is supported by recent studies that have demonstrated that 15–20% of term SGA fetuses with normal UA Doppler have reduced impedance in MCA blood flow, and that this sign is associated with poorer perinatal outcome [39,40] and neurobehavior, both at birth [41,42] and at 2 years of age [43,44]. Furthermore, the cerebroplacental ratio (CPR), which combines the pulsatility index of the middle cerebral and umbilical arteries, has proven a more sensitive proxy for hypoxia than its individual components [45], and it correlates better with adverse outcome [46,47]. In addition to these brain Doppler parameters, abnormal uterine artery (UtA) Doppler has been associated with an increased risk of intrapartum fetal distress, emergency cesarean delivery, and admission to an intensive care unit [48,49]. Finally, evidence also exists that very low estimated fetal weight (EFW) centile by itself predicts a higher risk of adverse perinatal outcome in term SGA fetuses without Doppler signs of brain redistribution and normal umbilical and uterine artery Doppler [16,50].

The clinical relevance of using a combined model is the significant improvement in prediction over using a single predictor (a detection rate for adverse outcome of 83% for a 48% of false positives) [51] without excessive technical sophistication; the estimation of the fetal weight is an integrated part of the third-trimester echography and Doppler interrogation of the UA, MCA, and UtA, and is easily accomplished in the great majority of cases. Such algorithm allows profiling of the general population of late SGA fetuses in two risk-differing groups. While SGA fetuses with moderate growth restriction (>3rd centile) and normal placental function on both the fetal (normal CPR) and maternal (normal uterine Doppler) sides could be considered low risk and managed as constitutionally small babies, those with either severe growth restriction or evidence of placental dysfunction (abnormal uterine arteries) should be considered high risk. In the studies from the Barcelona group, constitutional smallness accounted for 40% of the population, in which only 17% of adverse outcomes occurred, whereas late FGR represented the remaining 60% of the population, which concentrated 83% of instances of adverse outcome.

It is likely that in future years maternal blood biomarkers will be incorporated as a diagnostic criterion of FGR in composite algorithms, as a marker of placental involvement [52–54]. Indeed, it has been shown in late-onset FGR that angiogenic factors correlate with placental findings secondary to underperfusion [55,56].

Pathophysiological Issues

Over the past decade, two different patterns of clinical presentation, determined primarily by the gestational age at disease onset and the pattern of umbilical artery Doppler, have been more clearly characterized [34,57,58].

FGR has a different phenotypic expression, evolution, and outcome when it starts early in gestation. The typical pattern of deterioration progresses from escalating abnormalities in UA, MCA, and venous Doppler parameters to abnormal biophysical parameters. The rate of deterioration of Doppler parameters determines the overall speed of deterioration in early-onset FGR, often necessitating preterm delivery. In addition, there is a high association with preeclampsia and perinatal mortality [57–59].

In contrast, late-onset FGR is normally associated with less severe placental disease, so that normal or minimally elevated UA Doppler indices are usually observed. Overt cardiovascular adaptation does not extend beyond the cerebral circulation, manifesting as decreased CPR. The association between late-onset FGR with preeclampsia is minimal in comparison with early-onset forms [60].

A recent study [61] aimed at setting the optimal cut-off to differentiate early and late forms has shown that a cut-off of 32 weeks at diagnosis or 34 weeks at delivery maximizes differences between early- and late-onset FGR, but results in substantial overlapping of cases with similar characteristics. Umbilical artery Doppler discriminated better than gestational age two groups with different timing, natural history, and rate of adverse outcome.

Clinical Management of Growth-Restricted and SGA Fetuses

There is evidence from one randomized trial [62] that when compared with monitoring every 2 weeks, twice-a-week monitoring results in more inductions without any improvement in the perinatal outcomes. Thus, the standard of care for those low-risk SGA would be the former regime. However, in late-onset FGR such definition of low-risk SGA could not be reliably trusted on the umbilical Doppler, and, therefore, some other markers are needed.

Amniotic Fluid

In a large study on late SGA [63], it was found that about one third of the pregnancies had oligohydramnios, as defined by an amniotic fluid index below 5. However, it could be argued that such a substantial proportion of cases does not represent fetuses at higher risk of progression but an overdiagnosis. In fact, evidence [64] shows that compared with the single deepest vertical pocket, the amniotic fluid index results in more inductions and cesarean sections without any improvement in the perinatal outcomes.

A meta-analysis [65] of 18 randomized studies demonstrated that a reduced amniotic fluid index is associated with an abnormal 5-minute Apgar score, but failed to demonstrate an association with acidosis or perinatal death in those cases associated with SGA (RR 1.6 [95% CI 0.9–2.6]).

Because evidence is limited on the role of oligohydramnios to predict perinatal complications in SGA fetuses already managed with umbilical artery Doppler and MCA, its inclusion in management protocols is doubtful.

Doppler Parameters

Middle Cerebral Artery

Longitudinal studies in late-onset SGA cases have shown that while UA Doppler remains virtually unchanged from diagnosis to delivery, MCA becomes abnormal in about 15% of the cases [34]. It has been shown that in near-term SGA fetuses, Doppler evaluation of the middle cerebral artery could be useful to predict adverse outcome, independently of the umbilical artery [39,66]. Remarkably, when labor is induced, SGA babies with abnormal MCA-PI had six times higher probability of emergency cesarean section due to fetal distress, and a fourfold increment in the risk of neonatal metabolic acidosis when compared with SGA fetuses with normal MCA-PI Doppler evaluation [66]. This is a relevant finding because, according to the evidence from a recent randomized study, labor induction at term is the current standard of care of late-onset SGA [63,67]. At birth, late-SGA children presenting abnormal MCA-PI before delivery have poorer neurobehavioral competence, and, at 2 years of age, significantly lower scores in communication, problem solving, and personal-social areas [68]. Therefore, there is an association between abnormal MCA-PI and adverse perinatal and neurological outcome in late-onset FGR fetuses. This sign is rather a late manifestation, with acceptable specificity but low sensitivity for clinical applicability. Other cerebral Doppler parameters have been proposed to overcome such limitation.

Cerebroplacental Ratio (CPR)

In the early days of Doppler, a ratio of the umbilical artery resistance divided by cerebral resistance (U/C ratio) was proposed [69]. An increased U/C ratio was considered abnormal and was related to poor outcome in FGR fetuses [70]. However, for the Doppler evaluation of the late FGR, the more recently universally accepted ratio is the cerebroplacental ratio (CPR). Due to increased impedance in the placental vasculature in combination with a decrease in cerebral resistance secondary to vasodilation, the ratio between the middle cerebral artery and umbilical artery is decreased even when the UA-PI and MCA-PI values are within normal range [46].

Consistently, animal models have demonstrated that CPR is better correlated with hypoxia than its individual components [45]. In late-SGA fetuses, abnormal CPR is present before delivery in 20% of the cases, being more sensitive than MCA [66]. In these fetuses, abnormal CPR is associated with a higher risk of adverse outcome at induction, although to a lesser degree than MCA [39]. There are no long-term studies evaluating the neurobehavioral or neurodevelopmental consequences in the specific group of late SGA with abnormal CPR. However, it is relevant that even in the general population, an abnormal CPR during the third trimester of pregnancy is associated with neurobehavioral problems at 18 months of age [71]. Interestingly, the anterior cerebral artery-CPR rather than the MCA-CPR showed the stronger association, demonstrating differential impact of regional alterations in cerebral blood flow impedance on development, which is consistent with findings in early-FGR [44,68].

A recent study has pointed out that the predictive value of abnormal cerebral Doppler for poor outcome in late FGR is strictly dependent from the moment the investigation is performed [72].

Uterine Artery

Some evidence shows that Doppler evaluation of uterine artery is also more sensitive than umbilical artery to detect mild forms of placental insufficiency and therefore to identify many instances of adverse outcome in term SGA fetuses [40,48,49]. In a recently reported longitudinal series [73], approximately one-third of abnormal third-trimester uterine Doppler studies occurred in women with normal scans during the second trimester, suggesting that a segment of placental disease emerges late in pregnancy. Hence, the potential advantage of a third-trimester Doppler scan is the ability to detect MUP of differing pathways.

Severi and colleagues [40] described that the combination of MCA and UtA Doppler abnormalities showed an exponential effect in the risk of adverse pregnancy outcome. Thus, cases with MCA vasodilation (MCA PI below -2 z-scores) and increased UtA (resistance index above 0.5 and bilateral notch) showed an 86% probability of developing distress and being delivered by cesarean section in comparison with a 4% probability when both parameters were normal. Aside from the prediction of adverse perinatal outcome, some other evidence [74] suggests that uterine artery Doppler abnormalities could play an additional role in offering an early prediction of later appearance of brain sparing. Thus, in the presence of abnormal uterine artery Doppler, brain redistribution appeared 2 weeks earlier and in up to 63% of the cases.

This finding is consistent with previous observations in high-risk pregnancies complicated by pregnancy-induced hypertension or FGR, in which the degree of increased placental vascular resistance was reflected in the brain-sparing phenomenon by a negative correlation between MCA PI and CPR values with the UtA PI and by a linear increase in the proportion of MCA and CPR abnormalities across the severity scores of increased UtA impedance [75].

Placental Pathology in Late-Onset Fetal Growth Restriction

Placentae from FGR delivered at term show significantly increased frequencies of uteroplacental vascular lesion such as infarcts, compared to normal fetuses, although many cases do not present specific placental pathologies [76]. Placental lesions in late-onset growth restriction may partly overlap with those seen in early GR [77]. Commonly reported villous lesions in term growth restriction are fibrosis, hypovascularity, and avascularity, suggestive of fetal thrombotic events. Other nonvascular pathologies, such as chronic villitis, are also common in late growth restriction [78]. In two-thirds of these placentae, hypoxic/ischemic injuries due to placental underperfusion are observed, and they are correlated with abnormal uterine artery and umbilical vein Doppler in prenatal life and with an increased neonatal morbidity [36].

This suggests that abnormal uterine artery flow profiles and abnormal umbilical venous flow, more than UA Doppler, may alert clinicians to the possible risks of placental underperfusion.

Management and Delivery

As the only treatment of restricted intrauterine growth is delivery, the main consideration needs to be the appropriate timing of delivery, balancing the risk of continuing exposure to an unfavorable intrauterine environment and potential iatrogenic morbidity due to a preterm delivery. However, added into the equation is the awareness that leaving pregnancies with FGR to deliver at term may also lead to perinatal mortality, morbidity, and delayed effects such as cerebral palsy [79]. In a recent large population study of 1,170,534 pregnancies in the Netherlands, about half of the late stillbirths occurred after 37 weeks, of which 88% were fetuses with birth weights between the 50th and P2,3 c. The frequency increased from 2.6% of the

fetuses with birth weight between the P50–P20 to 20.15% of those with birth weight below P2,3 [30].

One randomized equivalence trial exists, comparing the effect of induction of labor or expectant monitoring in women after 37 weeks' gestation with suspected SGA. The authors found negligible differences in perinatal and neonatal outcomes between induction of labor and expectant monitoring [63,67]. At 2 years of age, about half of the cohort was evaluated for neurodevelopmental and neurobehavioral assessment, with no differences between both strategies [80]. Based on these results, it seems reasonable to offer delivery after 37 weeks in SGA infants on the rationale of preventing those infrequent but devastating instances of stillbirth, which are more common after this gestational age [30,81].

However, with such a strategy, a large fraction of constitutionally and healthy SGA babies is unnecessarily induced, which has the potential to result in lower satisfaction and poorer fulfillment with the birth experience [63]. An algorithm based on the growth centile and Doppler parameters (middle cerebral and uterine arteries) has been proposed to identify those cases at the lowest risk for expectant management, with a good capacity to rule out adverse outcome [51].

As far as the monitoring parameters are concerned, once a small fetus (EFW <10th centile) has been identified and other causes such as malformations or infections have been ruled out, an attempt should be made to classify FGR versus SGA. Abnormal uterine artery flow is indicative of inadequate placentation, but this is a rare finding in late-onset GR. Biometry should be repeated at 2-week intervals, and special attention should be paid to the trajectory of growth or deflecting growth, even when the growth falls within normal ranges. Doppler parameters should include the C/P ratio repeated twice weekly if the growth is below the 10th centile or if there is a deflecting growth. The frequency should be intensified if growth slows down (flow chart). Maternal awareness of fetal movements remains of pivotal importance [82], although the optimal method to quantify movements remains elusive.

In the absence of serial growth assessment revealing deflecting growth late in gestation, reduced fetal movements is the only resource to identify apparently normally grown fetuses that failed to reach their endowed growth potential and therefore are at risk of fetal distress or stillbirth.

In the absence of indications for an earlier delivery in pregnancies with SGA fetuses, delivery should

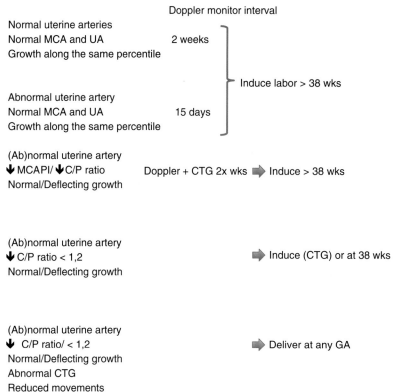

Figure 23.1 Proposed monitoring interval and management protocol for the late (GA ≥34 weeks) SGA = AC <P10 or deflecting growth.
Parameters to be monitored: Ut. arteries repeat once after 30 weeks.
Biometry every 10 days.

be considered starting from 38 weeks. In an economic evaluation of the DIGITAT study, costs are lower in the expectant monitoring group before 38 weeks' gestation and after 38 weeks in the induction of labor group. So if induction of labor is considered to preempt possible stillbirth in suspected FGR, it is reasonable to delay until 38 weeks, with watchful monitoring [83].

The optimum mode of induction of labor for these infants may be with a Foley catheter, as this reduces the risk of uterine hyper-stimulation leading to fetal heart changes [84], which the SGA fetus may not tolerate as well as an appropriately grown fetus.

Key Points

- Identification of late FGR remains challenging.
- Late FGR is not generally accompanied by preeclampsia.
- A single biometric assessment is not very effective in identifying fetuses that failed to reach their endowed growth potential.

- Screening for FGR by biometrical assessment is best accomplished around 37 weeks.
- Umbilical artery Doppler is not effective in identifying fetuses at risk of fetal distress/stillbirth.
- Serial MCAPI/UA PI ratio (CPR) until late in the third trimester seems the best parameter to identify these fetuses.
- Maternal awareness of fetal movements is of pivotal importance.
- In case of small fetuses, induction of labor should be considered at 38 weeks.
- Induction by Foley catheter is the method of choice.

References

1. Hepburn M, Rosenberg K. An audit of the detection and management of small-for-gestational age babies. *BJOG* 1986;93(3):212–16.

2. Sharp AN, Alfirevic Z. First trimester screening can predict adverse pregnancy outcomes. *Prenat Diagn* 2014 Jul;34(7):660–7.

3. Halscott TL, Ramsey PS, Reddy UM. First trimester screening cannot predict adverse outcomes yet. *Prenat Diagn* 2014 Jul;34(7):668–76.

4. Backe B, Nakling J. Effectiveness of antenatal care: A population based study. *BJOG* 1993;100(8):727–32.

5. Lindqvist PG, Molin J. Does antenatal identification of small-for-gestational age fetuses significantly improve their outcome? *Ultrasound Obstet Gynecol* 2005;25(3):258–64.

6. Gardosi J, Madurasinghe V, Williams M, Malik A, Francis A. Maternal and fetal risk factors for stillbirth: Population based study. *BMJ* 2013;346:f108.

7. Richardus JH, Graafmans WC, Verloove-Vanhorick SP, Mackenbach JP, EuroNatal International Audit P, EuroNatal Working G. Differences in perinatal mortality and suboptimal care between 10 European regions: Results of an international audit. *BJOG* 2003;110(2):97–105.

8. Cnossen JS, Morris RK, Ter Riet G, Mol BW, Van der Post JA, Coomarasamy A, et al. Use of uterine artery Doppler ultrasonography to predict pre-eclampsia and intrauterine growth restriction: A systematic review and bivariable meta-analysis. *Cmaj* 2008;178(6):701–11.

9. Yu CK, Khouri O, Onwudiwe N, Spiliopoulos Y, Nicolaides KH: Fetal Medicine Foundation Second-Trimester Screening Group. Prediction of pre-eclampsia by uterine artery Doppler imaging: Relationship to gestational age at delivery and small-for-gestational age. *Ultrasound Obstet Gynecol* 2008;31:310–13.

10. Kean L, Liu D. Antenatal care as a screening tool for the detection of small for gestational age babies in the low risk population. *Journal of Obstetrics and Gynaecology* 1996;16:77–82.

11. Monier I, Blondel B, Ego A, Kaminiski M, Goffinet F, Zeitlin J. Poor effectiveness of antenatal detection of fetal growth restriction and consequences for obstetric management and neonatal outcomes: A French national study. *BJOG* 2015 Mar;122(4):518–27.

12. Clausson B, Gardosi J, Francis A, Cnattingius S. Perinatal outcome in SGA births defined by customized versus population-based birthweight standards. *BJOG* 2001;108(8):830–4.

13. Moraitis AA, Wood AM, Fleming M, Smith GC. Birth weight percentile and the risk of term perinatal death. *Obstet Gynecol* 2014;124(2 Pt 1):274–83.

14. Baschat AA, Cosmi E, Bilardo CM, Wolf H, Berg C, Rigano S, et al. Predictors of neonatal outcome in early-onset placental dysfunction. *Obstet Gynecol* 2007;109(2 Pt 1):253–61.

15. Trudell AS, Cahill AG, Tuuli MG, Macones GA, Odibo AO. Risk of stillbirth after 37 weeks in pregnancies complicated by small-for-gestational-age fetuses. *Am J Obstet Gynecol* 2013;208(5):376 e1–7.

16. Savchev S, Figueras F, Cruz-Martinez R, Illa M, Botet F, Gratacos E. Estimated weight centile as a predictor of perinatal outcome in small-for-gestational-age pregnancies with normal fetal and maternal Doppler indices. *Ultrasound Obstet Gynecol* 2012;39(3):299–303.

17. Clausson B, Cnattingius S, Axelsson O. Preterm and term births of small for gestational age infants: A population-based study of risk factors among nulliparous women. *Br J Obstet Gynaecol* 1998;105(9):1011–17.

18. Souka AP, Papastefanou I, Pilalis A, Michalitsi V, Kassanos D. Performance of third-trimester ultrasound for prediction of small-for-gestational-age neonates and evaluation of contingency screening policies. *Ultrasound Obstet Gynecol* 2012;39(5):535.

19. Bricker L, Neilson JP, Dowswell T. Routine ultrasound in late pregnancy (after 24 weeks' gestation). *Cochrane Database Syst Rev* 2008(4):CD001451.

20. Skrastad RB, Eik-Nes SH, Sviggum O, Johansen OJ, Salvesen KA, Romundstad PR, et al. A randomized controlled trial of third-trimester routine ultrasound in a non-selected population. *Acta Obstet Gynecol Scand* 2013;92(12):1353–60.

21. McKenna D, Tharmaratnam S, Mahsud S, Bailie C, Harper A, Dornan J. A randomized trial using ultrasound to identify the high-risk fetus in a low-risk population. *Obstet Gynecol* 2003;101(4):626–32.

22. Duff GB. A randomized controlled trial in a hospital population of ultrasound measurement screening for the small for dates baby. *Aust N Z J Obstet Gynaecol* 1993;33(4):374–8.

23. Neilson JP, Munjanja SP, Whitfield CR. Screening for small for dates fetuses: A controlled trial. *BMJ* (Clin Res Ed) 1984;289(6453):1179–82.

24. Roma E.,Arnau A.,Berdala R., Bergos C., Montesinos J., Figueras F. *Ultrasound Obstet Gynecol* 2015;46(4):391–7.

25. Stirnemann JJ, Benoist G, Salomon LJ, Bernard JP, Ville Y. Optimal risk assessment of small-for-gestational-age fetuses using 31–34-week biometry in a low-risk population. *Ultrasound Obstet Gynecol* 2014 Mar;43(3):311–16. doi: 10.1002/uog.13288. Epub 2014 Feb 12. PubMed PMID: 24357451

26. Alfirevic Z, Neilson JP. Doppler ultrasonography in high-risk pregnancies: Systematic review with meta-analysis. *Am J Obstet Gynecol* 1995;172(5):1379–87.

27. Clausson B, Gardosi J, Francis A, Cnattingius S. Perinatal outcome in SGA births defined by

customized versus population-based birthweight standards. *BJOG* 2001;108(8):830–4.

28. Trudell AS, Cahill AG, Tuuli MG, Macones GA, Odibo AO. Risk of stillbirth after 37 weeks in pregnancies complicated by small-for-gestational-age fetuses. *Am J Obstet Gynecol* 2013;208(5):376e1–7.

29. Papageorghiou AT, Ohuma EO, Altman DG, Todros T, Cheikh Ismail L, Lambert A, Jaffer YA, Bertino E, Gravett MG, Purwar M, Noble JA, Pang R, Victora CG, Barros FC, Carvalho M, Salomon LJ, Bhutta ZA, Kennedy SH, Villar J; International Fetal and Newborn Growth Consortium for the 21st Century (INTERGROWTH-21st). International standards for fetal growth based on serial ultrasound measurements: The Fetal Growth Longitudinal Study of the INTERGROWTH-21st Project. *Lancet* 2014 Sep 6;384(9946):869–79.

30. Vasak B, Koenen SV, Koster MP, Hukkelhoven CW, Franx A, Hanson MA, Visser GH. Human fetal growth is constrained below optimal for perinatal survival. *Ultrasound Obstet Gynecol* 2015 Feb;45(2):162–7.

31. Gardosi J, Clausson B, Francis A. The value of customised centiles in assessing perinatal mortality risk associated with parity and maternal size. *BJOG* 2009 Sep;116(10):1356–63.

32. Kiserud T, Johnsen SL. Biometric assessment. *Best Pract Res Clin Obstet Gynaecol* 2009 Dec;23(6):819–31.

33. Chang TC, Robson SC, Spencer JA, Gallivan S. Prediction of perinatal morbidity at term in small fetuses: Comparison of fetal growth and Doppler ultrasound. *Br J Obstet Gynaecol* 1994;101(5):422–7.

34. Oros D, Figueras F, Cruz-Martinez R, Meler E, Munmany M, Gratacos E. Longitudinal changes in uterine, umbilical and fetal cerebral Doppler indices in late-onset small-for-gestational age fetuses. *Ultrasound Obstet Gynecol* 2011;37(2):191–5.

35. Parra-Saavedra M, Crovetto F, Triunfo S, Savchev S, Parra G, Sanz M, et al. Added value of umbilical vein flow as a predictor of perinatal outcome in term small-for-gestational-age fetuses. *Ultrasound Obstet Gynecol* 2013.

36. Parra-Saavedra M, Crovetto F, Triunfo S, Savchev S, Peguero A, Nadal A, Gratacós E, Figueras F. Association of Doppler parameters with placental signs of underperfusion in late-onset small-for-gestational-age pregnancies. *Ultrasound Obstet Gynecol*. 2014 Sep;44(3):330–7.

37. Morrow RJ, Adamson SL, Bull SB, Ritchie JW. Effect of placental embolization on the umbilical arterial velocity waveform in fetal sheep. *Am J Obstet Gynecol* 1989;161(4):1055–60.

38. Thompson RS, Stevens RJ. Mathematical model for interpretation of Doppler velocity waveform indices. *Med Biol Eng Comput* 1989;27(3):269–76.

39. Hershkovitz R, Kingdom JC, Geary M, Rodeck CH. Fetal cerebral blood flow redistribution in late gestation: Identification of compromise in small fetuses with normal umbilical artery Doppler. *Ultrasound Obstet Gynecol* 2000;15(3):209–12.

40. Severi FM, Bocchi C, Visentin A, Falco P, Cobellis L, Florio P, et al. Uterine and fetal cerebral Doppler predict the outcome of third-trimester small-for-gestational age fetuses with normal umbilical artery Doppler. *Ultrasound Obstet Gynecol* 2002;19(3):225–8.

41. Cruz-Martínez R, Figueras F, Hernandez-Andrade E, Oros D, Gratacos E. Fetal brain Doppler to predict cesarean delivery for nonreassuring fetal status in term small-for-gestational-age fetuses. *Obstet Gynecol* 2011 Mar;117(3):618–26.

42. Morales-Roselló J, Khalil A, Morlando M, Bhide A, Papageorghiou A, Thilaganathan B. Poor neonatal acid-base status in term fetuses with low cerebroplacental ratio. *Ultrasound Obstet Gynecol* 2015 Feb;45(2):156–61.

43. Eixarch E, Meler E, Iraola A, Illa M, Crispi F, Hernandez-Andrade E, et al. Neurodevelopmental outcome in 2-year-old infants who were small-for-gestational age term fetuses with cerebral blood flow redistribution. *Ultrasound Obstet Gynecol* 2008;32(7):894–9.

44. Figueras F, Cruz-Martinez R, Sanz-Cortes M, Arranz A, Illa M, Botet F, Costas-Moragas C, Gratacos E. Neurobehavioral outcomes in preterm, growth-restricted infants with and without prenatal advanced signs of brain-sparing. *Ultrasound Obstet Gynecol* 2011 Sep;38(3):288–94.

45. Arbeille P, Maulik D, Fignon A, Stale H, Berson M, Bodard S, et al. Assessment of the fetal PO2 changes by cerebral and umbilical Doppler on lamb fetuses during acute hypoxia. *Ultrasound Med Biol* 1995;21(7):861–70.

46. Gramellini D, Folli MC, Raboni S, Vadora E, Merialdi A. Cerebral-umbilical Doppler ratio as a predictor of adverse perinatal outcome. *Obstet Gynecol* 1992;79(3):416–20.

47. Bahado-Singh RO, Kovanci E, Jeffres A, Oz U, Deren O, Copel J, et al. The Doppler cerebroplacental ratio and perinatal outcome in intrauterine growth restriction. *Am J Obstet Gynecol* 1999;180(3 Pt 1):750–6.

48. Ghosh GS, Gudmundsson S. Uterine and umbilical artery Doppler are comparable in predicting perinatal outcome of growth-restricted fetuses. *BJOG* 2009;116(3):424–30.

49. Vergani P, Roncaglia N, Andreotti C, Arreghini A, Teruzzi M, Pezzullo JC, et al. Prognostic value of uterine artery Doppler velocimetry in growth-restricted fetuses delivered near term. *Am J Obstet Gynecol* 2002;187(4):932–6.

50. Fratelli N, Valcamonico A, Prefumo F, Pagani G, Guarneri T, Frusca T. Effects of antenatal recognition and follow-up on perinatal outcomes in small-for-gestational age infants delivered after 36 weeks. *Acta Obstet Gynecol Scand* 92(2):223–9.

51. Figueras F, Savchev S, Triunfo S, Crovetto F, Gratacos E. An integrated model with classification criteria to predict small-for-gestational fetuses at risk of adverse perinatal outcome. *Ultrasound Obstet Gynecol* 2014.

52. Aviram R, T BS, Kidron D. Placental aetiologies of foetal growth restriction: clinical and pathological differences. *Early Hum Dev* 2010;86(1):59–63.

53. Lobmaier SM, Figueras F, Mercade I, Perello M, Peguero A, Crovetto F, Ortiz JU, Crispi F, Gratacós E. Angiogenic factors vs Doppler surveillance in the prediction of adverse outcome among late-pregnancy small-for-gestational-age fetuses. *Ultrasound Obstet Gynecol* 2014 May;43(5):533–40.

54. Bakalis S, Gallo DM, Mendez O, Poon LC, Nicolaides KH. Prediction of small-for-gestational-age neonates: Maternal biochemical markers at 30–34 weeks. *Ultrasound Obstet Gynecol* 2015.

55. Benton SJ, Hu Y, Xie F, Kupfer K, Lee SW, Magee LA, et al. Angiogenic factors as diagnostic tests for preeclampsia: A performance comparison between two commercial immunoassays. *Am J Obstet Gynecol* 2011;205(5):469 e1–8.

56. Triunfo S, Lobmaier S, Parra-Saavedra M, Crovetto F, Peguero A, Nadal A, et al. Angiogenic factors at diagnosis of late-onset small-for-gestational age and histological placental underperfusion. *Placenta* 2014;35(6):398–403.

57. Hecher K, Bilardo CM, Stigter RH, Ville Y, Hackeloer BJ, Kok HJ, et al. Monitoring of fetuses with intrauterine growth restriction: A longitudinal study. *Ultrasound Obstet Gynecol* 2001;18(6):564–70.

58. Turan OM, Turan S, Gungor S, Berg C, Moyano D, Gembruch U, et al. Progression of Doppler abnormalities in intrauterine growth restriction. *Ultrasound Obstet Gynecol* 2008;32(2):160–7.

59. Lees C, Marlow N, Arabin B, Bilardo CM, Brezinka C, Derks JB, et al. Perinatal morbidity and mortality in early-onset fetal growth restriction: Cohort outcomes of the trial of randomized umbilical and fetal flow in Europe (TRUFFLE). *Ultrasound Obstet Gynecol* 2013;42(4):400–8.

60. Crovetto F, Crispi F, Scazzocchio E, Mercade I, Meler E, Figueras F, et al. First-trimester screening for early and late small-for-gestational-age neonates using matern

61. Savchev S, Figueras F, Sanz-Cortes M, Cruz-Lemini M, Triunfo S, Botet F, et al. Evaluation of an optimal gestational age cut-off for the definition of early- and late-onset fetal growth restriction. *Fetal Diagn Ther* 2014;36(2):99–105.

62. McCowan LM, Harding JE, Roberts AB, Barker SE, Ford C, Stewart AW. A pilot randomized controlled trial of two regimens of fetal surveillance for small-for-gestational-age fetuses with normal results of umbilical artery Doppler velocimetry. *Am J Obstet Gynecol* 2000;182(1 Pt 1):81–6.

63. Boers KE, Vijgen SM, Bijlenga D, Van der Post JA, Bekedam DJ, Kwee A, et al. Induction versus expectant monitoring for intrauterine growth restriction at term: Randomised equivalence trial (DIGITAT). *BMJ* 2010;341:c7087.

64. Nabhan AF, Abdelmoula YA. Amniotic fluid index versus single deepest vertical pocket as a screening test for preventing adverse pregnancy outcome. *Cochrane Database Syst Rev* 2008(3):CD006593.

65. Chauhan SP, Sanderson M, Hendrix NW, Magann EF, Devoe LD. Perinatal outcome and amniotic fluid index in the antepartum and intrapartum periods: A meta-analysis. *Am J Obstet Gynecol* 1999;181(6):1473–8.

66. Cruz-Martinez R, Figueras F, Hernandez-Andrade E, Oros D, Gratacos E. Fetal brain Doppler to predict cesarean delivery for nonreassuring fetal status in term small-for-gestational-age fetuses. *Obstet Gynecol* 2011;117(3):618–26.

67. Boers KE, Van Wyk L, Van der Post JA, Kwee A, Van Pampus MG, Spaanderdam ME, et al. Neonatal morbidity after induction vs expectant monitoring in intrauterine growth restriction at term: A subanalysis of the DIGITAT RCT. *Am J Obstet Gynecol* 2012;206(4):344 e1–7.

68. Oros D, Figueras F, Cruz-Martinez R, Padilla N, Meler E, Hernandez-Andrade E, et al. Middle versus anterior cerebral artery Doppler for the prediction of perinatal outcome and neonatal neurobehavior in term small-for-gestational-age fetuses with normal umbilical artery Doppler. *Ultrasound Obstet Gynecol* 2010;35(4):456–61.

69. Arduini D, Rizzo G. Prediction of fetal outcome in small for gestational age fetuses: Comparison of Doppler measurements obtained from different fetal vessels. *J Perinat Med* 1992;20(1):29–38.

70. Hecher K, Spernol R, Stettner H, Szalay S. Potential for diagnosing imminent risk to appropriate- and small-for-gestational-age fetuses by Doppler sonographic examination of umbilical and cerebral arterial blood flow. *Ultrasound Obstet Gynecol* 1992 Jul 1;2(4):266–71.

71. Roza SJ, Steegers EA, Verburg BO, Jaddoe VW, Moll HA, Hofman A, et al. What is spared by fetal brain-sparing? Fetal circulatory redistribution and behavioral problems in the general population. *Am J Epidemiol* 2008;168(10):1145–52.

72. Akolekar R. Syngelaki A, Gallo DM, Poon LC, Nicolaides KH. Umbilical and fetal middle cerebral artery Doppler at 35–37 weeks' gestation in the prediction of adverse perinatal outcome. *Ultrasound Obstet Gynecol* 2015 Jul;46(1):82–92.

73. Figueroa-Diesel H, Hernandez-Andrade E, Acosta-Rojas R, Cabero L, Gratacos E. Doppler changes in the main fetal brain arteries at different stages of hemodynamic adaptation in severe intrauterine growth restriction. *Ultrasound Obstet Gynecol* 2007;30(3):297–302.

74. Llurba E, Turan O, Kasdaglis T, Harman CR, Baschat AA. Emergence of late-onset placental dysfunction: Relationship to the change in uterine artery blood flow resistance between the first and third trimesters. *Am J Perinatol* 2013;30(6):505–12.

75. Cruz-Martinez R, Savchev S, Cruz-Lemini M, Mendez A, Gratacos E, Figueras F. Clinical utility of third trimester uterine artery Doppler in the prediction of brain hemodynamic deterioration and adverse perinatal outcome in small-for-gestational-age fetuses. *Ultrasound Obstet Gynecol* 2014.

76. Mifsud W, Sebire NJ. Placental pathology in early-onset and late-onset fetal growth restriction. *Fetal Diagn Ther* 2014;36(2):117–28.

77. Apel-Sarid L, Levy A, Holcberg G, Sheiner E: Term and preterm (<34 and <37 weeks' gestation) placental pathologies associated with fetal growth restriction. *Arch Gynecol Obstet* 2010;282:487–92.

78. Cheema R, Dubiel M, Gudmundsson S. Fetal brain sparing is strongly related to the degree of increased placental vascular impedance. *J Perinat Med* 2006;34(4):318–22.

79. Jacobsson B, Ahlin K, Francis A, Hagberg G, Hagberg H, Gardosi J. Cerebral palsy and restricted growth status at birth: Population-based case-control study. *BJOG* 2008;115(10):1250–5.

80. Van Wyk L, Boers KE, Van der Post JA, Van Pampus MG, Van Wassenaer AG, Van Baar AL, et al. Effects on (neuro)developmental and behavioral outcome at 2 years of age of induced labor compared with expectant management in intrauterine growth-restricted infants: long-term outcomes of the DIGITAT trial. *Am J Obstet Gynecol* 2012;206(5):406e1–7.

81. Vijgen SM, Boers KE, Opmeer BC, Bijlenga D, Bekedam DJ, Bloemenkamp KW, de Boer K, Bremer HA, le Cessie S, Delemarre FM, Duvekot JJ, Hasaart TH, Kwee A, Van Lith JM, Van Meir CA, Van Pampus MG, Van der Post JA, Rijken M, Roumen FJ, Van der Salm PC, Spaanderman ME, Willekes C, Wijnen EJ, Mol BW, Scherjon SA. Economic analysis comparing induction of labour and expectant management for intrauterine growth restriction at term (DIGITAT trial). *Eur J Obstet Gynecol Reprod Biol* 2013 Oct;170(2):358–63.

82. Scala C, Bhide A, Familiari A, Pagani G, Khalil A, Papageorghiou A, Thilaganathan B. Number of episodes of reduced fetal movements at term: Association with adverse perinatal outcome. *Am J Obstet Gynecol* 2015 Jul 20. pii: S0002-9378(15)00751-6.

83. Pilliod RA, Cheng YW, Snowden JM, Doss AE, Caughey AB. The risk of intrauterine fetal death in the small-for-gestational-age fetus. *Am J Obstet Gynecol* 2012;207(4):318e1–6.

84. Jozwiak M, Ten Eikelder M, Oude Rengerink K, de Groot C, Feitsma H, Spaanderman M, Van Pampus M, de Leeuw JW, Mol BW, Bloemenkamp K; PROBAAT Study Group. Foley catheter versus vaginal misoprostol: Randomized controlled trial (PROBAAT-M study) and systematic review and meta-analysis of literature. *Am J Perinatol* 2014 Feb;31(2):145–56.

Severe Fetal Growth Restriction: Pregnancy Management at the Limits of Viability

Aris T. Papageorghiou and J. W. Ganzevoort

Background

In normal pregnancy, physiological remodeling of the maternal spiral arteries by extravillous trophoblast (EVT) converts these narrow, high-resistance arteries into wide, low-resistance vessels with high flow circulation, which are unresponsive to normal regional vascular control. The series of vascular transformations of the spiral arteries normally ensures a more than tenfold increase in blood supply to the intervillous space in normal pregnancy. In some pregnancies, this transformation is incomplete, and such defective trophoblastic invasion of the spiral arteries is associated with subsequent development of fetal growth restriction (FGR), preeclampsia, and intrauterine death. In these pregnancies, the uteroplacental circulation remains in a state of high resistance, which causes generalized endothelial cell injury, compromising vascular integrity and causing an arthrosis-like process in the small arteries, resulting in vessel occlusion, local ischemia, and necrosis. This high resistance of the uteroplacental circulation can be observed using Doppler ultrasound of the uterine artery [1,2].

Very early-onset FGR, in the absence of a fetal abnormality or congenital infection, is most often the result of such abnormal placentation, and is highly associated with preeclampsia. Essentially, the poor placental implantation leads to reduced exchange between mother and fetus across the placenta, and in turn leads to poor growth and ultimately hypoxia and fetal death. Such severe early FGR is rare, affecting about 0.4% of all pregnancies, but represents an important burden of disease due to the high risks of iatrogenic preterm birth, Survival rates for severely growth-restricted fetuses born very remote from term (<28 weeks' gestation) are less than 50% and there are very high rates of morbidity [3–8]. In addition, there is an association between severe early FGR and adverse long-term health effects, including increased risks of persistent short stature, poor intellectual and psychological performance, neurodevelopment disabilities, and increased cardiovascular complications in later life [9–13].

Management

At present there is no treatment for early-onset FGR due to placental insufficiency, and the only current option is elective preterm delivery in order to "rescue" the baby from an adverse intrauterine environment. FGR and the associated indicated preterm birth expose the fetus and neonate to significant mortality and morbidity, posing an important management dilemma: early delivery causes extreme prematurity with all its sequelae, while delivering the baby too late risks intrauterine death or morbidity secondary to critical fetal hypoxia.

This balanced approach between delivery and expectant management is of course influenced by gestational age: at late gestational ages, the main problem is identification of small babies and the decision to deliver is taken more lightly (see Chapter 23), while at early gestational ages, the high perinatal risks of mean intensive fetal surveillance are indicated with elective delivery performed when there is evidence of presumed fetal acidosis/distress (see Chapter 22).

The key determinants of death and both short-term and long-term morbidity in severe early-onset FGR are gestational age at birth and birth weight. At lower and lower gestational ages, such iatrogenic delivery is associated with higher and higher risks. An increase in neonatal survival of 2% is reported for each additional day in utero up to 32 weeks. Intact survival is less than 25% for an infant weighing 600g born at 25 completed weeks' gestation, and is still only approximately 50% up to 28 weeks' gestation [14].

Management

The aim of management of pregnancies in the previable period is different from that in the period thereafter. Obviously, in all cases, management is aimed at optimizing chances of healthy survival of the fetus while minimizing maternal risks and disadvantages. The balance of risks of prolonged intrauterine hypoxia versus the complications associated with preterm birth is clearly shifted toward a non-intervention strategy. By definition, delivery as an intervention does not improve fetal outcome in the period deemed previable.

The transition from previable to viable is subject to change over time, and is concurrently different between and within countries. As experience with postnatal management increases and results improve, the previable period is shifted toward lower gestational ages. Management of these cutting-edge situations involves difficult balancing of the postnatal risks and chances of delivery for a fetus (and its mother). For that reason, and due to the fact that the absolute number of these cases is limited, management and counseling should take place in highly specialized fetal and neonatal centers. In these centers, a perinatal team, consisting of obstetrician gynecologists/maternal fetal medicine specialists/perinatologists, and neonatologists, is recommended. Referral should be as early as possible, also if the problem is identified weeks before what is considered the viable period.

Following careful evaluation and exclusion of other causes of FGR (see Chapter 3), parents should be counseled to encompass the fetal situation, and this should be informed in the light of relevant information from prospective studies. Depending on the individual situation, possible scenarios need to be sketched out to parents, and these will vary from a policy of non-intervention with a high likelihood of fetal demise to possible delivery after reaching a viable gestational age and estimated weight. Relevant information will be based on studies that report outcomes of all babies seen at referral centers at a given gestational age, including those with fetal demise and not just those that survive until delivery [15–18]; studies restricted to babies alive at delivery may be less relevant at this stage in counseling [19–22].

One of the largest studies [18] focused specifically on singleton fetuses presenting with FGR in the periviable period, using data from three large London teaching hospitals. The periviable FGR was defined here as an abdominal circumference ≤3rd percentile for gestational age between 22+0 and 25+6 weeks. The cases were subcategorized into *uteroplacental* (uterine

artery PI>95th percentile for gestational age and/or bilateral notches and/or reduced amniotic fluid); *placental* (ultrasound evidence of placental abnormality (thickened placenta, extensive lakes, or jelly-like appearance) with the presence of normal uterine artery Doppler assessment); *congenital infection* (not considered further here) or as *unclassified* (cases that did not fulfill the criteria for the other defined categories and where there was no antenatal cause identified). The outcomes for the categories are shown in the table.

It is noteworthy that in this cohort of severely growth-restricted fetuses, overall survival was 41%. This ranged from 13% if delivery was <28 weeks up to >90% if delivery was after 36 weeks. There was a wide range of gestational age at birth, with some pregnancies having a long diagnosis-to-delivery interval; overall, 15% of these cases diagnosed at such an early GA were delivered beyond 36 weeks, and had good short-term outcomes (though no long-term assessment was carried out in this study).

Notwithstanding that the primary focus lies with the fetus, the mother must be clearly counseled that there is a significant risk of development of maternal hypertensive disorders after the diagnosis of FGR [17], and that FGR is very common in women with very early-onset hypertensive disorders of pregnancy [21].

In terms of management choices, the main focus should lie on helping the parents understand the factors that determine decisions. All relevant outcomes, including the high burden of long-term sequelae, should be discussed. It should be taken into account that with progression in time, outcomes are gradually improving [18]. The managing clinician needs to get a view on how the parents weigh up these factors, and which adverse outcomes they are more or less likely to accept. Finally, in early gestation far from the viability threshold, termination of pregnancy may also be an option, depending on the legal circumstances in each country. Some perspective of the relatively good outcomes in future pregnancy may be helpful [23].

After counseling, the management team in consultation with the parents should come to a clear decision on whether expectant or active management will be followed; it must be clear that active management is an option only if the gestation and weight are beyond the limits of viability. Once a decision has been made to manage actively, there is an intent to deliver once

Table 24.1 Outcomes of 244 cases of fetuses with a diagnosis of an abdominal circumference <3rd centile at 22+0 to 25+6 weeks, adapted from [18]

Category	Survival, n (%)	NND, n (%)	IUFD, n (%)	Fetocide / ToP, n (%)	Median GA at delivery, weeks (range)	Median diagnosis-to delivery Interval in liveborn babies, weeks (range)	Incidence of PE, n (%)
Uteroplacental, n = 201	78 (39)	19 (10)	77 (38)	27 (13)	27.5 (22.3–40.3)	6.6 (0–16)	49/145 (34)
Placental, n = 13	7 (54)	0 (0)	2 (15)	4 (31)	27.0 (22.6–38.3)	7.1 (2.3–15.9)	2/12 (17)
Unclassified, n = 30	16 (53)	3 (10)	9 (30)	2 (7)	34.9 (22.3–41.3)	13.6 (3.3–18.1)	2/18 (11)
Total, n = 244	**101 (41)**	**22 (9)**	**88 (36)**	**33 (14)**	**27.7 (22.3–41.3)**	**7.6 (0–18.1)**	**53/175 (30)**

NND, neonatal death; IUFD, intrauterine fetal death; TOP, termination of pregnancy; GA, gestational age; PE, pre-eclampsia

the fetal condition deteriorates to the extent that risks of fetal demise increase; if these estimated risks outweigh the estimated risks of postnatal death, the baby should be delivered. This management is described in full in Chapter 22.

Does Anything Else Work?

At present, there are no known therapies for early-onset severe fetal growth restriction. Lifestyle modifications, such as reducing or stopping work, stopping aerobic exercise, resting at home, and hospital admission for rest and surveillance, are not supported by evidence of efficacy and are based on the hypothesis that rest may reduce "vascular steal" from the uteroplacental circulation.

A number of experimental treatments for severe early-onset FGR are currently under investigation. Sildenafil potentiates the effect of nitrous oxide (NO) and thus causes vasodilatation of vessels responsive to NO – such as incompletely remodeled maternal spiral arteries. Thus, Sildenafil has the theoretical potential to increase uteroplacental circulation and perfusion, resulting in improved gaseous and nutrient exchange and one small non-randomized study suggested improved growth in severe early FGR [24]. Whether this can be replicated or improves perinatal outcomes is the subject of a number of ongoing randomized trials that are part of an international collaboration [25].

As placental oxidative damage is an important feature in FGR and preeclampsia, antioxidants have also been tested. Despite the initial promise of antioxidant vitamin supplementation (mainly vitamins C and E), larger studies have failed to treat preeclampsia or FGR [26]. Melatonin is also a strong antioxidant; in vitro studies show that melatonin treatment protects the villous trophoblast against hypoxia-reperfusion injury and apoptosis, and in animals, it inhibits middle cerebral artery constriction while it induces umbilical vasodilation. In humans, it has not been used in FGR, but a randomized study is now under way [27]. Other mimetics of free radical scavengers, such as tempol (a superoxide dismutase (SOD) mimetic that has improved maternal blood pressure and increased fetal weight in mouse models) and resveratrol, a plant polyphenol, are in the early stages of assessment [28]. The prospect of gene therapy for the condition is discussed in Chapter 16.

After Pregnancy

Investigations after birth should include careful placental pathology, in particular looking for chronic intervillositis of the placenta, which carries a high risk of recurrence [29]. In the case of fetal or neonatal death, a postmortem to assess for other possible causes should also be encouraged.

In early-onset fetal growth restriction (and hypertensive disorders of pregnancy), the incidence of underlying hemostatic abnormalities is increased [30–32]. The extreme phenotype of overt FGR in the previable period warrants further investigation, because it may influence management in a subsequent pregnancy. This is particularly true for the antiphospholipid syndrome. It is defined by obstetric complications, and its diagnosis impacts future pregnancies.

Key Points

- At present there is no treatment for early-onset FGR, and decisions about delivery are based on weighing up the risks between early delivery versus expectant management.

- The definition of the periviable period is subject to change due to advances in medical care.

- Management and counseling in the periviable period are recommended to take place in highly specialized fetal and neonatal centers.

- Relevant information for counseling women should report the outcomes of all babies seen at referral centers at the given gestational age – including those with fetal demise and not just those that survive until delivery.

- The mother must be clearly counseled that there is a significant risk of development of maternal hypertensive disorders after the diagnosis of FGR.

- Investigations after birth should include placental pathology, in particular looking for chronic intervillositis of the placenta, which carries a high risk of recurrence. In the absence of this, the chances of a good outcome in the next pregnancy are high.

References

1. Papageorghiou AT, Leslie K. Uterine artery Doppler in the prediction of adverse pregnancy outcome. *Curr Opin Obstet Gynecol* 2007;19(2):103–9.

2. Papageorghiou AT, Yu CK, Nicolaides KH. The role of uterine artery Doppler in predicting adverse pregnancy outcome. *Best Pract Res Clin Obstet Gynaecol* 2004;18(3):383–96.

3. Ananth CV, Vintzileos AM. Maternal-fetal conditions necessitating a medical intervention resulting in preterm birth. *Am J Obstet Gynecol* 2006;195(6):1557–63.

4. Lee MJ, Conner EL, Charafeddine L, Woods JR, Jr., Del Priore G. A critical birth weight and other determinants of survival for infants with severe

intrauterine growth restriction. *Ann N Y Acad Sci* 2001;943:326–39.

5. Petersen SG, Wong SF, Urs P, Gray PH, Gardener GJ. Early onset, severe fetal growth restriction with absent or reversed end-diastolic flow velocity waveform in the umbilical artery: Perinatal and long-term outcomes. *Aust N Z J Obstet Gynaecol* 2009;49(1):45–51.

6. Batton DG, DeWitte DB, Espinosa R, Swails TL. The impact of fetal compromise on outcome at the border of viability. *Am J Obstet Gynecol* 1998;178(5):909–15.

7. Lees CC, Marlow N, Van Wassenaer-Leemhuis A, Arabin B, Bilardo CM, Brezinka C, et al. 2 year neurodevelopmental and intermediate perinatal outcomes in infants with very preterm fetal growth restriction (TRUFFLE): A randomised trial. *Lancet* 2015;385(9983):2162–72.

8. Baschat AA, Cosmi E, Bilardo CM, Wolf H, Berg C, Rigano S, et al. Predictors of neonatal outcome in early-onset placental dysfunction. *Obstet Gynecol* 2007;109(2 Pt 1):253–61.

9. Strauss RS. Adult functional outcome of those born small for gestational age: Twenty-six-year follow-up of the 1970 British Birth Cohort. *JAMA* 2000;283(5):625–32.

10. Hediger ML, Overpeck MD, Maurer KR, Kuczmarski RJ, McGlynn A, Davis WW. Growth of infants and young children born small or large for gestational age: Findings from the Third National Health and Nutrition Examination Survey. *Arch Pediatr Adolesc Med* 1998;152(12):1225–31.

11. Lundgren EM, Cnattingius S, Jonsson B, Tuvemo T. Intellectual and psychological performance in males born small for gestational age with and without catch-up growth. *Pediatr Res* 2001;50(1):91–6.

12. Sung IK, Vohr B, Oh W. Growth and neurodevelopmental outcome of very low birth weight infants with intrauterine growth retardation: Comparison with control subjects matched by birth weight and gestational age. *J Pediatr* 1993;123(4):618–24.

13. Stein CE, Fall CH, Kumaran K, Osmond C, Cox V, Barker DJ. Fetal growth and coronary heart disease in south India. *Lancet* 1996;348(9037):1269–73.

14. Bernstein IM, Horbar JD, Badger GJ, Ohlsson A, Golan A. Morbidity and mortality among very-low-birth-weight neonates with intrauterine growth restriction. The Vermont Oxford Network. *Am J Obstet Gynecol* 2000;182(1 Pt 1):198–206.

15. Van Wassenaer AG, Westera J, Van Schie PE, Houtzager BA, Cranendonk A, De Groot L, et al. Outcome at 4.5 years of children born after expectant

management of early-onset hypertensive disorders of pregnancy. *Am J Obstet Gynecol* 2011;204(6):510 e1–9.

16. Lees C, Marlow N, Arabin B, Bilardo CM, Brezinka C, Derks JB, et al. Perinatal morbidity and mortality in early-onset fetal growth restriction: Cohort outcomes of the trial of randomized umbilical and fetal flow in Europe (TRUFFLE). *Ultrasound Obstet Gynecol* 2013;42(4):400–8.

17. Rep A, Ganzevoort W, Van Wassenaer AG, Bonsel GJ, Wolf H, De Vries JI. One-year infant outcome in women with early-onset hypertensive disorders of pregnancy. *BJOG* 2008;115(2):290–8.

18. Lawin-O'Brien AR, Dall'Asta A, Knight C, Sankaran S, Scala C, Khalil A, et al. Short-term outcome of periviable small-for-gestational-age babies: Is our counseling up to date? *Ultrasound Obstet Gynecol* 2016;48(5):636–41.

19. Zeitlin J, El Ayoubi M, Jarreau PH, Draper ES, Blondel B, Kunzel W, et al. Impact of fetal growth restriction on mortality and morbidity in a very preterm birth cohort. *J Pediatr* 2010;157(5):733–9 e1.

20. Morsing E, Asard M, Ley D, Stjernqvist K, Marsal K. Cognitive function after intrauterine growth restriction and very preterm birth. *Pediatrics* 2011;127(4):e874–82.

21. Ganzevoort W, Rep A, Bonsel GJ, De Vries JI, Wolf H, for the Pi. Dynamics and incidence patterns of maternal complications in early onset hypertension of pregnancy. *BJOG* 2007;114(6):741–50.

22. Visser GHA, Bilardo CM, Lees C. Fetal growth restriction at the limits of viability. *Fetal Diag Ther* 2014;36:162–5.

23. Van Oostwaard MF, Langenveld J, Schuit E, Papatsonis DN, Brown MA, Byaruhanga RN, et al. Recurrence of hypertensive disorders of pregnancy: An individual patient data metaanalysis. *Am J Obstet Gynecol* 2015;212(5):624 e1–17.

24. Von Dadelszen P, Dwinnell S, Magee LA, Carleton BC, Gruslin A, Lee B, et al. Sildenafil citrate therapy for severe early-onset intrauterine growth restriction. *BJOG* 2011;118(5):624–8.

25. Ganzevoort W, Alfirevic Z, Von Dadelszen P, Kenny L, Papageorghiou A, Van Wassenaer-Leemhuis A, et al. STRIDER: Sildenafil Therapy In Dismal prognosis Early-onset intrauterine growth Restriction –a protocol for a systematic review with individual participant data and aggregate data meta-analysis and trial sequential analysis. *Syst Rev* 2014;3:23.

26. Rumbold A, Duley L, Crowther CA, Haslam RR. Antioxidants for preventing pre-eclampsia. *Cochrane Database Syst Rev* 2008(1):CD004227.

27. Alers NO, Jenkin G, Miller SL, Wallace EM. Antenatal melatonin as an antioxidant in human pregnancies complicated by fetal growth restriction – a phase I pilot clinical trial: Study protocol. *BMJ Open* 2013;3(12):e004141.

28. Cottrell EC, Sibley CP. From pre-clinical studies to clinical trials: Generation of novel therapies for pregnancy complications. *Int J Mol Sci* 2015;16(6):12907–24.

29. Man J, Hutchinson JC, Heazell AE, Ashworth M, Jeffrey I, Sebire NJ. Stillbirth and intrauterine fetal death: Role of routine histopathological placental findings to determine cause of death. *Ultrasound Obstet Gynecol* 2016.

30. Kupferminc MJ, Many A, Bar-Am A, Lessing JB, Ascher-Landsberg J. Mid-trimester severe intrauterine growth restriction is associated with a high prevalence of thrombophilia. *BJOG* 2002;109(12):1373–6.

31. Brenner B, Kupferminc MJ. Inherited thrombophilia and poor pregnancy outcome. *Best Pract Res Clin Obstet Gynaecol* 2003;17(3):427–39.

32. Ganzevoort W, Rep A, De Vries JI, Bonsel GJ, Wolf H, Investigators P. Relationship between thrombophilic disorders and type of severe early-onset hypertensive disorder of pregnancy. *Hypertens Pregnancy* 2007;26(4):433–45.

25 Fetal Growth Restriction in Twin Pregnancies

Isabel Couck, Kurt Hecher, and Liesbeth Lewi

Introduction

The widespread use of assisted reproductive technologies has led to a dramatic increase in the incidence of twin pregnancies worldwide. In some Western countries, nowadays 1 in every 30 births involves a twin instead of the expected 1 in 90 after natural conceptions [1]. Problems of fetal growth occur more commonly in twin pregnancies because in humans the womb seems less well adapted to nurture two fetuses to term [2]. As such, about one in four twins has a birth weight below the 10th percentile [3], which contributes greatly to the poorer outcome known to multiple births.

Twin growth is quite similar to that of singletons up to 30 weeks' gestation. From 30 weeks onward, the growth velocity of twins starts to decline, so that by 38 weeks, twins will on average be small for dates and have a birth weight at or below the 10th centile according to singleton standards. Some consider this growth restriction physiological and therefore advocate for the use of twin-specific nomograms [3,4]. However, twins who are small for dates according to singleton standards are at equal risk of a poor outcome as small-for-dates singletons [5]. The concept that being small is "normal" for twins thus creates a false sense of security, which may have deleterious consequences. Therefore, the clinical management of twin pregnancies is best based on singleton growth charts.

In twin pregnancies, one twin may grow normally, whereas the other may be small for dates. The degree of discordant growth, expressed in percentages, is calculated as (weight heavier-weight lighter)*100/weight heavier. The average growth discordance for a twin pregnancy is 10%. Although several definitions are used in the literature, there is general consensus that a 20% difference in estimated weight (EFW) best identifies those pregnancies at risk for adverse outcome. Such weight discordance of 20% or more is found in about one in six twin pregnancies [6].

In this chapter, we will focus on discordant growth, because the problem is unique to twin pregnancies and highlights the challenge to balance the opposite interests of each twin. An elective preterm birth will rescue the smaller twin, but will expose the larger twin to the risks of a very preterm birth. Growth discordance also better predicts adverse outcome than individual twin growth [6,7]. Finally, even if both twins are appropriate for dates, discordant growth still confers an added risk, especially if it concerns a monochorionic twin pregnancy [8].

Although incidences of discordant growth are similar, we will address monochorionic and dichorionic twins separately, because the pathophysiology, management, and outcome differ considerably. About one in four twin pregnancies is monochorionic. These twins are monozygotic and share a single placenta with vascular anastomoses connecting the two fetal circulations. Nearly all have separate amniotic sacs, though, and they are therefore denoted as monochorionic diamniotic (MCDA) twins. On the other hand, about three out of four twin pregnancies are dichorionic. They are dizygotic in about 90% of cases, have separate placentas and amniotic sacs without vascular anastomoses, and therefore are also designated as dichorionic diamniotic (DCDA) twins. Although we will focus our attention to the "starved" small twin, it is important always to exclude congenital infections, chromosomal anomalies, and genetic syndromes as a cause of discordant growth in the small twin, as this will obviously require a different management. Usually, "abnormal" small twins show additional ultrasound features suggesting an underlying infectious, genetic, or chromosomal cause and lack the abnormal Doppler findings typical for the diminished perfusion of the starved small twin [9].

Ultrasound scanning plays a key role in the diagnosis and management of poor growth in twins. However, ultrasound assessment is technically more

(a)

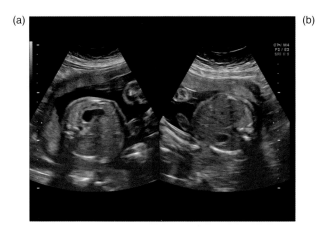

(b)

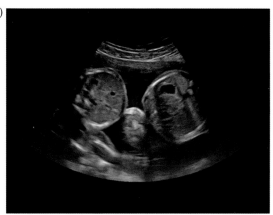

Figure 25.1 Sonographic image of the abdominal circumferences of concordant and discordant growth pairs.

challenging than in singletons and the error in growth discordance estimation may be doubled because of the combination of two measurements. Nevertheless, if well-trained sonographers with good-quality equipment perform the scans, fetal growth as well as growth discordances can be estimated accurately, also in the setting of twins. As such, estimated growth discordance is usually within 15% of the actual birth weight discordance and for a 25% discordant pair, the estimation would thus be between 21% and 29% [10]. The advantage of a twin pregnancy is also that the other twin may serve as a control. So, if in doubt about any significant discordance, it is often helpful to put the two images of both abdominal circumferences next to one another to rule out or confirm any important differences (Figure 25.1).

Discordant Growth in Monochorionic Diamniotic Twin Pregnancies

As mentioned earlier, MCDA twins are monozygotic and thus discordant growth cannot usually be attributed to genetic differences in growth potential. Discordant growth in an MCDA twin pair is thus by definition abnormal and related either to a diminished nutrition toward the smaller twin because of unequal placental sharing, to an unbalanced inter-twin blood exchange or to placental dysfunction of the placental part of the smaller twin. MCDA twins are more commonly growth restricted than DCDA twins and discordant growth is also associated with poorer outcomes [11]. Because of the shared circulation, not only must we take into account the opposing interests of both the growth-restricted and appropriately grown

twin, but also the fact that their well-being is inter-related. More specifically, if the growth-restricted twin dies, the larger twin may exsanguinate in its demised co-twin across the vascular anastomoses and die as well or sustain brain damage. Meta-analysis shows that, in the event of single intrauterine fetal demise in monochorionic twins, the risk of co-twin death is 15% and the risk of neurodevelopmental morbidity in the co-twin is 26% [12].

Although monochorionic twins are monozygotic, discordant chromosomal and genetic syndromes can occur in very rare instances. They may arise either because of errors in mitotic division in the early embryo, differential gene activation, or even more rarely because the monochorionic twin pregnancy is in fact dizygotic. In the setting of discordant growth, one may thus encounter very rare cases, in which trisomy 18, triploidy, or Beckwith-Wiedemann syndrome affects only one of a monochorionic pair [13,14]. Similarly, in a monochorionic twin pregnancy, congenital infections will not usually cause discordant growth, as transmission to both fetuses is expected through the shared circulation, although one twin may be more affected than the other.

Definition and Diagnosis

Isolated discordant growth in MCDA twins must be distinguished from twin-twin transfusion syndrome (TTTS) and twin anemia polycythemia sequence (TAPS). Both conditions are complications of the shared circulation and commonly associated with discordant growth. The differential diagnosis between TTTS, TAPS, and isolated discordant growth is very easy. TTTS is characterized by a severe amniotic fluid discordance, defined as a deepest vertical pocket of less than 2 cm in one twin and more than 8 cm in the other prior to 20 weeks and more than 10 cm after 20 weeks. TAPS, on the other hand, is characterized by a severe discordance in hemoglobin between the twins, diagnosed as middle cerebral artery-peak systolic velocity (MCA-PSV) above 1.5 multiples of the median (MoM) in one twin and below 1 MoM in the other [15]. A more than 20% difference in EFW is thus only called isolated discordant growth if the amniotic fluid and MCA-PSV discordance do not meet the criteria required for the diagnosis of TTTS or TAPS. As such, the diagnosis of isolated discordant growth can be made only in retrospect after birth, because as long as the twins remain undelivered, TTTS or TRAP may still occur [16].

The literature reporting on the outcome of isolated discordant growth in MCDA twins uses several definitions: a discordance of more than 20% or 25% with or without one twin below the 10th or 5th centile, or one twin below the 10th or 5th centile regardless of any discordance. As mentioned earlier, a cut-off of 20% best defines discordant growth, especially in an MCDA setting where any discordance is by definition abnormal, regardless of whether the smaller twin is small for dates or not.

Discordance in the First Trimester

The 12-week ultrasound scan is the ideal time to determine chorionicity and identify the MCDA twin pairs at risk for inter-twin transfusion imbalances. Every diagnosis of a twin pregnancy should, therefore, specify whether it involves an MCDA or a DCDA pair. MCDA twins are separated by two thin amniotic membranes only, which can easily be identified as two thin layers separating the two fetal poles [16].

Discordant growth may already be present in the first trimester as a difference in crown rump length (CRL), which confers a significantly increased risk of adverse outcome [17]. As such, a discordance in CRL of 12 mm or more is associated with an adverse outcome in about 80% of MCDA twins and with a survival rate of only 50%, whereas in cases of a difference in CRL less than 12 mm, the chance for an uncomplicated outcome was 80% with 93% survival rate [18]. CRL discordance, despite being very specific (low false positive rate), poorly predicts adverse outcome, once chromosomal and structural anomalies have been excluded, because most cases that ultimately result in adverse outcome do not present with a discordant CRL at 12 weeks (high false negative rate or low sensitivity). CRL difference in the first trimester thus identifies a subgroup of MCDA twin pregnancies at especially high risk of a complicated outcome and patients should be referred to a fetal medicine center if discordance in CRL is ≥ 10%.

In contrast to CRL discordance at 12 weeks, a discordance of 19% or more in CRL between 7 to 10 weeks may be an excellent predictor of subsequent single loss at 12 weeks (sensitivity 87% for a 5% false positive rate). Conversely, with lesser degrees of discordance, there is a 99% chance of survival of both twins to the first trimester scan, which can be used to reassure parents [19]. If the CRL is discordant in spontaneously conceived twins, the CRL of the larger twin should be used for dating to avoid any false reassurance that the larger twin is too large and the smaller is appropriate for dates, whereas in reality the smaller twin is growth restricted.

Classification

For TTTS, there are clear guidelines as to the management of affected pregnancies, based on randomized controlled trials. For discordant growth, management is less well defined. A first step toward an evidence-based management is to establish a good classification system to identify pregnancies at highest risk of adverse outcome. Both the gestational age at first diagnosis and Doppler studies have now been incorporated in the classification of discordant growth.

Classification According to Gestational Age at First Diagnosis

Discordant growth can be divided into early-onset (present before 26 weeks) and late-onset (present after 26 weeks) discordant growth. Especially early-onset discordant growth is a challenge for clinicians, as it occurs at a pre-viable gestational age when delivery is not yet an option. Early-onset discordant growth, defined as a birth weight discordance of more than 25% and an EFW discordance of more than 20% prior to 26 weeks, occurs in about 8% of MCDA twins, and the survival rate for this group is 83%. Late-onset discordant growth is present in another 7% of MCDA twins and results in a survival rate of 96%. The outcome and placental characteristics of early- versus late-onset discordant growth is summarized

Table 25.1 Outcome and placental characteristics in monochorionic diamniotic twin pregnancies based on early- or late-onset discordant growth [20]

Data are expressed as % and mean ± SD

	Early-onset (N = 15)	Late-onset (N = 13)	Concordant (N = 150)	P-value
Survival rate (%)	83	96	99	<0.0001
Pregnancies with IUFD (%)	27	8	1	<0.0001
Pregnancies with TAPS (%)	0	38	3	<0.0001
Abnormal UA Doppler (%)	73	0	3	<0.0001
GA at delivery (weeks)	33 ± 2	35 ± 2	35 ± 2	<0.001
Birth weight (BW) ratio (± SD)	1.43 ± 0.06	1.44 ± 0.14	1.11 ± 0.08	<0.0001
Placental territory (PT) ratio (± SD)	2.55 ± 0.76	1.59 ± 0.36	1.38 ± 0.35	<0.0001
BW/PT ratio (± SD)	0.60 ± 0.17	0.95 ± 0.27	0.88 ± 0.17	<0.0001
Diameter of AA anastomoses (mm) (± SD)	3.66 ± 1.83	1.34 ± 1.15	2.15 ± 1.46	<0.01
Total anastomotic diameter (mm) (± SD)	13.97 ± 7.07	5.83 ± 5.24	8.86 ± 6.30	= 0.01

IUFD = intrauterine fetal death; TAPS = twin anemia polycythemia sequence; UA = umbilical artery; GA = gestational age; AA = arterio-arterial

in Table 25.1. Intrauterine demise occurs more frequently in the early-onset group. When imminent intrauterine demise of the smaller twin is diagnosed, an invasive procedure can be offered in the early-onset group to protect the larger twin, which often results in the demise of the smaller twin. In contrast, in the late-onset group, an elective preterm birth will salvage both twins. This largely explains the lower survival rate in the early-onset group. Twins with early-onset discordant growth are also delivered earlier and an abnormal umbilical artery Doppler pattern in the cord of the growth-restricted twin is rarely seen in the late-onset group, whereas it occurs in the majority of early-onset cases [20].

The underlying mechanism of growth restriction also seems to be different in early- and late-onset discordant growth. As such, the main cause of early-onset discordant growth is not so much a transfusion imbalance, but rather unequal sharing of the placenta between the twins [20–23]. The degree of unequal sharing is higher in cases of early-onset discordant growth, as demonstrated in Table 25.1. Furthermore, the total diameter of artery-to-artery anastomoses is higher in these placentas, as is the total diameter of all anastomosing vessels. The circulations of the fetuses are thus linked more tightly in early-onset, as compared to late-onset and concordant-growth twins. The discordance in birth weight in the early-onset group is also smaller than expected based on placental sharing alone. This suggests that the more elaborate blood exchange in the early-onset placentas benefits the twin on the smaller placental share and at least partially compensates for the high degree of unequal placental sharing [20].

A velamentous cord insertion is more often present in the smaller twin of a discordant pair, and is associated with growth restriction. At the moment, we cannot predict the degree of unequal placental sharing antenatally. However, a combination of an eccentric or velamentous cord insertion may be a good indicator of unequal sharing. This combination of cord insertions is three times more common in MCDA (18%) than in DCDA twins (6%) and discordant growth is seen in nearly half of these cases. Determining the cord insertions antenatally may serve as a surrogate marker for unequal sharing and helps us to identify a subgroup of twins at increased risk of discordant growth [24–28].

On the other hand, late-onset discordant growth seems more often associated with transfusion imbalance earlier defined as TAPS, demonstrated by the fact that 38% of these twin pairs are born with discordant hemoglobin levels. These late-onset discordant growth placentas do not show a marked difference from placentas of concordant-growth twins. However, in pregnancies that are complicated by TAPS, the typical finding is an equally shared placenta with only very small unidirectional anastomoses, resulting in a net transfusion of red blood cells and a difference in birth weight that is larger than expected, given the equally shared placenta [20].

Next to unequal sharing and vascular anastomoses, placental implantation may also influence growth. Growth-restricted twins of an MCDA pair have increased vascular resistance in the spiral arteries compared to their appropriately grown co-twins, suggesting a role for impaired endovascular trophoblast invasion in the pathogenesis [29]. On the other hand, uterine artery Doppler in the mid-trimester has not proven useful in predicting fetal growth restriction in both monochorionic and dichorionic twins [30–32]. Mean uterine artery pulsatility index is significantly lower in twins compared to singleton pregnancies, irrespective of chorionicity. Focally defective trophoblastic invasion in the placental share of the growth-restricted twin can be masked by a decrease in pulsatility index caused by the correct implantation of the placental part of the appropriately grown twin, explaining why uterine artery Doppler is a less sensitive method to predict poor growth in twins compared to singletons [33].

Classification According to the Umbilical Artery Blood Flow in the Smaller Twin

Umbilical artery Doppler in MCDA twins does not only reflect the vascular resistance as in singletons, but it is also influenced by the direction and shunting of blood flow across the inter-twin anastomoses, and the results can therefore not be interpreted in the same way as in singletons. Based on the umbilical artery Doppler pattern in the smaller twin, Gratacos and colleagues developed a staging system for discordant growth [34].

A positive end-diastolic flow (EDF) pattern, with or without increased pulsatility index (PI), is described as type I. Type II is defined as a continuous absent or reversed end-diastolic flow (AREDF) pattern. When an absent or reversed end-diastolic flow is observed over a short period, rapidly alternating with positive flow, it is labeled as intermittent AREDF (iAREDF), and this is classified as type III. The iAREDF pattern is unique to MCDA twins and reflects the colliding of the two circulations within a large arterio-arterial anastomosis.

The clinical evolution of type I is the most favorable, followed by type III, with the worst outcomes for type II. As such, overall survival with expectant management is 96%, 59%, and 81% for types I, II, and III, respectively [35]. Type I is also associated with a lower birth weight discordance compared to type II and III (29% versus 38% and 36%,

respectively). Further, in type I, fetal deterioration requiring active management is rare. On the contrary, 90% of type II cases will deteriorate at some stage. For type III, 11% will show signs of deterioration. Fetal deterioration with imminent demise of the growth-restricted twin can be diagnosed by one of the following criteria, which are the same as for singletons: persistent reversed EDF, ductus venosus pulsatility index above two standard deviations for gestational age, oligohydramnios with DVP <2 cm, and after viability: persistently abnormal fetal heart rate tracing or persistent abnormal biophysical profile. Unexpected fetal demise is rarely seen in type I and type II (3% and 0%, respectively), but occurs in about 15% of pregnancies with type III [34]. When the growth-restricted twin dies in type III, there is also a 50% chance of demise of the larger twin. Fetal demise is unpredictable in this group, as it occurs in fetuses with previous normal Doppler findings [36]. Parenchymal brain damage is rare in type I, but can occur in type II and type III. However, in type II, it is typically seen in the smaller twin (14% of cases) and it is less common in the larger twin (3% of cases). Conversely, in type III, it is the larger that is more often affected by parenchymal brain damage (20% of cases, versus only 2% of the smaller twins). This type of brain damage is not limited to pregnancies complicated by single demise, but on the contrary, it occurs frequently in cases where both survive [34].

As summarized in Table 25.2 and represented in Figure 25.2, placentas differ greatly between the different types. Unequal sharing is present in all of them, but is less pronounced in type I and is most severe in type III. The fetal weight ratio/placental territory ratio decreases from type I to type III, showing that type III growth-restricted twins partially compensate for their very small placental share. Indeed, type III placentas have more and larger artery-to-artery anastomoses, allowing for bidirectional blood flow. This tight link between the circulations allows the smaller twin to survive and grow thanks to blood exchange with the larger twin. However, blood flow in these large bidirectional anastomoses can change very suddenly, which explains the higher incidence of unexpected demise or parenchymal brain damage in these cases. In pregnancies with single demise, the large anastomoses allow for a rapid exsanguination of the larger twin, explaining why double demise is more often seen in this category. Double demise is more rare in type II, which

Table 25.2 Outcome and placental characteristics of monochorionic diamniotic twin pregnancies according to umbilical artery Doppler pattern in the smaller twin [34]

Data are expressed as % and mean

	Uncomplicated (N = 76)	Type I (N = 39)	Type II (N = 30)	Type III (N = 65)
Umbilical artery Doppler	NA	Positive EDF	Continuous AREDF	Intermittent AREDF
Fetal weight (FW) ratio	1.1	1.4	1.6	1.6
Placental territory (PT) ratio	1.3	1.8	2.6	4.4
FW ratio/PT ratio	0.94	0.79	0.71	0.44
AA anastomoses (%)	80	78	73	100
large AA anastomoses >2 mm (%)	55	70	18	98

NA = not applicable; EDF = end diastolic flow; AREDF = absent reversed end-diastolic flow; AA = arterioarterial

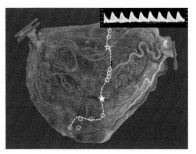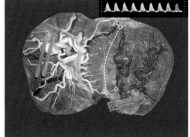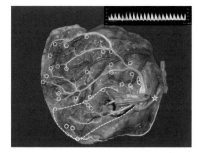

Figure 25.2 Typical monochorionic diamniotic twin placentas of types I, II, and III cases with their respective Doppler patterns.

is understandable given the fact that these placentas have smaller anastomoses that make rapid exsanguination less likely [34].

Management and Outcome

Management is different in MCDA as compared to DCDA twins, since the fetal circulations are linked and the well-being of the larger twin depends on the condition of the growth-restricted twin. As in DCDA twins, we have to take preterm birth into account: when the smaller needs to be delivered prematurely, this preterm birth can cause problems for the appropriately grown twin. But on the other hand, unlike in DCDA twins, if the smaller twin dies in utero, the larger twin can lose large volumes of blood through the intertwin anastomoses, which can result in demise or brain damage for the larger. It is thus more difficult to find the right balance.

The management also differs for early- and late-onset discordant growth, simply because delivery is not yet an option in early pregnancy. The presence of abnormal Doppler patterns further complicates management. Discordant-growth MCDA twins can be divided into three categories that each has to be managed differently:

Early-Onset Discordant Growth with Positive End-Diastolic Flow (Type I)

As mentioned previously, type I has a good prognosis. When managed expectantly, the survival rate is 96% [35]. Intervention is therefore usually not needed in these cases. Weekly follow-up is warranted, however, since evolution to TTTS, TAPS, or stage II can occur. Therefore it is advised to evaluate these cases weekly for amniotic fluid assessment and umbilical and middle cerebral artery Doppler examination. Fetal growth should be assessed every 2 weeks. Weekly cardiotocography (CTG) and/or biophysical profile scores can be added once viability has been reached. The aim is to prolong the pregnancy as much as possible, and to plan elective delivery between 34 and 35 weeks [37]. In type I, routine prophylactic administration of corticosteroids for lung maturity is usually not indicated, but of course they should be administered when preterm delivery seems likely, especially whenever an elective preterm cesarean section is planned.

Early-Onset Discordant Growth with Continuous or Intermittent Absent End-Diastolic Flow (Types II and III)

Early-onset types II and III are most challenging for clinicians as there is a real risk of single or double fetal demise. Overall survival with expectant management is 59% for type II and 81% for type III [35,36]. This in contrast to TTTS, where the natural course is associated with a nearly 100% mortality rate. However, when imminent demise of the growth-restricted twin is suspected, an intervention may become necessary to protect the larger twin from acute shifts in blood volume that can cause demise or brain damage of the larger twin. As mentioned earlier, fetal deterioration with imminent demise of the growth-restricted twin can be diagnosed by the same criteria as in singletons. Growth discordance of more than 35% and growth stop of the smaller twin have also been suggested as criteria for invasive therapy [34–42]. There are, however, no formal recommendations at the moment, and it is at the discretion of the clinician to decide when to intervene. Two types of interventions can be performed to isolate the circulation of the larger twin and unlink the shared circulation: either cord occlusion of the growth restricted twin, or laser coagulation of the inter-twin anastomoses. In type II, intervention can be offered when demise of the growth-restricted twin is imminent. However, in type III, demise is often sudden and unexpected, making it more difficult to decide when to intervene.

The outcome of expectant management versus cord occlusion and laser surgery can be found in Table 25.3. After cord occlusion, the survival for the growth-restricted twin is obviously 0%, but it allows for survival of the larger twin in 93% of cases. However, the gestational age at birth in this series was 36 weeks, which is later than with expectant management or after laser surgery. Also, it has to be noted that laser surgery is not possible in all cases due to technical difficulties. Indeed, there is no polyhydramnios in the co-twin, as in TTTS, which makes it more difficult to access the vascular equator. Ultimately, the choice between cord occlusion or laser surgery will be determined by technical aspects, severity of the disease, and the preference of the patients.

Before 28 weeks, these patients are followed up weekly (Doppler and amniotic fluid assessment) with growth assessment every 2 weeks similar to type I, although ductus venosus Doppler examination is performed as an additional exam. From 28 weeks on, intensive follow-up of these pregnancies is warranted. We advise inpatient management with CTG, Doppler monitoring, and biophysical profile. Corticosteroids for lung maturity can be administered at this time. In the absence of early fetal deterioration, we advise to deliver these pregnancies between 32 and 33 weeks in case of expectant management, to prevent late in-utero complications. A repeat dose of corticosteroids might be given immediately before delivery. However, if laser therapy or cord occlusion has been performed, it is possible to prolong the pregnancy because there is no longer a shared circulation in these cases. We recommend delivery by cesarean section in case of survival of the growth-restricted twin, since this twin is already compromised and might not tolerate labor well. Figure 25.3 represents the flow chart for the management of early-onset discordant growth in MCDA twins.

Late-Onset Discordant Growth (Usually Type I)

Late-onset discordant growth develops only after 26 weeks, when the twins are already viable. This means that in case of deterioration of the condition of one or both fetuses, they can be delivered and there is no need for an intrauterine intervention. As mentioned previously, the expected survival rate is around 96% in case of late-onset growth discordance and they reach a gestational age of 35 weeks on average, which is not significantly different from MCDA twins with concordant growth. The discordance in birth weight is not different from that in early-onset discordant growth, but umbilical artery Doppler abnormalities are rare in this group. TAPS, however, is seen in 38% of these cases. Monitoring of the MCA velocities in these pregnancies is thus a must [20].

Again, weekly monitoring of Doppler patterns and amniotic fluid is recommended, with growth estimation every 2 weeks similar as for type I. CTG and BFP can also be performed weekly, once viability has been reached. Delivery should be considered whenever signs of fetal deterioration (as mentioned earlier) are present, and can otherwise be planned between 34 and 35 weeks.

Neonatal Outcome for Discordant Twins

Discordant twin pairs are at risk of severe preterm birth and the associated complications thereof, such as respiratory distress, bronchopulmonary dysplasia,

Table 25.3 Summary of reported outcome of monochorionic diamniotic twin pregnancies according to type of discordant growth and management
Data are expressed as % and median (ranges)

		Expectant Management			Laser		Cord Occlusion	
		Type I	Type II	Type III	Type II	Type III	Type II	Type III
Reference		Ishii [35] (N = 23)	Ishii [35] (N = 27)	Gratacos [36] (N = 31)	Peeva [40] (N = 142)	Gratacos [36] (N = 18)	Parra [41] (N = 41)	Parra [41] (N = 49)
Survival (%)	Overall	96	59	85	53	64	46	47
	Small	96	52	81	39	33	0	0
	Large	96	67	90	68	94	93	93
GA at birth (weeks)		36 (26–38)	28 (18–40)	31 (26–33)	32 (24–41)	32.6 (23–38)	36.4 (29–41)	36.5 (26–41)
Reference		Gratacos [36] (N = 39)*	Gratacos [36] (N = 30)*	Gratacos [36] (N = 65)*	Chalouhi [39] (N = 23)**		Chalouhi [39] (N = 22)**	
Early neurological morbidity in survivors (%)	Small	0	29	8	14		NA	
	Large	0	7	23	0		5	
Reference		Ishii [35] (N = 23)	Ishii [35] (N = 27)	Ishii [35] (N = 13)	NA		NA	
Neurological morbidity at 6 months in survivors (%)***	Small	5	29	27	NA		NA	
	Large	0	17	50	NA		NA	

GA=gestational age
* Intraventricular hemorrhage and parenchymal brain damage, as assessed by transcranial ultrasound at 4 days of life and 1 month.
** Cerebral lesions were assessed by transcranial ultrasound before discharge and included intraventricular hemorrhage grades III and IV, flares or cystic periventricular leukomalacia, lissencephaly, schizencephaly, and heterotopias.
*** Any significant abnormal findings on transcranial ultrasound or MRI at 6 months of age (including intraventricular hemorrhage grades III or IV and cystic periventricular leukomalacia, blindness, or deafness).

patent ductus arteriosus, and necrotizing enterocolitis. There are some differences in neonatal outcome between MCDA and DCDA twins, most importantly the higher neurological morbidity in MCDA twins due to the shared circulation. Furthermore, the birth weight of MCDA twins tends to be lower than in dichorionic twins and they have a longer hospital stay. However, Apgar scores, respiratory complications, infectious complications, and incidence of necrotizing enterocolitis are comparable in both groups [43].

Importantly, in discordant MCDA twins where both are live born, severe neonatal morbidity is seen more in the larger (38%) as compared to the smaller twin (19%). Especially the risk of respiratory distress syndrome is increased in the larger twin, 32% versus 6% in the growth-restricted twin. This can be explained by the fact that the growth-restricted twin has experienced more stress in utero and is therefore better able to cope with the demands of an early birth [44].

When managed expectantly, discordant growth monochorionic twins are also more at risk of parenchymal brain damage than non-discordant monochorionic twins or dichorionic twins born at the same gestational age. This is most commonly seen in the larger twin. As mentioned previously, brain damage in the larger twin can occur even when the growth-restricted twin is live born [45]. The average incidence of severe cerebral injury in cases of discordant growth seems to be about 8%. However, the incidence is higher in studies that include cases of single intrauterine demise and in studies with a median gestational age at birth of 32 weeks or less. The risk seems to be

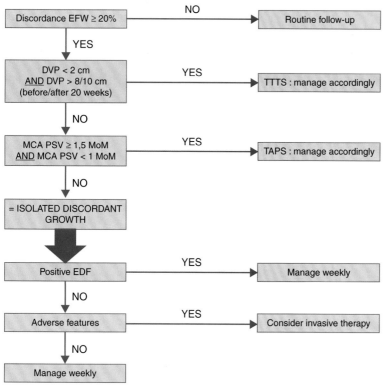

Figure 25.3 Flow chart for the evaluation and management of early-onset discordant growth.
EFW = estimated fetal weight;
DVP = deepest vertical pocket; MCA PSV middle cerebral artery peak systolic velocity;
EDF = end-diastolic flow
Adverse features include one of the following prior to viability: ductus venosus pulsatility index above two standard deviations for gestational age, stuck twin phenomenon with DVP <2 cm, growth discordance of more than 35%, and growth stop of the smaller twin

higher in pregnancies with abnormal umbilical artery Doppler studies (13.5% vs. 2.5%) and in larger twins (9% vs. 5%) [46]. As yet, there are no data on long-term developmental outcome in these children.

In 20% of cases with type III discordant growth, the larger twin presents antenatally with cardiomegaly and increased ventricular wall thickness. However, this does not seem to be associated with poorer neonatal outcome. Most likely, these changes are reactive to the increased strain on the heart of the larger twin [47]. Also in these pregnancies there can be an association of pulmonary artery stenosis in the larger twin and aortic coarctation in the smaller twin.

Discordant Growth in Dichorionic Twin Pregnancies

DCDA twins differ from monochorionic twins, since in essence they are singletons who share the same womb. Their placentas are not linked and their well-being is not as interrelated as in monochorionic twins. This makes management somewhat less complicated; however, there are still two fetuses to consider when contemplating delivery.

First Trimester Discordance

As for MCDA twins, CRL discordance of ≥10% at the time of the first trimester scan is a highly specific predictor for a poor pregnancy outcome; however, the sensitivity is very low. If CRL discordance is picked up in the first trimester, this pregnancy is at higher risk of adverse outcome and needs to be followed up more closely [17]. Also similar to MCDA twins, CRL discordance of ≥19% between 7 and 10 weeks is highly predictive of early fetal loss at the time of the first trimester scan, whereas concordant growth in the early first trimester is a reassuring feature [19].

Definition and Diagnosis

As in monochorionic twins, several cut-off values have been used to describe discordant growth in DCDA twins ranging from 15 to 30%. However, there is a general consensus that a cut-off of 20% discordance best predicts poor outcome also in DCDA twins.

We do not know the zygosity of DCDA twins antenatally, unless they are different-sex twins or result from a single embryo transfer. In contrast to MCDA twins (100% monozygotic), only 10% of DCDA twins are monozygotic, the remaining 90% being dizygotic. In the latter group, genetic differences often explain why one twin is bigger than the other. The smaller twin may thus well be constitutionally smaller instead of growth restricted.

Twins are generally smaller than singletons, but the difference with singletons is less pronounced in DCDA than in MCDA twins. For all twins, fetal growth decreases after 30 weeks compared to singletons [4]. Parity and gender of the fetuses have little impact on fetal growth and should therefore not be taken into account when assessing whether fetal growth is appropriate [3]. About 95% of twins after assisted conception are DCDA. These twins have similar risks of developing growth restriction and the complications hereof as spontaneously conceived twins [48].

Management

Management of DCDA discordant twins differs greatly from that of MCDA twins, since demise of the growth-restricted twin usually does not affect its co-twin. This means birth can be delayed until an acceptable gestational age is reached with a good chance of intact survival for both twins. Even if the growth-restricted twin deteriorates or dies, delivery can be delayed to provide the best chances for survival of the larger twin. Essentially, DCDA twins behave as singletons that occupy the same space, but they have opposing interests in case of discordant growth and the main question is when to deliver the babies for the benefit of the growth-restricted twin, without causing too much harm to the larger twin.

The cut-off to define a viable gestational age may differ between centers and also depends on the wishes of the parents. It can range from 28 to 32 weeks. Biweekly sonographic follow-up before 28 weeks is sufficient to follow growth, umbilical artery, and middle cerebral artery Doppler. In case of abnormal umbilical artery and middle cerebral artery Dopplers of the smaller twin, additional Doppler evaluation of the ductus venosus Doppler should be performed. If the smaller twin has an abnormal Doppler of the umbilical artery, steroids and inpatient management may be considered once the cut-off of a viable gestational age is reached. Also, daily CTG and a biweekly ultrasound evaluation should be performed in these severe cases. If all remains stable, steroids can be administered and delivery may be planned after completion of steroids between 32–35 weeks depending

on the severity. In case of absent or reversed ductus venosus a-wave or abnormal CTG, immediate delivery is indicated. Unfortunately, there is no clear guidance on how to manage and when to deliver these pregnancies, and these recommendations are largely based on expert opinion. Recently, both EFW and cerebroplacental ratio discordance were shown to be independent predictors of fetal loss, and the combination of both parameters identifies most twin pregnancies at risk of fetal loss [49].

As mentioned before, cesarean section is likely the preferred mode of delivery, depending on the severity of the pathology, fetal position, parity, and parental wishes [50]. In exceptional circumstances, selective feticide of the FGR twin can be considered in dichorionic twins, e.g., in case of severe early-onset preeclampsia, selective feticide of the growth-restricted twin may improve the maternal condition and prolong the pregnancy for the benefit of the larger twin [51].

Outcome

In contrast with MCDA twins, the absence of inter-twin anastomoses protects the larger twin from demise or brain damage in case of demise of the growth-restricted twin. The outcome of the larger twin is thus determined by the degree of preterm birth and not by the condition of the smaller twin. Otherwise, as mentioned before, the risks to the neonates are comparable in MCDA and DCDA twins [43]. When discordant DCDA twins are born preterm and the smaller twin has a birth weight below the 10th centile, the smaller twin also seems to have fewer respiratory problems than the co-twin. They experience less respiratory distress and apnea and require less respiratory support than the appropriately grown twin [52].

Conclusion

Discordant growth affects both MCDA and DCDA twins, but its management and outcome differ significantly. Management in MCDA twins is complicated by the presence of inter-twin vascular anastomoses, which make their well-being interrelated and account for the increased perinatal mortality and neurologic morbidity of growth-discordant MCDA as compared to DCDA pairs. However, in both MCDA and DCDA twins, ultrasound and Doppler evaluation play a key role in the follow-up of these high-risk pregnancies and the prediction of perinatal outcome. The aim in managing these pregnancies is to deliver them at the optimal time so that the growth-restricted twin is born alive and well, without causing too much harm to its larger twin due to preterm birth. This chapter aimed to provide clinicians with updated information on how best to achieve this goal.

Key Points

- Discordant growth in monochorionic twins represents a risk for both fetuses, owing to placental vascular anastomoses.

- Discordant growth in monochorionic twin pregnancies may be isolated or it may occur in combination with TTTS or TAPS.

- Measurement of the deepest vertical pockets and Doppler ultrasound investigation of the middle cerebral artery are mandatory to distinguish isolated discordant growth from TTTS and TAPS.

- The main cause for early-onset discordant growth in monochorionic twin pregnancies is unequal placental sharing, and severely abnormal umbilical artery Doppler waveforms are typical. Multiple anastomoses may compensate for this situation.

- Late-onset discordant growth in monochorionic twin pregnancies is more often associated with TAPS, which is characterized by markedly different peak systolic blood flow velocities in the middle cerebral arteries of both fetuses.

- Early-onset discordant growth in monochorionic twin pregnancies may be managed expectantly or invasively (laser or bipolar cord coagulation of the smaller twin to prevent damage to the larger twin) and late-onset discordant growth by elective delivery in case of deterioration of one or both fetuses.

- Dichorionic twins behave as singletons due to the separate placental masses and can be followed up accordingly.

- In dichorionic twins, demise of the smallest twin does not usually affect the larger twin. Therefore, active management can be delayed until an appropriate gestational age for delivery is reached, as to maximize the chances of intact survival of the larger twin.

References

1. Three decades of twin births in the USA, 1980–2009. NCHS Data Briefs 2012. www.cdc.gov/nchs/data/databriefs/db80.htm

2. Blickstein I. Normal and abnormal growth of multiples. *Semin Neonatol* 2002;7:177–85.

3. Ananth CV, Vintzileos AM, Shen-Schwarz S, Smulian JC, Lai Y-L. Standards of birth weight in twin gestations stratified by placental chorionicity. *Obstet Gynecol* 1998;91:917–24.

4. Stirrup OT, Khalil A, D'Antonio F, Thilaganathan B; Southwest Thames Obstetric Research Collaborative (STORK). Fetal growth reference ranges in twin pregnancy: Analysis of the Southwest Thames Obstetric Research Collaborative (STORK) multiple pregnancy cohort. *Ultrasound Obstet Gynecol* 2015;45:301–7.

5. Hamilton EF, Platt RW, Morin L, Usher R, Kramer M. How small is too small in a twin pregnancy? *Am J Obstet Gynecol* 1998;179:682–5.

6. Breathnach FM, McAuliffe FM, Geary M, Daly S, Higgins JR, Dornan J, Morrison JJ, Burke G, Higgins S, Dicker P, Manning F, Mahony R, Malone FD; Perinatal Ireland Research Consortium. Definition of intertwin birth weight discordance. *Obstet Gynecol* 2011;118:94–103.

7. Khalil AA, Khan N, Bowe S, Familiari A, Papageorghiou A, Bhide A, Thilaganathan B. Discordance in fetal biometry and Doppler are independent predictors of the risk of perinatal loss in twin pregnancies. *Am J Obstet Gynecol* 2015;213:222. e1–222.e10.

8. Harper LM, Weis MA, Odibo AO, et al. Significance of growth discordance in appropriately grown twins. *Am J Obstet Gynecol* 2013;208:393.e1–5.

9. Lewi L, Devlieger R, De Catte L, Deprest J. Growth discordance. *Best Pract Res Clin Obstet Gynaecol* 2014;28:295–303.

10. Van Mieghem T, Deprest J, Klaritsch P, Gucciardo L, Done' E, Verhaeghe J, Lewi L. Ultrasound prediction of intertwin birth weight discordance in monochorionic diamniotic twin pregnancies. *Prenat Diagn* 2009;29:240–4.

11. Victoria A, Mora G, Arias F. Perinatal outcome, placental pathology, and severity of discordance in monochorionic and dichorionic twins. *Obstet Gynecol* 2001;97:310–15.

12. Hillman S, Morris R, Kilby M. Co-twin prognosis after single fetal death: A systematic review and meta-analysis. *Obstet Gynecol* 2011;118(4):928–40.

13. Lewi L, Blickstein I, Van Schoubroeck D, et al. Diagnosis and management of heterokaryotypic

monochorionic twins. *Am J Med Genet A* 2006;140:272–5.

14. Weksberg R, Shuman C, Caluseriu O, et al. Discordant KCNQ1OT1 imprinting in sets of monozygotic twins discordant for Beckwith-Wiedemann syndrome. *Hum Mol Genet* 2002;11:1317–25.

15. Slaghekke F, Kist W, Oepkes D, Pasman S, Middeldorp J, Klumper F, Lopriore E et al. Twin anemia-polycythemia sequence: diagnostic criteria, classification, perinatal management and outcome. *Fetal Diagn Ther* 2010;27(4):181–90.

16. Lewi L, Gucciardo L, Van Mieghem T, de Koninck P, Beck V, Medek H, Van Schoubroeck D, Devlieger R, De Catte L, Deprest J. Monochorionic diamniotic twin pregnancies: Natural history and risk stratification. *Fetal Diagn Ther* 2010;27:121–33.

17. D'Antonio F, Khalil A, Pagani G, Papageorghiou AT, Bhide A, Thilaganathan B. Crown-rump length discordance and adverse perinatal outcome in twin pregnancies: Systematic review and meta-analysis. *Ultrasound Obstet Gynecol* 2014;44:138–46.

18. Lewi L, Lewi P, Diemert A, Jani J, Gucciardo L, Van Mieghem T, Doné E, Gratacós E, Huber A, Hecher K, Deprest J. The role of ultrasound examination in the first trimester and at 16 weeks' gestation to predict fetal complications in monochorionic diamniotic twin pregnancies. *Am J Obstet Gynecol* 2008;199:493. e1–7.

19. D'Antonio F, Khalil A, Mantovani E, Thilaganathan G. Embryonic growth discordance and early fetal loss: The STORK multiple pregnancy cohort and systematic review. *Human Reprod* 2013;28:2621–7.

20. Lewi L, Gucciardo L, Huber A, Jani J, Van Mieghem T, Doné E et al. Clinical outcome and placental characteristics of monochorionic diamniotic twin pairs with early- and late-onset discordant growth. *Am J Obstet Gynecol* 2008;199:511-e1.

21. Fick A, Feldstein V, Norton M, Fyr C, Caughey A, Machin G. Unequal placental sharing and birth weight discordance in monochorionic diamniotic twins. *Am J Obstet Gynecol* 2006;195:178–83.

22. Lewi L, Cannie M, Blickstein I, Jani J, Huber A, Hecher K et al. Placental sharing, birthweight discordance, and vascular anastomoses in monochorionic diamniotic twin placentas. *Am J Obstet Gynecol* 2007;197:587-e1.

23. Hack K, Nikkels P, Koopman-Esseboom C, Derks J, Elias S, Van Gemert M, Visser G. Placental characteristics of monochorionic diamniotic twin pregnancies in relation to perinatal outcome. *Placenta* 2008;29:976–81.

24. Lopriore E, Pasman S, Klumper F, Middeldorp J, Walther F, Oepkes D. Placental characteristics in growth-discordant monochorionic twins: A matched case-control study. *Placenta* 2012;33:171–4.

25. De Paepe M, Shapiro S, Young L, Luks F. Placental characteristics of selective birth weight discordance in diamniotic-monochorionic twin gestations. *Placenta* 2010;31:380–6.

26. Kent E, Breathnach F, Gillan J, McAuliffe F, Geary M, Daly S et al. Placental cord insertion and birthweight discordance in twin pregnancies: Results of the national prospective ESPRiT Study. *Am J Obstet Gynecol* 2011;205:376-e1.

27. Machin G. Velamentous cord insertion in monochorionic twin gestation. An added risk factor. *J Reprod Med* 1997;42:785–9.

28. Hanley M, Ananth C, Shen-Schwarz S, Smulian j, Lai Y, Vintzileos A. Placental cord insertion and birth weight discordancy in twin gestations. *Obstet Gynecol* 2002;99:477–82.

29. Matijevic R, Ward S, Bajoria R. Non-invasive method of evaluation of trophoblast invasion of spiral arteries in monochorionic twins with discordant birthweight. *Placenta* 2002;23:93–9.

30. Yu C, Papageorghiou A, Boli A, Cacho A, Nicolaides K. Screening for pre-eclampsia and fetal growth restriction in twin pregnancies at 23 weeks of gestation by transvaginal uterine artery Doppler. *Ultrasound Obstet Gynecol* 2002;20:535–40.

31. Geipel A, Berg C, Germer U, Katalinic A, Krapp M, Smrcek J, Gembruch U. Doppler assessment of the uterine circulation in the second trimester in twin pregnancies: Prediction of pre-eclampsia, fetal growth restriction and birth weight discordance. *Ultrasound Obstet Gynecol* 2002;20:541–5.

32. Geipel A, Hennemann F, Fimmers R, Willruth A, Lato K, Gembruch U, Berg, C. Reference ranges for Doppler assessment of uterine artery resistance and pulsatility indices in dichorionic twin pregnancies. *Ultrasound Obstet Gynecol* 2011;37:663–7.

33. Sebire N. Routine uterine artery Doppler screening in twin pregnancies?. *Ultrasound Obstet Gynecol* 2002;20:532–4.

34. Gratacos E, Lewi L, Munoz B, Acosta-Rojas R, Hernandez-Andrade E, Martinez J et al. A classification system for selective intrauterine growth restriction in monochorionic pregnancies according to umbilical artery Doppler flow in the smaller twin. *Ultrasound Obstet Gynecol* 2007;30:28–34.

35. Ishii K, Murakoshi T, Takahashi Y, Shinno T, Matsushita M, Naruse H et al. Perinatal outcome of monochorionic twins with selective intrauterine growth restriction and different types of umbilical artery Doppler under expectant management. *Fetal Diagn Ther* 2009;26:157–61.

36. Gratacós E, Antolin E, Lewi L, Martínez J, Hernandez-Andrade E, Acosta-Rojas R et al. Monochorionic twins with selective intrauterine growth restriction and intermittent absent or reversed end-diastolic flow (Type III): Feasibility and perinatal outcome of fetoscopic placental laser coagulation. *Ultrasound Obstet Gynecol* 2008;31:669–75.

37. Gratacos E, Ortiz J, Martinez J. A systematic approach to the differential diagnosis and management of the complications of monochorionic twin pregnancies. *Fetal Diagn Ther* 2012;32:145–55.

38. Quintero R., Bornick P, Morales W, Allen M. Selective photocoagulation of communicating vessels in the treatment of monochorionic twins with selective growth retardation. *Am J Obstet Gynecol* 2001;185:689–96.

39. Chalouhi G, Marangoni M, Quibel T, Deloison B, Benzina N, Essaoui M et al. Active management of selective intrauterine growth restriction with abnormal Doppler in monochorionic diamniotic twin pregnancies diagnosed in the second trimester of pregnancy. *Prenat Diagn* 2013;33:109–15.

40. Peeva G, Bower S, Orosz L, Chaveeva P, Akolekar R, Nicolaides K. Endoscopic placental laser coagulation in monochorionic diamniotic twins with type II selective fetal growth restriction. *Fetal Diagn Ther* 2015; 38:86–93.

41. Parra M, Bennasar M, Martinez J, Eixarch E, Torres X, Gratacos E. Cord occlusion in monochorionic twins with early selective intra-uterine growth restriction and abnormal umbilical artery Doppler: A consecutive series of 90 cases. *Fet Diagn Ther* DOI: 10.1159/000439023

42. Ishii K, Murakoshi T, Hayashi S, Saito M, Sago H, Takahashi Y et al. Ultrasound predictors of mortality in monochorionic twins with selective intrauterine growth restriction. *Ultrasound Obstet Gynecol* 2011;37:22–6.

43. De Cassia Alam Machado R, De Lourdes Brizot M, Liao A, Krebs V, Zugaib M. Early neonatal morbidity and mortality in growth-discordant twins. *Acta Obstet Gynecol Scand* 2009;88:167–71.

44. Lopriore E, Sluimers C, Pasman S, Middeldorp J, Oepkes D, Walther F. Neonatal morbidity in growth-discordant monochorionic twins: Comparison between the larger and the smaller twin. *Twin Res Hum Genet* 2012;15:541–6.

45. Gratacos E, Carreras E, Becker J, Lewi L, Enriquez G, Perapoch J et al. Prevalence of neurological damage in monochorionic twins with selective intrauterine growth restriction and intermittent absent or reversed end-diastolic umbilical artery flow. *Ultrasound Obstet Gynecol* 2004;24:159–63.

46. Inklaar M, Klink J, Stolk T, Zwet E, Oepkes D, Lopriore E. Cerebral injury in monochorionic twins with selective intrauterine growth restriction: A systematic review. *Prenat Diagn* 2014;34(3):205–13.

47. Muñoz-Abellana B, Hernandez-Andrade E, Figueroa-Diesel H, Ferrer Q, Acosta-Rojas R, Cabero L, Gratacos E. Hypertrophic cardiomyopathy-like changes in monochorionic twin pregnancies with selective intrauterine growth restriction and intermittent absent/reversed end-diastolic flow in the umbilical artery. *Ultrasound Obstet Gynecol* 2007;30:977–82.

48. Helmerhorst FM, Perquin DA, Donker D, Keirse MJ. Perinatal outcome of singletons and twins after assisted conception: A systematic review of controlled studies. *BMJ* 2004;328:261.

49. Khalil A, Khan N, Bowe S, Familiari A, Papageorghiou A, Bhide A, Thilaganathan B. Discordance in fetal biometry and Doppler are independent predictors of the risk of perinatal loss in twin pregnancies. *Am J Obstet Gynecol* 2015;213:222-e1.

50. Kingdom J, Nevo O, Murphy K. Discordant growth in twins. *Prenatal Diagn* 2005;25:759–65.

51. Heyborne K, Porreco R. Selective fetocide reverses preeclampsia in discordant twins. *Am J Obstet Gynecol* 2004;191:477–80.

52. Halmovich Y, Ascher-Landsberg J, Azem F, Mandel D, Mimouni F, Many A. Neonatal outcome of preterm discordant twins. *J Perinat Med* 2011;39:317–22.

Fetal Growth Restriction and Neonatal Outcomes

Rashmi Gandhi and Neil Marlow

Introduction

Fetal growth restriction (FGR), as defined in previous chapters, may be summarized as failure to reach a fetus's genetic growth potential. This may result from a range of pathological factors. Much of the obstetric and neonatal literature confuses the two concepts of FGR and being small for gestational age (SGA), further complicated by the use of different definitions in different studies [1].

SGA is a statistical concept. The World Health Organization (WHO 1995) has used 10th percentile or -2SD of the population-based growth curves as arbitrary cut-off points for identifying SGA [2]. Within this group up to 70% of SGA fetuses are constitutionally small and healthy. This definition is thus not useful for screening for FGR and fails to identify the fetus with growth restriction whose estimated fetal weight has not dropped to below the 10th percentile [3].

In contrast, FGR requires the presence of subnormal growth velocity and is associated with high risk of mortality and morbidity, both in the neonatal period and beyond. FGR is the most common cause of stillbirth and is the second leading cause of perinatal mortality after preterm birth.

Customized growth charts have been used in the past to help differentiate FGR from constitutionally small fetuses. These charts take into consideration anthropometric variables of mother and fetus, ethnicity, and parity [4]. Use of these charts along with population-based growth curves can improve the identification of the small fetus or newborn at risk of adverse outcomes [5]. Other studies have tried to use different weight cut-offs to produce better prediction of adverse outcome as a result of FGR. Zhang in 2010 proposed a <5th percentile cut-off as better predicting adverse neurodevelopmental outcome [6], whereas the PORTO study proposes EFW <3rd percentile in addition to abnormal umbilical artery Doppler flow

and oligohydramnios to be most consistently associated with adverse outcome [7].

In the past it was thought that relative sparing of head growth was an important parameter to determine outcome. For example, Tolsa and colleagues described a significant reduction in intracranial volume and in cerebral cortical grey matter in preterm newborns with FGR [8]. However, ultrasound measurement of head size depends on skull dimensions: brain growth slows before skull growth and so the concept of "brain sparing" based on skull measurement is incorrect [9]. FGR presenting later in pregnancy is likely to have less effect on head and presumably brain growth. A small and symmetrical head size may likewise be due to external factors – such as intrauterine infections – or to early placental insufficiency and poor brain growth, with significant effect on outcomes as demonstrated in the classic studies of Parkinson and colleagues [10]. Other measurements, such as body "fatness" as variously defined, have also been used: for example, a low ponderal index (<10th percentile) is better associated with adverse perinatal outcome compared to birth weight alone [11]. This is less popular because of the inherent error in measurement of neonatal length, which is then multiplied by 10^3 in the calculation [12].

Thus there is little substitute for careful screening of fetal size and investigation of at risk pregnancies to evaluate fetal condition and growth to identify FGR. Furthermore the identification and prospective follow-up of fetuses by experts may significantly reduce the risk of long-term problems; thus data derived from population studies, comprising fetuses with identified and unidentified FGR, may have worse outcomes than, for example, focused studies – for example, GRIT and TRUFFLE – where women with identified FGR are carefully monitored and delivery planned based on fetal health [13,14].

Populations of babies born after FGR undeniably have increased risk of a range of adverse outcomes

237

Table 26.1 Results of meta-regression, data from Damodaram et al. [1], and TRUFFLE data, calculated from Lees et al. [14]

Parameter	Group	24–27w * Percent (95%CI)	28–31 * Percent (95%CI)	32–36w * Percent (95%CI)
Neonatal death	FGR	21.8 (19.7–24)	15.5 (13.6–17.4)	9.5 (8–11.1)
	AGA	6.1 (5.8–6.3)	2.8 (2.7–2.9)	0.6 (0.5–0.7)
	TRUFFLE FGR	*11 (7–19)*	*5 (3–9)*	*1 (0.1–5)*
Intraventricular hemorrhage	FGR	32 (29.5–34.6)	14.8 (12.9–16.7)	2.1 (1.4–3.0)
	AGA	19.6 (19.1–20.2)	6.2 (6.1–6.4)	0 (0–0)
	TRUFFLE FGR	*5*	*3*	*1*
Sepsis	FGR	42.1 (32.7–51.9)	40.3 (35.1–45.7)	34.9 (26.6–43.7)
	AGA	16.9 (11.5–23.1)	15.5 (11.8–19.7)	12 (5.7–9.6)
	TRUFFLE FGR	*21*	*18*	*15*
Necrotizing enterocolitis	FGR	20.5 (18.1–23.1)	11.6 (9.7–13.7)	4.1 (3.0–5.5)
	AGA	8.1 (7.7–8.5)	2.8 (2.7–2.9)	0.1 (0–0.1)
	TRUFFLE FGR	*5 (2–10)*	*2 (1–5)*	
Respiratory complications	FGR	75.6 (71.7–79.2)	53.4 (49–57.7)	26.7 (23–30.6)
(Early)	AGA	41.3 (40.6–42)	20 (19.7–20.2)	3.5 (3.3–3.6)
(Later)	*TRUFFLE FGR*	*71*	*38*	*23*
	Ventilated	*33 (35–51)*	*16 (11–21)*	*4 (2–8)*
	BPD at 28d	*27 (20–35)*	*7 (4–11)*	*1 (0.1–5)*
	BPD at 36w			

* all meta-regression results FGR v AGA p<0.001 and gestational age effect p<0.001

as described in this chapter, but there are frequently challenges in ascribing such outcomes to FGR or to prematurity. In a recent meta-analysis, Damodaram and colleagues reported neonatal outcomes following FGR, which is a valuable starting point and demonstrates increased risk over the range of neonatal outcomes [1]. Table 26.1 shows their findings and the contrasting prevalence from TRUFFLE, as a contemporary cohort of FGR babies born after a tightly managed prenatal period:

Neonatal Mortality

Estimates of neonatal mortality due to FGR differ widely and are likely to depend on the population considered and the degree of fetal surveillance offered. Whereas the risk of fetal and neonatal death may be increased, there is uncertainty about the quantum of increased neonatal mortality in this group, and the data cited previously seem to show an unusually low mortality for AGA babies of 27 weeks or less. Many studies are small and not powered to identify an increased risk of a rare event such as neonatal death. In population studies the number of babies born

after true FGR, as opposed to being SGA, is relatively small. Birth weight standards for preterm children are derived usually from births rather than a whole fetal population and often these identify fewer SGA babies compared to populations defined using either fetal weight standards or customized growth charts. The study demonstrating this difference most clearly demonstrated that among VLBW babies, the relationship between cerebral palsy and small size for gestation is revealed only when fetal growth standards as opposed to birth weight standards are used [15]. Hence without careful population studies based on fetal growth standards and identifying prospectively identified and monitored FGR, it is difficult to identify increased mortality, and the identification of FGR itself may reduce mortality. Furthermore neonatal survival, particularly at very low gestations, is continuing to increase [16], and thus without prospective large and controlled studies, making firm conclusions about the quantum of increased risk is difficult.

It has generally held that the application of Doppler assessment of the circulation in an at-risk fetus has had a significant impact on reducing perinatal mortality [17]. In the meta-analysis by Damodaram, growth-restricted fetuses with both arterial and venous abnormalities had a higher risk of neonatal death and intracranial hemorrhage as compared to those with just arterial Doppler abnormalities.

In terms of recent data, Brodszki and colleagues reported a case series from a single center, demonstrating 90% survival to discharge home in babies born <30 weeks' gestation after FGR and long-term survival to 2 years, which was similar to their AGA background population [18]. In the PORTO study of more than 1,116 fetuses with an identified FGR (EFW <10th percentile), there were eight (0.7%) deaths, of which there were four neonatal deaths [7]. All mortalities in this study were of fetuses with EFW of <3rd percentile. Among the GRIT trial population (n = 587), the number of fetal/neonatal deaths overall did not differ between the immediate (12%) and delayed (11%) delivery groups, but the relative proportion of deaths before and after delivery was altered, early delivery was associated with more neonatal deaths, and delayed delivery with a greater proportion of fetal deaths [13]. Hence there may be a trade-off between more facilitative approaches to delivering the at-risk fetus compared to more conservative approaches complicating the quantification of neonatal mortality due to FGR alone. In the TRUFFLE cohort, intrauterine death was uncommon, neonatal mortality was related to gestational age at birth, being 12% at 26–27 weeks, 6% at 28–29 weeks, and 2% at 30–31 weeks [14]. This was substantially lower than the results of the meta-regression [1], thus it would seem that time and improving fetal surveillance may be producing better outcomes for this group.

Fetal mortality appears to be higher for twins affected by growth restriction as compared to singletons, but once born alive, neonatal outcome seems to be more closely aligned with gestational age [19].

Hence it is difficult to tease out whether the baby born after FGR is at increased risk of neonatal death, and many recent studies report relatively low neonatal mortality regardless of how the population is collected.

Neonatal Complications

Key neonatal organ systems are sensitive to perinatal hypoxia and acidosis, such as the lung, gut, and brain, in each of which there is anxiety about excess morbidity among babies born following FGR. Furthermore, with increasing neonatal survival, the perinatal team has confidence in delivering the baby at relatively early gestations before critical hypoxia/acidosis ensues; this of course may alter previously held associations with later morbidity that were mediated by these variables. The potential for poor outcomes is discussed in each system:

Lung: Factors leading to improved lung outcomes for preterm babies are the avoidance of perinatal acidosis and hypoxia. In severe FGR there may be additional anxiety concerning pulmonary hypoplasia in association with poor somatic growth and oligohydramnios, partly offset by the induction of surfactant and antioxidant synthesis by antenatal steroids. Studies evaluating the prevalence of lung disease in babies following FGR have shown inconsistent results. In the studies reported in the meta-analysis [1], definition was variable and the increase in respiratory problems reflected a range of early interventions, which were more prevalent in the FGR group and of a similar frequency to those in TRUFFLE. In the Lund FGR cohort of babies born before 30 weeks' gestation, the prevalence of bronchopulmonary dysplasia, as indicated by use of supplemental oxygen at 36 weeks post-menstrual age, was 65% compared to 37–40% in non-FGR groups [18], associated with longer periods on respiratory support and longer stay in neonatal care. This is probably a more important outcome as it reflects serious respiratory morbidity. In attempt to tease out FGR effects, Garite and colleagues evaluated outcomes following antenatal recognition of fetal growth restriction (FGR) and SGA [20]. Similar outcomes were observed with an increased need for respiratory support at 28 days in their large database. In contrast the prevalence of BPD (supplemental oxygen at 36 weeks) in the TRUFFLE group was 27% for births 26–27 weeks, 7% at 28–29 weeks, and 1% at 30–31 weeks. Thus older reports from large population studies do demonstrate increased risk of neonatal lung disease with FGR in various definitions, but the most recent study points to lower prevalence, which is highly dependent on gestation at delivery, as it is in the wider population. Thus the picture may change as fetal and neonatal care improves. There are no data to support the use of antenatal steroid in the face of FGR, but good practice usually includes treating such pregnancies when very preterm delivery is anticipated.

Gut: Necrotizing enterocolitis (NEC) is a condition characterized by a triad of gut hypoxia, infection, and feeding. Prevalence in different centers varies widely. Following FGR there is circulatory redistribution of blood flow, increasing flow to essential organs (e.g., brain, heart) and reducing flow to less critical tissues (e.g., muscle, gut, and kidney). Evidence of renal impairment is shown by oligohydramnios, but effects on other tissues are less obvious and it is likely that in babies born following FGR there has been exposure to gut hypoxia, fulfilling the first of the triad. Gut hypoxia may manifest as the clinical symptoms of increased gastric aspirates (residuals), delayed passage of meconium and persisting bowel distension, a pattern not infrequently seen following FGR, and one that tends to occur in the first 24 hours after birth. Clinical management of this situation is challenging: it is clear that administration of minimal enteral nutrition, particularly colostrum, may be prophylactic against NEC, but in the face of early symptoms, most neonatologists withhold feeds until distension settles. In a meta-analysis by Tyson and Kennedy, minimal enteral feeding (MEF) led to shorter duration of stay and shorter duration to full enteral feeding, but the rates of NEC were similar in MEF group as compared to the control group [21]. The ADEPT trial randomized growth-restricted infants to early and late feeding protocol, but found no difference in the NEC outcomes in both groups. The NEC risk increased with decreasing gestational age, and infants <29 weeks' gestation achieved full feeds later compared to those >28 weeks [22]. Withholding early feeds probably disrupts the normal endocrinological adaptation process after birth, which appears to follow the first feed and reduces the stimulus for gut growth and coordination of peristalsis [23]. Large trials are continuing to investigate this area, which is as controversial for extremely preterm babies as it is following FGR.

A range of studies have trialed various feeding practices to prevent or minimize the risk of feed intolerance or NEC in this population. To date no single strategy appears more effective, although the simple expedient of having an agreed feeding policy appears to be associated with a reduced risk of NEC. Some groups have focused on the use of pre- or probiotics. To date this area too remains controversial. Most probiotic trials have used different preparations, at varying doses, and most trials until recently have been relatively small. Current trials powered on a reduction in the prevalence of NEC have produced different effects, adding to the confusion as to whether probiotics are effective and what preparation and schedule

is effective [24–26]. Small early prebiotic trials using lactoferrin are encouraging [27].

Classical NEC has been associated with antenatal markers of FGR in a range of studies, and through a series of population analyses [1]. The relative risk of NEC rises in parallel with gestation, although it falls as an absolute risk, which suggests a real association with FGR, most complications of prematurity being less prevalent as gestation increases. (Table 26.1) The recent TRUFFLE data suggest that the prevalence may also be now even lower, being 5% (95%CI 2–10%) <28 weeks and only 2% (1–5%) at 28–31 weeks [14].

Brain: Fetal acidosis has been associated with a greater risk of irreversible developmental delay [28]. Prevention of fetal hypoxia and acidosis has been the central hypothesis of management of FGR. Absent or reversed end-diastolic flows through the umbilical arterial and venous systems have been associated with adverse neonatal outcomes. Various studies have used Doppler ultrasound to assess fetal circulation and effect of redistribution of flow through the umbilical venous and arterial systems, thus causing brain-sparing effect. Scherjon studied this effect of selective brain sparing in neonates born at 26–33 weeks' gestation. He used the ratio between umbilical and cerebral artery pulsatility index as a marker of redistribution of flow as a result of placental insufficiency. At 3 years of age, he did not find any difference in the neurodevelopmental outcome, suggesting fetal brain sparing as a benign adaptive mechanism to prevent severe brain damage [29].

Gestational age at delivery has a confounding negative effect on developmental outcome until 32–34 weeks' gestation. Several recent studies have shown impairments in general cognitive and a range of other quantitative scores of motor performance and childhood outcomes. Vossbecks evaluated 40 infants with absent and reversed end-diastolic flows (AREDF) in <30 weeks of gestation and demonstrated a higher incidence of severe motor impairment and lower general cognitive scores after 2.5 years, compared to gestational age-matched controls [30]. Similarly, Morsing demonstrated lower verbal and full-scale intelligence quotients following FGR compared to AGA controls before 29 weeks' gestation [31]. Similar findings were seen in a study by Shand of fetuses born <32 weeks with abnormal Doppler velocities. This study also reported that fetuses with abnormal AREDF delivered at 32–34 weeks' gestation had lower fine motor and neuropediatric scores, seemingly negating the protective effect of delivery at higher gestation [32].

However, in GRIT, 2-year and school-age outcomes did not differ between the allocated groups, suggesting delayed delivery had little effect on long-term outcome compared to immediate delivery [13]. This contrasts with TRUFFLE, which did demonstrate lower rates of neurodevelopmental impairment among survivors delivered in the late ductal venosus changes arm, offset by slightly higher mortality in the primary composite outcome [14]. Close surveillance and expectant management of FGR pregnancies may be one of the reasons for these outcomes.

Fetuses who develop late-onset FGR are at higher risk of perinatal mortality and are the highest cause of term stillbirth [33]. They are also at a higher risk to suffer long-term detrimental outcomes. In a study by Figueras of neonates with FGR in the third trimester with normal umbilical artery Doppler examination was associated with decreased scores in attention, habituation and motor, social-interactive, and state-regulation domains [34]. Leitner and colleagues followed the children with late-onset FGR until 10 years of age and demonstrated significant difference in the neurodevelopmental scores, intelligent quotient and school achievements [35].

There seems little doubt that cognitive development may be somewhat impaired in children born after identified FGR, and that this is irrespective of the gestational age at delivery, but early identification and close monitoring as specified in the TRUFFLE protocol late ductal changes arm may be associated with reduced rates of moderate or severe impairment.

Other Short- and Long-Term Systemic Effects of FGR

Cardiovascular: A FGR neonate is at high risk of suffering from neonatal hypotension due to myocardial dysfunction. Subclinical cardiac dysfunction occurs very early in the disease process and increases across all stages of fetal compromise. Assessment of fetal cardiac dysfunction can be achieved by fetal echocardiography. Modified myocardial performance index, blood B-type natriuretic peptide, and early-to-late diastolic filling ratios are all important prognostic indicators and increase in a stage-dependent manner. These indicators have been described as being raised in the FGR fetus with increased mortality [36,37].

Following FGR, the newborn baby can experience hypotension early in the postnatal period, due to myocardial dysfunction, but can later have hypertension and hypervolemia due to hemodynamic redistribution and adaptation to hypoxia. Molecular changes in the cardiac myocyte contractility machinery have also been demonstrated due to chronic hypoxia. These changes are similar to changes seen in dilated cardiomyopathy [38]. Nilsson studied the relationship of birth weight to systolic blood pressure at 18 years of age in Swedish boys and found statistically significant relationship of hypertension to low birth weight, which supports the effect of early molecular changes and altered programming as a result of growth restriction. This effect was more pronounced in subjects who were growth restricted and then had a rapid catch-up growth and were then at the highest BMI centile at 18 years of age [39].

Hematology: Chronic hypoxia leads to an increase in erythropoietin production, which in turn may increase red cell mass. This complication is seen in up to 5% of the growth-restricted neonates [40]. This in turn may lead to polycythemia with high hematocrit levels >70%, and this may be associated with plasma hyperviscosity, increased red cell "sludging," which manifest as free hemoglobin, and clinical syndrome thought to be associated with hypoglycemia, respiratory distress, and neurological symptoms. It remains unclear as to the benefit of the use of exchange transfusion in the face of high hematocrit.

Thrombocytopenia is also commonly seen in FGR neonates. In one study, approximately 51% of neonates suffered from mild to moderate thrombocytopenia and 9% severe. This may be due to increase in erythropoietin, which suppresses the megakaryocyte or due to decrease in the liver perfusion as a result of decrease ductus venosus flow, which is the main site for production of platelets in fetal life [41,42].

Thrombocytopenia can be due to other causes that need to be ruled out, e.g., congenital viral infections. In very few instances does this need active platelet transfusion, and mild-to-moderate thrombocytopenia can be reversed as soon as the hypoxic state is reversed.

Immunology and infection: Intrauterine hypoxia may lead to immune abnormalities in the growth-restricted fetus. FGR as a result of pregnancy-induced hypertension is associated with neutropenia in early postnatal life, which may affect susceptibility to infective factors.

241

Troger compared the white cell counts, neutrophil counts, and interleukin production of FGR infants <32 weeks' gestation and compared with age-matched AGA infants and found significantly lower WCC and neutrophil counts on day 0 and day 3 for FGR infants. This effect disappeared by day 7. He also found lower pro-inflammatory cytokine levels of IL-6 and IL-8 in SGA infants [43]. Although this theoretically can lead to higher susceptibility to infections, it has not been shown to be consistent, as quantitative deficiencies of the immune system are not directly linked to functional deficiencies.

In the PROGRAMS trial, neonates born less than 31 completed weeks of gestation and birth weight less than 10th centile were enrolled. Twenty-one percent of the neonates had a low neutrophil count of $<1.1 \times 10^9$/L at birth. Trial of granulocyte-monocyte colony-stimulating factor (GM-CSF) overall increased the neutrophil count in the treated arm, but this did not lead to direct reduction in sepsis episodes or survival, thus supporting the aforementioned fact [44].

Metabolic: FGR is associated with a range of endocrinological and consequent metabolic changes such as insulin resistance, hypoglycemia, and metabolic syndrome. Insulin, like growth factor-1, has an important role in the growth of the fetus. Studies have demonstrated that the levels of IGF-1 are reduced in an FGR fetus. These levels are also dependent on maternal nutritional status. Other hormonal factors that affect the growth-restricted fetus are decreases in the levels of insulin and thyroid-stimulating hormone, whereas there is an increase in growth hormone. Along with the endocrine changes, a growth-restricted fetus also demonstrates low glucose, albumin and cholesterol concentrations, and elevated concentrations of lactate and non-esterified fatty acid [45].

Hypoglycemia, especially fasting, is very common in growth-restricted infants. The greatest risk is seen in the first 3 days of life. This is mainly due to decrease in the liver glycogen stores and decrease in gluconeogenesis because of inactive enzyme systems and co-factors. There is also a decrease in the counter-regulatory response. Close monitoring of the glucose levels in the blood is mandated in the management of severely growth-restricted infants.

Long-term studies have shown that growth-restricted infants show metabolic alterations like insulin resistance and reduced glucose tolerance. They are at higher risk of developing type 2 diabetes mellitus, hypertension, and altered lipid metabolic profile, also termed as metabolic syndrome [46]. The etiological basis of adult disease as a result of growth restriction has not been completely delineated. One of the hypotheses for this has been the "thrifty genotype hypothesis," also termed as the "Barker hypothesis," which hypothesizes activation of particular genes for fetal growth and survival in an unfavorable environment [47].

Studies have also observed an early-onset insulin resistance as early as 1 year of age [48]. Visceral fat excess has also been shown to be present by the age of 6 in this group, thus enhancing insulin resistance.

Adult follow-up studies at 22–30 years of age tend to have higher insulin levels, arterial blood pressure, and higher metabolic prevalence than the AGA counterparts [49].

Growth: FGR can significantly impact the long-term growth outcomes [50]. Bocca-Tjeertes studied preterm neonates born with symmetrical and asymmetrical growth restriction and compared them with non-growth-restricted neonates. At 4 years of age, both symmetric and asymmetric growth-restricted neonates were shorter and lighter as compared to the AGA counterparts. There was a catch-up of growth of head circumference in symmetric growth-restricted infants, but this did not impact their long-term neurodevelopmental outcome [51].

Conclusion

Fetal growth restriction remains one of the leading causes of significant neonatal morbidity both in terms of immediate outcomes and of long-term development. As many of these babies deliver preterm, gestational age at birth and markers of vascular adaptation appear to remain important predictors for long-term outcome in this population [52]. Detection and close monitoring of pregnancies complicated by FGR may have an important impact on these important outcomes. Advances in perinatal and neonatal care have enabled fetuses with early-onset growth restriction to be delivered at an earlier gestational age before fetal compromise becomes irreversible, although the place and value of antenatal steroid in this group is unclear and the cost-effectiveness of early screening, close management, and delivery has not been systematically studied.

Prevention of growth restriction must remain the underlying strategy to reduce adverse long-term outcomes in this population. Important changes in fetal development occur before deterioration in growth and physiology are evident, and most fetuses with growth restriction are identified at a relatively late stage. Hence intervention and delivery may occur too late to alter the long-term outcome of these pregnancies.

Key preventive strategies to improve neonatal outcomes are still required and better markers of fetal health are necessary to determine the point at which the benefit from delivery is apparent.

Key Points

- The neonatal outcomes in small for gestational age babies are quite different to those of fetal growth restriction: SGA is a statistical construct based usually on a 10th percentile cut-off.

- The major systems affected by fetal growth restriction include brain, lung, cardiovascular and gut.

- No feeding regime has proven to reduce the incidence of necrotising enterocolitis.

- The magnitude of the effect of fetal growth restriction on mortality at very preterm gestation is probably over estimated.

- The value of antenatal steroids in fetal growth restriction is unproven.

- Most fetuses with growth restriction are identified late, and though timing of delivery is important in minimizing perinatal mortality, it may be too late to materially improve neurodevelopmental outcome.

References

1. Damodaram M, Story L, Kulinskaya E, et al. Early adverse perinatal complications in preterm growth-restricted fetuses. *Aust N Z J Obstet Gynaecol* 2011;51:204–9.

2. WHO 1995, *Expert Committee Report: Physical Status: The Use and Interpretation of Anthropometry*. Technical report series 854. World Health Organization, Geneva.

3. Lin CC, Santolaya-Forgas J. Current concepts of fetal growth restriction. Part 1. Causes, classification and pathophysiology. *Obstet Gynecol* 1998;92:1044–55.

4. Wilcox M, Gardosi J, Mongelli M, et al. Birth weight from pregnancies dated by ultrasonography in a multicultural British population. *BMJ* 1993 Sep 4; 307(6904):588–91.

5. Gardosi J, Chang A, et al. Customised antenatal growth charts. *Lancet* 1992;339:283–7.

6. Zhang J, Mikolajczyk R, et al. Prenatal application of the individualised fetal growth reference. *Am J Epidemiol* 2011;173:539–43.

7. Unterscheider J, Daly S, et al. Optimising the definition of intrauterine growth restriction: The multicentre prospective PORTO study. *Am J Obstet Gynecol* 2013;208:290,e1–6.

8. Tolsa CB, Zimine S, Warfield SK et al. Early alteration of structural and functional brain development in premature infants born with intrauterine growth restriction. *Pediatr Res* 2004 Jul;56(1):132–8.

9. Duncan KR, Issa B, Moore R et al. A comparison of fetal organ measurements by echo-planar magnetic resonance imaging and ultrasound. *BJOG* 2005 Jan;112(1):43–9.

10. Parkinson C, Wallis S, Harvey D School achievement and behaviour of children who were small-for-dates at birth develop. *Med Child Neurol* 1981;23:41–50.

11. Walther F, Ramaekers L, et al. The ponderal index as a measure of the nutritional status at birth and its relation to some aspects of neonatal morbidity. *J Perinat Med* 1982;10:42–7.

12. Williams MC, O'Brien WF. Cerebral palsy in infants with asymmetric growth restriction. *Am J Perinatol* 1997 Apr 14;(4):211–15.

13. The GRIT Study group. Infant wellbeing at 2 years of age in the growth restriction intervention trial (GRIT): Multicentred randomised controlled trial. *Lancet* 2004;364:513–20.

14. Lees C, Marlow N, et al. Perinatal morbidity and mortality in early-onset fetal growth restriction: Cohort outcomes of the trial of randomised umbilical and fetal flow in Europe (TRUFFLE). *Ultrasound Obstet Gynecol* 2013;42:400–8.

15. Jarvis S, Glinianaia SV, Torrioli MG, et al. Cerebral palsy and intrauterine growth in single births: European collaborative study. *Lancet* 2003;362:1106–11.

16. Moore T, Hennessy EM, Myles J, et al. Neurological and developmental outcome in extremely preterm children born in England in 1995 and 2006: The EPICure studies. *BMJ* 2012 Dec 4;345:e7961.

17. Morris RK, Malin G, at el. Fetal umbilical artery Doppler predict compromise of fetal/neonatal wellbeing in a high risk population: Systematic review and bivariate meta-analysis. *Ultrasound Obstet Gynecol* 2011;37:135–42.

18. Brodszki J, Morsing E, et al. Early intervention in management of very preterm growth-restricted fetuses: 2-year outcome of infants delivered in fetal indication before 30 gestational weeks. *Ultrasound Obstet Gynecol* 2009;34:288–96.

19. Manzanares S, Sanchez M, et al. Perinatal outcomes in preterm growth-restricted twins: Effects of gestational age and fetal condition. *Twin Res Hum Genet* 2013 Jun;16(3):727–31.

20. Garite T, Clark R, Thorp J. Intrauterine growth restriction increases morbidity and mortality among premature neonates. *AJOG* 2004;191:481e7.

21. Tyson JE, Kennedy KA. Minimal enteral nutrition for promoting feeding tolerance and preventing morbidity in parenterally fed infants. *Cochrane Database Syst Rev* 2000;(2):CD000504.

22. Kempley S, Gupta N, Linsell L, et al. Feeding infants below 29 weeks' gestation with abnormal antenatal Doppler: Analysis from a randomised trial. *Arch Dis Child Fetal Neonatal* Ed. 2014 Jan;99(1):F6–F11.

23. Dorling J, Kempley S, Leaf A. Feeding growth restricted preterm infants with abnormal antenatal Doppler results. *Arch Dis Child Fetal Neonatal* Ed. 2005;90:F359–F363.

24. Manzoni P, Meyer M, Stolfi I, et al. Bovine lactoferrin supplementation for prevention of necrotizing enterocolitis in very-low-birthweight neonates: A randomized clinical trial. *Early Hum Dev* 2014;90 Suppl 1:S60–5.

25. Costeloe K, Hardy P, Juszczak E, et al. Bifidobacterium breve BBG-001 in very preterm infants: A randomised controlled phase 3 trial. *Lancet* 2016 Feb 13; 387(10019):649–60.

26. Garland SM, Tobin JM, Pirotta M. The ProPrems trial: Investigating the effects of probiotics on late onset sepsis in very preterm infants. *BMC Infect Dis* 2011 Aug 4;11:210.

27. Barrington KJ, Assaad MA, Janvier A. The Lacuna Trial: A double-blind randomized controlled pilot trial of lactoferrin supplementation in the very preterm infant. *J Perinatol* 2016 Mar 3. doi: 10.1038

28. Soothill PW, Ajayi RA, Nicolaides KN. Fetal biochemistry in growth retardation. *Early Hum Dev* 1992 Jun–Jul;29(1–3):91–7.

29. Scherjon SA, Oosting H, Smolders-DeHaas H Neurodevelopmental outcome at three years of age after fetal "brain-sparing." *Early Hum Dev* 1998 Aug 28;52(1):67–79.

30. Vossbeck S, Kamargo OKD, et al. Neonatal and neurodevelopmental outcome in infants born before 30 weeks of gestation with absent or reversed end-diastolic velocities in the umbilical arteries. *Eur J Pediatr* 2001;160:128–34.

31. Morsing E, Asard M, et al. Cognitive function after intrauterine growth restriction and very preterm birth. *Pediatrics* 2011;127:e874–82.

32. Shand AW, Hornbuckle J, Nathan E. Small for gestational age preterm infants and relationship of abnormal umbilical artery Doppler blood flow to perinatal mortality and neurodevelopmental outcomes. *Aust N Z J Obstet Gynaecol* 2009 Feb;49(1):52–8.

33. Macdonald TM, McCarthy EA, Walker SP. Shining light in dark corners: Diagnosis and management of late onset fetal growth restriction. *Aust N Z J Obstet Gynaecol* 2015;55:3–10.

34. Figueras F, Gardosi J. Intrauterine growth restriction: New concepts in antenatal surveillance, diagnosis and management. *Am J Obstet Gynecol* 2011 Apr;204(4):288–300.

35. Leitner Y, Fattal-Valevski A, Geva R, et al. Neurodevelopmental outcome of children with intrauterine growth retardation: A longitudinal, 10-year prospective study. *J Child Neurol* May 2007;22(5):580–7.

36. Crispi F, Hernandez-Andrade E, et al. Cardiac dysfunction and cell damage across clinical stages of severity in growth-restricted fetuses. *Am J Obstet Gynecol* 2008 Sep;199(3):254.e1–8.

37. Comas M, Crispi F, et al. Usefulness of myocardial tissue Doppler vs conventional echocardiography in the evaluation of cardiac dysfunction in early-onset intrauterine growth restriction. *Am J Obstet Gynecol* 2010 Jul;203(1):45.e1–7.

38. Demicheva E, Crispi F. Long-term follow-up of intrauterine growth restriction: Cardiovascular disorders. *Fetal Diagn Ther* 2014;36:143–53.

39. Nilsson PM, Ostergren PO, Nyberg P, et al. Low birth weight is associated with elevated systolic blood pressure in adolescence: A prospective study of a birth cohort of 149,378 Swedish boys. *J Hypertens* 1997;15:1627–31.

40. Engineer N, Kumar S. Perinatal variables and neonatal outcomes in severely growth restricted preterm fetuses. *Acta Obstet Gynecol* 2010;89:1174–81.

41. Maruyama H, et al. Thrombocytopenia in preterm infants with intrauterine growth restriction. *Acta Med Okayama* 2008;62(5):313–17.

42. Vlug RD, Lopriore E, et al. Thrombocytopenia in neonates with polycythemia: Incidence, risk factors and clinical outcome. *Expert Rev Hematol* 2015; 8(1):123–9.

43. Tröger BM, Müller T, Faust K. Intrauterine growth restriction and the innate immune system in preterm infants of <32 weeks gestation. *Neonatology* 2013; 103:199–204.

44. Marlow N, Morris T, Brocklehurst P. A randomised trial of granulocyte-macrophage colony-stimulating factor for neonatal sepsis: Childhood outcomes at 5 years. *Arch Dis Child Fetal Neonatal Ed* 2015 Jul;100(4):F320–6.

45. Gluckman PD, Cutfield W, et al. Metabolic consequences of intrauterine growth retardation. *Acta Paediatr (suppl)* 1999;417:306.

46. Longo S, Bollani L, Decembrino L, et al. Short-term and long-term sequelae in intrauterine growth retardation (IUGR) *J Matern Fetal Neonatal Med* 2013;26(3):222–5.

47. Barker DJP, Eiksson JG, et al. Fetal origins of adult disease: Strength of effects and biological basis. *Int J Epidemiol* 2002;31:1235–9.

48. Soto N, Bazaes RA, et al. Insulin sensitivity and secretion are related to catch-up growth in small for gestational age infants at age 1 year: Results from a prospective cohort. *J Clin Endocrinol Metab* 2003;88:3645–50.

49. Meas T, Deghmoun S, Alberti C, et al. Independent effects of weight gain and fetal programming on metabolic complications in adults born small for gestational age. *Diabetologia* 2010 May;53(5):907–13.

50. Barker DJP. Adult consequences of fetal growth restriction. *Clin Obstet and Gynaecol* 49(2):270–83.

51. Bocca-Tjeertes I, Bos A, et al. Symmetrical and asymmetrical growth restriction in preterm-born children. *Pediatrics* 2014;133:e650–6.

52. Torrance HL, Bloemen MCT, et al. Predictors of outcome at 2 years of age after early intrauterine growth restriction. *Ultrasound Obstet Gynecol* 2010;36:171–7.

Chapter

27

Fetal Growth Restriction and Later Disease in the Mother and the Offspring

Birgit Arabin and Petra Arck

Introduction

The prevention of chronic illness is a major goal due to rising morbidity and mortality rates caused by non-communicable diseases (NCDs) worldwide. There are three times that a woman accesses the health care system: as an infant, during pregnancy and postpartum care, and in case of severe disease. For the majority, the peripartum period provides an early window of opportunity to identify risk factors improving not only the pregnancy outcome, but also the long-term health of herself and her offspring. The symptoms of chronic illnesses differ between men and women; many women die of cardiovascular disease (CVD) without prior warning, underlining that reducing illness should be addressed through improving awareness and prevention. Pregnancy complications such as preeclampsia (PE), gestational hypertension (GH), gestational diabetes mellitus (GDM), spontaneous preterm birth (SPB), and fetal growth restriction (FGR) are early identifiable markers for women's increased –yet still undiagnosed – risk of later disease and death [1–3].

Chronic diseases may originate prenatally. From the 1980s onward, David Barker and coworkers proposed that an adverse fetal environment may be a recipe for adult chronic disease, a claim referred to as the Barker Hypothesis [4–8] and even involving the placenta [9]. These studies correlated birth weight (BW) to the incidence of adult disease. Studies involving cohorts from the Dutch Hunger Winter have shown that, in addition to effects of prenatal food restriction on metabolism and CVD, there are gender-specific effects on age-associated cognitive functions. More recent publications highlight the disadvantageous effects of prenatal stress perception, medication, toxins, and infection for the future health of the unborn child [10]. The severity of diseases depends on critical periods when organs and tissues develop, catch-up growth, and the mismatch with the later environment.

Animal and human studies related to perfusion, endocrinology, immunology, and epigenetics start to evaluate the underlying mechanisms.

Unfortunately, health care providers and patients are still insufficiently aware of the associations between pregnancy-related problems and a woman's future health as well as of the associations of the fetal environment and future risks for the offspring. Accordingly, there are nearly no protocols connecting pregnancy risks with long-term follow-up of the infant or mother.

In this chapter, we highlight the epidemiology of under- or malnutrition and poor intrauterine growth, unrecognized and recognized maternal diseases combined with FGR and the impact for long-term maternal health, for individuals and society, and try to explain basic mechanisms linking FGR with underlying causes and long-term health of both mother and offspring. The issue of transition of care from the prenatal to the postpartum period for both mother and the offspring should lead to future health care concepts related to reduce the global long-term burden of chronic diseases across generations.

Epidemiology of Undernutrition: Impact for Mother and Child

On our planet, enough food is produced to supply everybody with around 2,400 kcal/day. Rice, wheat, and corn constitute roughly 30% of consumed calories in rich countries, in others up to 80% or more [11]. Even in industrialized countries, food containing essential micronutrients is likely to be more expensive [11], which impairs diet quality within low-income groups [12]. It has been shown that economic contraction in early pregnancy may be associated with FGR [13].

Adequate maternal nutrition related to workload and micronutrient density such as iron, copper, zinc, iodine, selenium, and vitamins A and D is prerequisite for healthy fetal growth. Even in countries with no absolute food shortage, such as Sri Lanka, a fourth of mothers and a third of all children were malnourished and thus at risk of anemia, mental illness, or poor immune system [14]. The 1,000-Day-Window (including 266 days of pregnancy) is a vulnerable period for physical and cognitive development, although the manifestation of visible symptoms may be late.

The eight Millennium Development Goals (MDGs) agreed to by all countries have been defined to meet the needs of the world's poorest. To **eradicate hunger and poverty** was the first MDG. The global poverty rate at $1.25/day (World Bank's definition), which is just enough to consume the daily minimum of 2,200 kcal/day, fell in 2010 to less than half the 1990 rate. Although the hunger reduction target was met in 2015, at the global level, 1.2 billion people are still living in extreme poverty, 842 million people and around 100 million children under the age of 5 are underweight [15], and 195 million are stunted (size not correlating with age) [16]. More than 90% of stunted children live in Africa and Asia, with around 10 countries (such as Afghanistan, Yemen, Guatemala, Burundi, and Ethiopia) having a stunting rate >50%! The fifth MDG, **to improve maternal health**, is the challenge not only to reduce maternal mortality rate, but also to improve maternal health care, which should decrease FGR and the resulting deficiencies. For girls, early chronic undernutrition can later lead to their children born with FGR and developing underweight or stunted growth. Thus a vicious circle of under- and malnutrition combined with risks of chronic diseases repeats itself (Figure 27.1).

The main goals of the Synthesis Report of the UN Secretary-General on the post-2015 agenda are to end poverty and fight inequality, including among women and children. To mobilize the political will to change will be easier when we know the roots and scientific and medical consequences of maternal malnutrition.

Cohort Studies Connecting Timely Regional Famine with the Health of Mothers and Children

Until recently, nothing had been known about the **vicious circle of malnutrition during pregnancy and its impact on the growth of fetal organs and the intellectual capacity of future generations within differently resourced societies** (Figure 27.1).

In 1977, Forsdhal described that children in Norway, raised in poor provinces in the early twentieth century and becoming prosperous thereafter, suffered as adults from excess rates of myocardial infarction [17].

In 1986, Barker and colleagues showed that the distribution of CVD in England was related to a person's birthplace [18]. A geographical relation was found between mortality rates from ischemic heart disease in 1968–78 and infant mortality in 1921–25. The hypothesis "*fetal origins of disease*" was proposed to explain associations between low birth weight (LBW) <2500 grams (g) and impaired glucose tolerance or CVD [19–23]. The authors proposed the **thrifty phenotype hypothesis** suggesting that fetal and early postnatal malnutrition induces poor development of pancreatic β-cell mass and program the metabolic syndrome [24,25]. LBW was related to high concentrations of split proinsulin, a sign of beta-cell dysfunction, linked to later high blood pressure [26,27] and to metabolic abnormalities in combination with low physical activity and/or high energy intake [28]. If hunger occurred in the first and second trimesters, the adult experienced high blood pressure and type-2 diabetes; hunger in the third trimester was associated with high blood pressure, high levels of low-density lipoprotein, cholesterol, and fibrinogen [29]. The British Maternal Nutrition Study correlated prenatal micronutrient deficiency with increased insulin resistance in childhood: the offspring of mothers with combined high folate and low vitamin B12 levels were most insulin resistant [30].

Vice versa, in the 1990s, it was demonstrated that a pregnancy with an LBW child indicates a risk for impaired maternal health or that predisposing risks affect the growth of her offspring: mothers delivering a child with FGR exhibited significantly lower early and late insulin, C-peptide, and proinsulin responses than controls. Insulin sensitivity was increased in the FGR compared to the control group [31].

Kannisto and colleagues analyzed cohorts during the **1866–1868 famine in Finland**, assessing survival from birth up to 80 years (!) and older. Survival from birth to 17 years of age was significantly lower in cohorts born before and during than in the cohorts born after the famine. Survival from 17 to 80 years and mean remaining lifetime were similar, suggesting that, after the crisis had passed, Finish people carried no further survival risks [32]. Similarly, the cohort mortality after the **1974–1975 Bangladesh famine** was

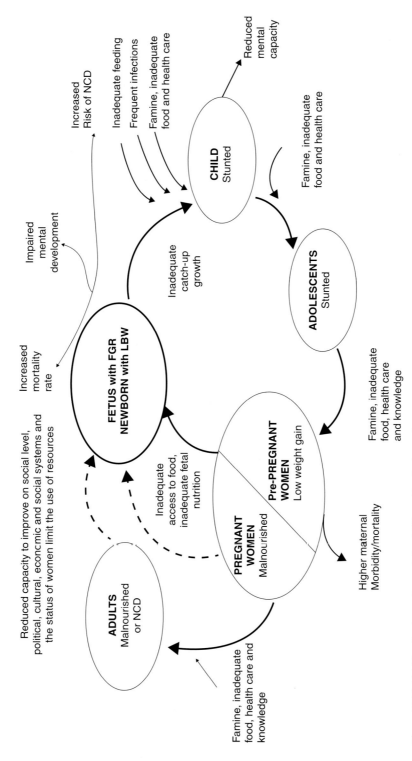

Figure 27.1 Nutrition, fetal growth retardation (FGR), and low birth weight (LBW) determining the life circle – a vicious circle for low-resourced countries. Adapted from UNICEF (1998) *The State of the World's Children* 1998. Oxford: Oxford University Press and the 4th Report – The World Nutrition Situation: Nutrition throughout the Life Cycle; 2000: Nutrition throughout the Life Cycle; United Nations, Sub–committee on Nutrition (ACC/SCN) in collaboration with International Food Policy Research Institute (IFPRI), (ACC/SCN) The UN System's Forum for Nutrition, United Nations.

examined, showing that famine-born cohorts continued to have a higher mortality in the second year of life, followed by a lower than usual mortality between 2 and 5 years [33]. Neonatal mortality was higher among infants conceived during the famine, whether it was malnutrition, lack of antenatal care, or stress, suggesting that in a chronically undernourished population, the impact of maternal famine on the age-specific mortality of the offspring is determined by a heterogeneous individual disposition.

The **Dutch Famine Birth Cohort Study** considers long-term effects of prenatal starvation among women born in Amsterdam before, during, or after the Hunger Winter [34]. Between August 1944 and April 1945, the average supply had been less than 1,000 calories/day from government food rations, and a later within-family analysis with siblings born between 1960 and 1985 revealed that BW was decreased when famine exposure of their mothers was in the third trimester, but not when it was in the first trimester. However, the expected increase in BW of the offspring with birth order was reversed after maternal exposure in the first trimester even after adjustment of other factors [35]. The results suggested that biologic effects depend on timing of gestational exposure and are still present in subsequent generations. Similarly, prenatal famine exposure during the Dutch Hunger Winter was associated with impaired glucose tolerance and insulin secretion in adulthood [36,37]. People who were conceived during the famine had doubled rates of CVD and atherogenic plasma lipid profiles, were at increased risk of schizophrenia, depression, or stress responsiveness, and performed worse on cognitive tasks correlated with accelerated ageing [38].

The 1959–1961 **Great Leap Forward Famine in China** has been a challenge to examine cohort mortality whereby the non-famine cohort caught up to and exceeded the famine cohort between 11 and 12 years, suggesting debilitating and selection effects [39]. Multilevel models revealed the underlying dynamic mortality convergence between famine and non-famine cohorts caused by differential excess infant mortality [39].

As in Dutch studies, it was shown that early gestational exposure to the famine in China was associated with a risk of schizophrenia in the offspring whereby micronutrient deficiencies were discussed [40]. Further studies identified a decline in sex ratio, followed by a compensatory rise 2 years after the famine ended, supporting the hypothesis that mothers in good condition are more likely to give birth to sons, mothers in poor condition to daughters [41].

In most of the studies, famine by itself cannot be clearly separated from stress and anxieties during pregnancy, mainly when hunger was combined with the trauma of war. Analogously, during the Chernobyl disaster, the perceived level of stress predicted the offspring's risk of cognitive disorders better than the actual exposure to radiation [42]. Conditions during and mainly after famine periods varied between countries, e.g., in the Netherlands, the Second World War was followed by a period of abundance, whereas in Russia, life conditions remained poor throughout adulthood – and no adverse effects on metabolic disorders have been found [43], suggesting that it is beneficial when the postnatal environment matches the prenatal environment.

However, there are individual differences in susceptibility toward hunger and stress dependent on the genetic background of the individual as recently summarized [44].

Maternal Diseases and Environmental Influences

Fetal growth restriction without maternal undernourishment has multifactorial origins. We here concentrate on diseases with bidirectional processes or already underlying maternal diseases and not on fetal syndromes. New studies imply that maternal well-being impacts fetal development in profound ways and that vice versa the pregnancy outcome may indirectly mirror subclinical and future maternal health risks.

Preeclampsia and Medical Complications Underlying Placental Disease

Risk factors of preeclampsia (PE) and FGR have been described, such as older maternal age, high BMI, primiparity, family history of preeclampsia, diabetes mellitus, chronic hypertension, renal disease, ethnicity, and socioeconomic status. Already in 2002 it was reported in *Nature* that first-trimester plasma levels of pregnancy-associated plasma protein-A (PAPP-A) are associated with placental nutrient transfer and highly correlated with BW [45]. Meanwhile, more complex first-trimester screening algorithms for PE and FGR offer individual risk prediction, a chance for a prevention of progression of the disease during pregnancy [46–48].

The clinical presentation of PE or FGR ranges from severe and rapidly progressing early-onset to late-onset. Endothelial dysfunction is the final common pathway of the two postulated entities. New guidelines support the use of signs of maternal organ dysfunction and placental soluble fms-like tyrosine kinase receptor-1 (sFlt-1), an antagonist of vascular endothelial and placental growth factor (PlGF) for surveillance [49].

The pathophysiological basis of PE and/or FGR can also be categorized into disease profiles such as "**personal** (maternal age, ethnicity, parity, tobacco use, history of pregnancy complications), **placental** (poor uterine Doppler profiles, a variety of serum biomarkers), **cardiovascular** (history of hypertension, renal disease, elevated blood pressure), **metabolic** (increased BMI, prior diabetes or gestational diabetes), and **prothrombotic** (thrombophilia), as summarized by Baschat for PE [50].

The retrospective evaluation of **cardiovascular, metabolic, and prothrombotic risk profiles** in women with a history of PE in the Netherlands revealed that 77% of patients had at least one risk profile whereby the CV one was most prevalent (66.1%), followed by hyperhomocysteinemia (18.7%), metabolic syndrome (15.4%), and thrombophilia (10.8%) [51]. Both **circulatory and metabolic risk** profiles were associated with earlier onset of PE and FGR. Delivery of an infant with FGR is more likely in patients with a diastolic blood pressure above 80 mm Hg [52]. The discussion whether early therapy of hypertension is beneficial since high blood pressure damages placental vessels or increases the risk of FGR due to uteroplacental underperfusion is still investigated [53,54]. Increased risk profiles and the combination of hypertensive disorders of pregnancy (HDP) and GDM raise the risk of premature maternal vascular disease not only during pregnancy. Therefore, the American Heart Association guidelines on female CV disease include GDM and HDP in their risk assessment [55]. Unfortunately, up to now, the surveillance of CV risk factors after pregnancy is underappreciated by women and their physicians. Although a balanced diet and physically active lifestyle reduce the risk for diabetes in women with GDM in the American Diabetes Prevention Program trial, adoption of these health behaviors is up to now low [56]. The parallel rise in PE rates and cardiovascular, renal, and metabolic complications further supports the importance of these risk profiles as being causative.

Thrombophilia and systemic lupus erythematosus (SLE) are associated with placental dysfunction, FGR, and PE. In patients with coagulation disorders, therapy with aspirin or heparin may decrease the rate of adverse outcome [57,58]. However, the generalized administration of anticoagulants for prevention of placental disease is not supported [57] until randomized trials show a benefit. In patients with **antiphospholipid syndrome (APS)** previous thrombosis, the presence of SLE and triple antiphospholipid antibody positivity (aPL) are independent risk factors for FGR. Women with thrombosis and triple APL positivity seem to have a higher live birth rate and less severe FGR when treated with additional second line therapy [59]. Complement system activation and inflammatory changes induce disorders in trophoblast invasion and placentation, indicating the use of prednisolone. The therapy of **hyperhomocysteinemia** with high-dose folic acid in all women or in women with elevated homocysteine levels is meanwhile being investigated [50].

A history of hypertension, renal disease, and GH preferably represents a cardiovascular risk; an increased BMI, diabetes, or GDM and a history of thrombophilia are indicative of prothrombotic risks. The parallel rise in PE, maternal long-term cardiovascular, renal, and metabolic complications, and first-trimester prediction concepts prior to the onset of PE/FGR support the assumption that risk profiles are causative [50].

The **placenta** modulates fetal responses to the environment. The described diseases may cause disturbances of perfusion and finally of diffusion. Placental invasion, size, and function are not only sensitive to undernutrition, but also to disturbances of maternal blood flow induced by the described maternal profiles, oxygen tension, and glucocorticoids. This "gateway" to the fetus modifies epigenetic marks and placental gene expression with sex-specific placental function leading to gender-specific diseases [60]. The placental vascular lesions of PE and severe FGR, such as "atherosis in the placental bed," are similar to observations in atherosclerosis, suggesting common genotypes and phenotypes. Research is now focusing on ways to reduce inflammation and oxidative stress in the placenta and the fetus.

The Impact of Pregnancy Complications on Later Maternal Health

Up to now, much less attention has been focused on the reciprocal relation between adverse pregnancy outcomes, such as PE, GDM, preterm birth, and FGR, and the mother's subsequent health. Interesting data are now linking maternal vascular, metabolic, and inflammatory complications of pregnancy and specifically FGR with an increased risk of NCDs in later life [2,61]. Women who had an LBW baby seem to be at around 10-fold risk of mortality from CVD compared to women with a baby of >3,500g [62,63]. These findings were not confounded by socioeconomic status or smoking.

Women who deliver babies that are both preterm *and* FGR **like in the Truffle study** appear to be at the greatest risk of later CVD! A Swedish national registry investigated women with first singleton births between 1983 and 2005 [64]. The reason for choosing 1983 as the start of the study was that information about mothers' smoking habits has been routinely collected since 1983. Follow-up of 923,586 women started at the first delivery and ended at December 31, 2005, or the date of first occurrence of the first CVD event, emigration from Sweden, or death. Incidence in CVD was defined as the first hospitalization or death caused by coronary heart disease (defined as unstable angina or acute myocardial infarction), cerebrovascular events (defined as cerebral infarction, cerebral hemorrhage, subarachnoid hemorrhage, transient ischemic attack, or other acute stroke), or heart failure. The hazard ratio of CVD ranged from 1.39 (95% CI: 1.22–1.58) to 2.57 (95% CI: 1.97–3.34) among mothers of moderately (32–37 weeks) and very preterm (28–31 weeks) infants, respectively. Among mothers of infants with severe FGR, the hazard ratio of CVD ranged from 1.38 (95% CI 1.15–1.65) to 3.40 (95% CI: 2.26–5.11) in mothers of term and very preterm (<32 weeks) infants, respectively. The highest rates of CVDs were found in mothers of very small and very preterm infants, also after adjustment for age as after adjustment for smoking! Maternal risks of CVD were not attenuated after BMI adjustment.

In another Swedish publication including 783,814 deliveries, offspring BW was inversely associated with cardiovascular and all-cause mortality even in both parents whereby the adjusted hazard ratio for cardiovascular mortality in mothers with 0.75 for each standard deviation was stronger than for fathers [65]. Low BW is even associated with increased mortality in grandparents [66]. This might mean that women at risk for CVD and FGR may carry genetic defects that contribute to both disease processes since a study looking at single nucleotide polymorphisms showed an association between variation in genes for cholesterol metabolism and decreased BW [67] cited in [61].

However, since the impact of the mother is stronger, other mechanisms are hypothesized: Women who are at high risk of CVD may not be able to mount an adequate hemodynamic response, leading to FGR and/or preeclampsia. The cardiac changes can be visualized by maternal echocardiography showing increases in chamber dimensions and left ventricular wall thickness consistent with hypertrophy. The likelihood of developing preeclampsia and/or FGR is increased by many maternal demographic and medical characteristics, such as hypertension, obesity, and age indicative of increased cardiovascular risk [68].

The possibility that maternal vascular risk factors are potentially "modifiable" before and after pregnancy [50], and correlate with increased risk of FGR and fetal programming, possibly impairing long-term cognitive development, requires further investigation. The mechanisms whereby women experiencing FGR later develop CVS are not yet sufficiently investigated. Nevertheless, the development of FGR may represent a unique opportunity to identify women at risk of long-term CVD before conventional symptoms become clinically apparent or before they might die from sudden insults. It is therefore an obligation for obstetricians to communicate these risks to general physicians for regular follow-up at a time where human "plasticity" still allows interventions for prevention (Figure 27.2) and might even be a future task for "the Truffle group" to follow not only the infants, but also their mothers, fathers, or grandparents.

Maternal Stress

Acute stress responses activate the hypothalamus-pituitary-adrenal axis (HPA) and the immune system, enabling the organism to deal with environmental threats. However, prolonged activation of the stress response may have adverse consequences for the individual.

Maternal stress, anxiety, and depression evoke immediate changes in blood flow to the uterus followed by fetal heart rate (FHR) or fetal movements (FM) patterns, but also induce fetal long-term changes in growth, metabolic disease, behavior, and cognition. Since there are no direct neural connections between mother and fetus, acute and chronic responses are elicited by neuroendocrine, autonomic, or vasodilatory input – partly in service of energy conservation.

251

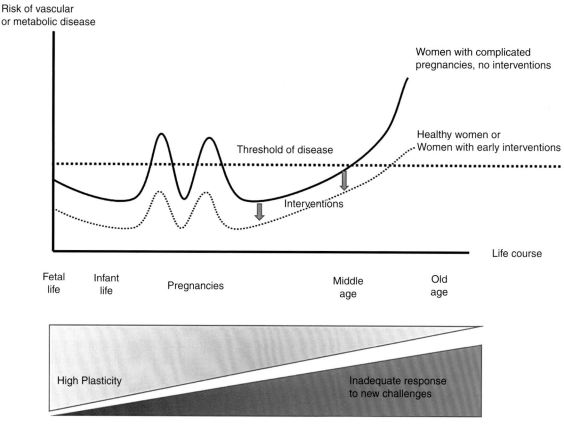

Figure 27.2 Effect of developmental environment on later maternal phenotype and pregnancy complications.
Risk for noncommunicable diseases (NCD) increases throughout a life course due to loss of plasticity, whereby the trajectory is set early. In women with increased underlying risk factors, pregnancy complications may be considered as the first "markers" and thus allow earlier surveillance and intervention strategies than waiting for first symptoms of chronic disease. Preventive measures require long-term investments, but are more likely to be effective after pregnancy than measures after the disease has manifested. Adapted from Sattar et al. [2] and Godfrey et al. [69]

Most results analyzing relationships of stressors are from well-educated women who volunteered to participate and may be different from women of other backgrounds.

Vice versa, FGR has been associated with "hostility" in adult life, e.g., a rival cynic personality with mistrust and negative affections, which again is combined with CVD [70].

Fascinating horizons arise if we imagine that even the fetus actively contributes to its own epigenesis: It was shown that FMs between 20 and 38 gestational weeks transiently stimulate maternal sympathetic arousal, whereby women did not become desensitized but were positively prepared for caretaking [71]. Listening to relaxing music has been shown to reduce pregnant women's experience of stress, anxiety, and depression and might also stimulate the fetus [72].

The interplay of maternal stress on metabolic disorders in the next generation has been investigated: Only 2/45 known type 2 diabetes susceptibility genes are associated with LBW, indicating that the association is mainly non-genetic. The developing fetal brain requires sufficient, but not overwhelming stress. In a univariate analysis and a logistic regression model, poor education, smoking, drinking habits, and social activities were associated with FGR [73]. Similarly, a threefold increase of FGR in relation to a poor social support has been reported. Even exposure to modern media "attacks" was found to reduce BW by 50g as compared to controls [74]. Maternal exposure to a death of a close relative is also correlated with LBW, whereby the effect was strongest during the second trimester when maternal spiral arteries invade the trophoblast cells whereby there is a dysregulation of the HPA [75].

Maternal endocrine factors such as ß-HCG or progesterone play a **gender-specific role** for poor growth and later diseases during critical periods. In a multivariable regression model, increase in maternal progesterone by 1 ng/ml during the first trimester increased girls' BW by 10.17 g (95% CI: 2.03–18.31); perceived worries (and smoking) during early pregnancy predicted FGR in boys irrespective of progesterone levels [76]. Fascinating new reviews of maternal stress and its implications as shown in animal and human research are available from Johns Hopkins University [44,77].

Smoking, Toxic Agents and Infection

Maternal smoking is one of the most frequent modifiable risk factors associated with FGR and adverse outcomes. It has been estimated that at least 20% of LBW infants are attributed to tobacco exposure during pregnancy and that exposure to passive smoking also has adverse effects [78]. FGR with BW <10th percentile was associated with smoking habits in a dose-dependent way (adjusted OR: 2.40 for 0–9, OR: 2.68 for 10–15, OR: 2.88 for >15 cigarettes daily).

Associations of parental smoking with offspring CVD have been demonstrated in pre-pubertal children [79]. After puberty, the effect of smoking at age 17 showed that parental smoking was positively associated with weight, height, and BMI (p <0.001) with a significant dose response for each additional 10 cigarettes smoked daily by both parents. The associations of maternal smoking were larger than for paternal smoking. At the age of 32, however, offspring of at least one smoking parent had higher weight, height, BMI, and waist circumference (WC) independent of characteristics at birth or of genetic variation, and there were significant associations between paternal smoking and these offspring variables for each additional 10 cigarettes/day. The associations between maternal cigarette numbers and offspring CVD tended to be smaller! Adjusted weight at age 17 was 63.2 kg for offspring of nonsmoking parents compared to 64.6 kg of at least one smoking parent and at age 32, 68.3 kg and 70.5 kg, respectively [80].

In many countries, pregnant mothers do not smoke but are exposed to **wood fuel smoke**, inducing placental hypoxia via carbon monoxide, which depresses energy-dependent processes and amino acid transport. It was shown that exposure to wood fuel smoke exhibits a reduction of infants' adjusted mean BW by -186 g [81]. Genetic variation in genes encoding enzymes that detoxify the products of cigarette smoking modify the associations between maternal cigarette smoking and BW, but the contribution of epigenetic mechanisms, rather than genetic, underlie the long-term effects of smoke exposure as shown in aberrant placental metabolism, syncytial knot formation, or markers of placental oxidative damage [82].

A variety of toxins has been investigated by two approaches to have an impact on FGR when pregnant mothers are exposed. **Exposure-type studies** include atomic bomb effects in Japan, patients with radio/chemotherapy, or mothers who have attempted suicide with large doses of chemicals. Babies born to self-poisoning females were found to have lower BWs than babies born before the suicide attempt [83]. **Cluster-type studies** include registries of mothers related to a common exposure to environmental or occupational toxins. We evaluated exposure to chemical substances (organic solvents, carbon tetrachloride, herbicides, chlorophenols, polychlorinated biphenyls, aromatic amines, lead and lead compounds, mercury and mercury compounds) and LBW using data from a prospective cohort study of 3,946 pregnant women in West Germany recruited between 15 and 28 gestational weeks by a job-exposure matrix weighted for working hours per week. The results of the dichotomous logistic regression analysis suggested that exposition to chlorophenols and aromatic amines were significantly associated with an LBW baby. Environmental toxins are ubiquitous and can affect the fetal epigenome; therefore screening for exposure is important in females of reproductive age.

As a result of **maternal inflammation**, the fetus is exposed to increased expression of cytokines, chemokines, and/or lipid mediators and it was speculated that reprogramming of the fetal immune response may predispose to diseases in adulthood [84]. In mice, impaired lung growth and pulmonary function are most severe after exposure to maternal inflammation and neonatal hyperoxia. As adults, these mice show systolic failure, increased left ventricular end systolic volumes, decreased posterior wall thickness, and decreased myocardial capillary density [85]. With younger gestational age infants surviving after maternal inflammatory conditions such as obesity or diabetes, the need to better understand these mechanisms is essential.

Malaria, especially when complicated by placental intervillositis, is a main contributor of FGR in endemic areas. Transplacental glucose transport by glucose transporter isoform 1 (GLUT-1), which impacts the syncytiotrophoblast microvillus and basal plasma membranes, is reduced in Plasmodium falciparum-positive placental specimens and correlated with LBW [86].

Mechanisms with an Impact for Health of Mother and Offspring

As outlined, FGR is a strong predictor for poor short- and long-term health outcomes. The identification of pathways causing FGR and placental insufficiency are and will be continuously evaluated by laboratory animal research and by correlating epidemiologic and epigenetic results. We here only summarize some underlying mechanisms.

First Steps to Correlate Placental Perfusion, Maternal Diet and Offspring Outcome

One of the first studies was conducted in guinea pigs, when unilateral uterine artery ligation resulted in FGR and hypertension in the offspring [87]. Feeding pregnant rats low-protein diets induced FGR during the last two gestational days, resulting in LBW and increased blood pressure; different protein compositions can have different effects on growth and later blood pressure or induce insulin resistance; a balanced maternal nutritional reduction had less distinct effects, suggesting that the balance of nutrients may be more critical than total amounts [88].

Endocrine Mechanisms

Maternal endocrine and immune markers synergistically maintain a tolerogenic niche in normally progressing pregnancies. This ensures decidualization, placentation, and ultimately proper placental function [10]. In eutherian mammals, the placenta ensures fetal supply with nutrients or oxygen and controls waste exchange between the fetal and maternal systems. Progesterone is crucial for pregnancy success, as it triggers decidualization of endometrial stromal cells at the onset of pregnancy and sustains uterine quiescence later during gestation. Reduced levels can affect the course of pregnancy and account for an increased risk for pregnancy complications, including LBW. Increasingly, heme oxygenase (HMOX)-1 – an enzyme catalyzing the degradation of heme into

carbon monoxide, biliverdin, and iron – is recognized as a critical mediator of pregnancy maintenance and placental function by promoting vasculature formation [89]. In mice and humans, the placenta expresses HMOX-1. Insights from genetically engineered mice reveal that implantations lacking HMOX-1 result in FGR [90]. The importance of HMOX-1 in human pregnancies is independently confirmed by a case report describing that HMOX-1 deficiency resulting from a spontaneous gene mutation in a male child is associated with FGR [91].

The maternal brain regulates reproduction via the physiological activation of the HPA axis [92]. Corticoid-releasing hormone (CRH) stimulates the maternal pituitary gland, leading to increasing levels of ACTH, which activates the release of cortisol from the adrenal gland. During pregnancy, cortisol also stimulates placental CRH synthesis [93,94] released into maternal blood during the second and third trimesters [95,96]. This physiological state of "hypercortisolism" during mammalian pregnancy is essential to meet the **maternal demand** for increased metabolism. Energy generation and pituitary-derived gonadotrophins stimulate the production of progesterone. In mice, similar endocrine adaptations occur, mirrored by a dramatic increase of plasma corticosterone in the second half of pregnancy. The fetus requires glucocorticoids to ensure growth and development of organs. Hence, glucocorticoids substantially prepare the fetus for postnatal adaptation and survival. Until late in gestation, the fetus is not capable of producing glucocorticoids. Corticosterone secretion by adrenal glands in fetal mice only commences at gestation day (gd) 15.5, peaks at 16.5 and declines before birth at 18.5 gd [97,98]. However, glucocorticoid receptors are expressed in the fetal lung, thymus, and liver prior to fetal glucocorticoid synthesis. Surprisingly, children born with the inability to make cortisol do not show impaired postnatal adaptation, e.g., abnormal lung development. Similarly in mice, normal fetal lung development is maintained in mutant mice that are unable to synthesize corticosterone. This explains that the transplacental glucocorticoid transfer sufficiently promotes fetal development even in the absence of its own production.

This transplacental transfer of glucocorticoids is regulated by two placental enzymes, 11β-hydroxysteroid dehydrogenase (HSD) type 1 (11βHSD-1) and type 2 (11βHSD-2) [99]. 11 βHSD-1 converts largely inert cortisone (11-dehydrocorticosterone in rodents) into active cortisol (corticosterone), whereas 11βHSD-2 converts active glucocorticoids into inactive glucocorticoids. Placental 11βHSD-1 is expressed at relatively low levels during early gestation and rises late in gestation. It is acknowledged that the role of placental 11βHSD-1 is to promote glucocorticoid transfer to the fetus. Placental glucocorticoid-inactivating 11βHSD-2 is highly expressed early to mid-gestation in normally progressing mammalian pregnancies, e.g., in the syncytiotrophoblast in humans and the labyrinth in rodents, and it declines late in gestation. Its functional role in normally progressing pregnancies includes the promotion of placental vascularization and nutrient transfer to the fetus. Moreover, placental 11βHSD-2 prevents the premature maturation of fetal organs by limiting the amount of glucocorticoid transferred to the fetus during early gestation. It may also protect the fetus from an excessive maternal glucocorticoid surge, e.g., in response to stress [100,101]. Hence, the fetal supply with glucocorticoids results from the spatial and temporal plasticity of placental 11βHSD-1 and 11βHSD-2 activity [99,102] whereby the plasticity of placental 11βHSD-2 acts as a "gatekeeper" according to fetal needs: its physiological decrease late in gestation facilitates the transplacental transfer of glucocorticoids when needed, e.g., to promote lung maturation. Vice versa, the high placental 11βHSD-2 activity seen during early to mid-gestation protects the fetus from excess maternal glucocorticoid levels, which may then interfere with the development of fetal organs such as the lung and immune system. The "gatekeeper" is vulnerable to excess fetal glucocorticoids found in undernutrition, infections, and inflammation, suggesting an insufficiency of placental 11βHSD-2 activity. Moreover, maternal anxiety is associated with excess fetal glucocorticoids, indicating that placental 11βHSD-2 activity may not suffice in response to stress. Overall, insufficient placental 11βHSD-2 activity and associated excess fetal glucocorticoid exposure results from high levels of free, biologically active maternal glucocorticoids and inflammation at the feto maternal interface, perpetuated by low progesterone levels. The maternal-fetal glucocorticoid gradient is physiologically approximately four times higher in late gestation. Fetal exposure to excess maternal glucocorticoids is hypothesized to be one of the most powerful links between fetal development and an impaired later health, as shown in animal experiments by an increase of maternal glucocorticoids resulting in LBW offspring with an activated HPA axis, adverse metabolic profile, and specific behavioral patterns in adulthood.

Epigenetic Mechanisms

The majority of genes are expressed by two parental alleles, but less than 1% are subject to parental imprinting. There is dynamic reprogramming of imprinting markers in primordial germ cells dependent on the gender during gamete maturation. The imprinted 11p15 region is essential for fetal growth; imprinted genes play a role in placental growth [103].

The term "epigenetic" was coined in the early 1940s by Conrad Waddington to explain "the interactions of genes with their environment, which bring the phenotype into being"; meanwhile, the term includes the field of phenotypes resulting from chromosomal changes without alterations in DNA sequence [104]. Epigenetic modifications include DNA methylation, histone modification, or non-coding RNA expression [105]. During early embryogenesis, the mammalian genome is "wiped clean" of epigenetic changes. Germ cells are de-methylated in the haploid genome and the preimplantation period in order to restore the genome to a pluripotent state; re-methylation occurs in anticipation of reproductive capability [106]; also DNA of somatic cells is de- and re-methylated during fetal development [107]. **Methylation of DNA** sequence of imprinted or non-imprinted genes, specifically in areas of CpG islands, is linked with long-term silencing of genes. In case of adverse nutritional status, such as a lack of folate, vitamin B12, and methionine, changes in the fetal epigenome are linked to FGR and later to obesity, insulin resistance, and hypertension in the offspring [107]. Positive correlations have been found between low methylation across the HSD2 region 1 and BW; DNA methylation at key genes in human peripheral blood at 40 years of life was associated with BW and later CVD [108]. Global DNA hypo-methylation was found in mothers with elevated bone lead stores; also metal-induced oxidative stress is thought to be a mechanism accounting for altered methylation and in humans exposed to cigarette smoke in utero [109]. **Histone modification** occurs in the context of short-term or flexible changes in gene expression [105]. Acetylation of lysine residues on the tails of histones correlates with chromatin and gene transcription and is accomplished by activities of histone acetyltransferases. Conversely, genes can be silenced by de-acetylation. Histone modifications have been linked to sustained pro-inflammatory responses in vascular smooth muscle and endothelial cells in animals [110]. Crosstalk between DNA methylation and histone modification occurs. **Non-coding RNAs**, especially **micro(mi)RNAs**, are likely to play a role in temporally controlled gene expression essential for normal development and were dramatically increased in mother and fetus in chorioamnionitis [111]. Recent studies have shown that human miRNAs can also induce chromatin remodeling, suggesting that DNA methylation, histone modification, and miRNAs may work in concert.

Epigenetic marks may be transmitted across generations, either by persisting through meiosis in primordial germ cells or through replication in the next generation [110]. Several reviews and a growing number of ongoing studies in animals and humans report on the environmental induction of the fetal genome, schematically summarized in Figure 27.3 [109,110].

Conclusions for Individual and Public Awareness as Well as Future Prevention

Poverty, poor education, and the lack of knowledge about adequate food intake and environmental factors increase the risks for mother and offspring. Deficits of nourishment may further reduce their physical and mental capacity for escaping poverty. As the post-MDG era approaches, reducing maternal and child undernutrition is gaining high priority on the international development agenda, both as a marker and as a maker of development. The concept of a mismatch between the early life and adult phenotype has been described in epidemiologic studies; research elucidating the mechanisms is still ongoing, specifying implications for the rise of NCDs throughout the globe and political concepts for pharmacological, lifestyle, and environmental interventions.

Concentrating on the "M" in maternal-fetal medicine in a sense that pregnancy not only determines fetal, but also maternal risks in later life is a young discipline. Maternal-fetal specialists and midwives should make the obstetric history available for primary health care providers. Algorithms could be applied not only for individualized risk profiles in ongoing pregnancies, but also for the identification of future maternal health problems and long-term risks of the offspring and their prevention. A life-course approach to health, commencing in early development, can

provide new opportunities for addressing this challenge across generations [114]. Health care interventions should be developed to reduce maternal stress, smoking of parents, and exposure to toxins and infections, but also to promote a healthy lifestyle in adolescents, young adults, and their children, for the prevention of immediate, but also of enduring complications related to cardio-metabolic and behavioral diseases of future generations. The dignity and political will for health care concepts dealing with preconceptional, pregnancy, and newborn care will be vital in the future.

Key Points

- A vicious circle of under- and malnutrition combined with risks of chronic diseases repeats itself.

- The concept of a mismatch between prenatal life and an adult phenotype of non communicable diseases has been described in several epidemiologic studies, creating the term "fetal origin of adult disease."

- In utero exposure to internal diseases, maternal stress, smoking, or chemicals is also combined with abnormal prenatal and postnatal development whereby the placenta functions as gatekeeper.

- Mothers with uncomplicated pregnancies have a lower incidence of subsequent hypertension than the general female population of similar age and race. Women with a history of PE and FGR have higher circulating concentrations of fasting insulin, lipid, and coagulation factors than controls matched for BMI and show defects of endothelial dependent function and correlated CVD.

- Thus similar algorithms could be applied for individualized risk profiles in ongoing pregnancies, and the identification of maternal health problems and long-term risks of the offspring.

- Nutritional and environmental exposures in utero play a role in gender-dependent developmental variation and disease susceptibility through vasculatory, endocrine, and epigenetic mechanisms.

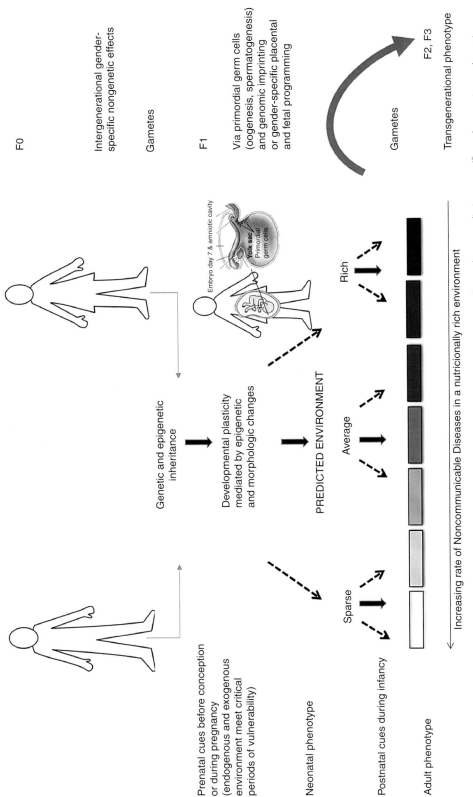

Figure 27.3 Gender-specific transmission of early nutrition and environmental exposure to subsequent generations. Prenatal cues predicting a specific environment cause impact epigenetic landscapes (F0) and cause a shift toward a phenotype matched to that environment (F1). Consequences of maternal F0 exposure during pregnancy can be transmitted via the placenta in a gender-specific manner and affect tissue development (F1). Primordial germ cells can be affected by F0 maternal environment and transfer information to the F2 generation. Maternal and paternal influences (F0) affect the transmission to F2 and F3 differently. Postnatal cues such as childhood nutrition can further shift the phenotype (dashed lines), all simplified in the diagram. Adapted from Gluckman et al. [112] and Gabory et al. [113].

- Specialists of maternal-fetal medicine have the potential to influence the incidence of both maternal and offspring's childhood and adult disease with appropriate maternal screening and counseling and by informing health care politicians about capacities of future concepts.

References

1. Rich-Edwards JW, McElrath TF, Karumanchi SA, Seely EW. Breathing life into the lifecourse approach: Pregnancy history and cardiovascular disease in women. *Hypertension* 2010;56(3):331–4.

2. Sattar N, Greer IA. Pregnancy complications and maternal cardiovascular risk: Opportunities for intervention and screening? *BMJ* 2002;325(7356):157–60.

3. Fleming K. Pregnancy: Window into women's future cardiovascular health. *Can Fam Physician* 2013;59(10):1033–5, 45–7.

4. Barker DJ, Gluckman PD, Robinson JS. Conference report: Fetal origins of adult disease –report of the First International Study Group, Sydney, 29–30 October 1994. *Placenta* 1995;16(3):317–20.

5. Barker DJ, Gluckman PD, Godfrey KM, Harding JE, Owens JA, Robinson JS. Fetal nutrition and cardiovascular disease in adult life. *Lancet* 1993;341(8850):938–41.

6. Barker DJ, Godfrey KM, Fall C, Osmond C, Winter PD, Shaheen SO. Relation of birth weight and childhood respiratory infection to adult lung function and death from chronic obstructive airways disease. *BMJ* 1991;303(6804):671–5.

7. Barker DJ, Osmond C, Golding J, Kuh D, Wadsworth ME. Growth in utero, blood pressure in childhood and adult life, and mortality from cardiovascular disease. *BMJ* 1989;298(6673):564–7.

8. Barker DJ. Intra-uterine programming of the adult cardiovascular system. *Curr Opin Nephrol Hypertens* 1997;6(1):106–10.

9. Barker DJ, Thornburg KL. Placental programming of chronic diseases, cancer and lifespan: A review. *Placenta* 2013;34(10):841–5.

10. Arck PC, Hecher K. Fetomaternal immune cross-talk and its consequences for maternal and offspring's health. *Nat Med* 2013;19(5):548–56.

11. Aggarwal A, Monsivais P, Drewnowski A. Nutrient intakes linked to better health outcomes are associated with higher diet costs in the US. *PloS One* 2012;7(5):e37533.

12. Darmon N, Drewnowski A. Does social class predict diet quality? *Am J Clin Nutr* 2008;87(5):1107–17.

13. Margerison-Zilko CE, Catalano R, Hubbard A, Ahern J. Maternal exposure to unexpected economic contraction and birth weight for gestational age. *Epidemiology* 2011;22(6):855–8.

14. UNICEF Ar. Drops of Life. Vitamin A supplementation for Child Survival. Progress and lessons learned in West and Central Africa. In: https://www.unicef.org/wcaro/WCARO_Pub_DropsLifeVitA.pdf, 2007.

15. Nations U. Millennium Goals United Nations: www.un.org/millenniumgoals/poverty, 2015.

16. (UNICEF) UNCsF. *Tracking Progress on Child and Maternal Nutrition: A Survival and Development Priority within Our Reach.* New York: United Nations Children's Fund (UNICEF) Publ., 2009.

17. Forsdahl A. Are poor living conditions in childhood and adolescence an important risk factor for arteriosclerotic heart disease? *Br J Prev Soc Med* 1977;31(2):91–5.

18. Barker DJ, Osmond C. Infant mortality, childhood nutrition, and ischaemic heart disease in England and Wales. *Lancet* 1986;1(8489):1077–81.

19. Barker DJ. The fetal and infant origins of adult disease. *BMJ* 1990;301(6761):1111.

20. Barker DJ. Fetal growth and adult disease. *BJOG* 1992;99(4):275–6.

21. Barker DJ. Intrauterine programming of adult disease. *Mol Med Today* 1995;1(9):418–23.

22. Barker DJ. Intrauterine programming of coronary heart disease and stroke. *Acta Paediatr Suppl* 1997;423:178–82; discussion 83.

23. Hales CN, Barker DJ, Clark PM, Cox LJ, Fall C, Osmond C, et al. Fetal and infant growth and impaired glucose tolerance at age 64. *BMJ* 1991;303(6809):1019–22.

24. Hales CN, Barker DJ. Type 2 (non-insulin-dependent) diabetes mellitus: The thrifty phenotype hypothesis. *Diabetologia* 1992;35(7):595–601.

25. Hales CN, Barker DJ. The thrifty phenotype hypothesis. *Br Med Bull* 2001;60:5–20.

26. Law CM, Shiell AW. Is blood pressure inversely related to birth weight? The strength of evidence from a systematic review of the literature. *J Hypertens* 1996;14(8):935–41.

27. Huxley RR, Shiell AW, Law CM. The role of size at birth and postnatal catch-up growth in determining systolic blood pressure: A systematic review of the literature. *J Hypertens* 2000;18(7):815–31.

28. Tappy L. Adiposity in children born small for gestational age. *Int J Obes (Lond)* 2006;30 Suppl 4:S36–40.

29. Barker DJ, Clark PM. Fetal undernutrition and disease in later life. *Rev Reprod* 1997;2(2):105–12.

30. Yajnik CS, Deshpande SS, Jackson AA, Refsum H, Rao S, Fisher DJ, et al. Vitamin B12 and folate concentrations during pregnancy and insulin resistance in the offspring: The Pune Maternal Nutrition Study. *Diabetologia* 2008;51(1):29–38.

31. Persson B, Pschera H, Binder C, Efendic S, Hanson U, Hartling S, et al. Decreased beta-cell function in women with previous small for gestational age infants. *Hormone Metab Res* 1993;25(3):170–4.

32. Kannisto V, Christensen K, Vaupel JW. No increased mortality in later life for cohorts born during famine. *Am J Epidemiol* 1997;145(11):987–94.

33. Razzaque A, Alam N, Wai L, Foster A. Sustained effects of the 1974–75 famine on infant and child mortality in a rural area of Bangladesh. *Popul Stud* 1990;44(1):145–54.

34. Lumey LH, Ravelli AC, Wiessing LG, Koppe JG, Treffers PE, Stein ZA. The Dutch famine birth cohort study: Design, validation of exposure, and selected characteristics of subjects after 43 years follow-up. *Paediatr Perinat Epidemiol* 1993;7(4):354–67.

35. Lumey LH, Stein AD. Offspring birth weights after maternal intrauterine undernutrition: A comparison within sibships. *Am J Epidemiol* 1997;146(10):810–19.

36. Roseboom T, de Rooij S, Painter R. The Dutch famine and its long-term consequences for adult health. *Early Hum Dev* 2006;82(8):485–91.

37. De Rooij SR, Painter RC, Phillips DI, Osmond C, Michels RP, Godsland IF, et al. Impaired insulin secretion after prenatal exposure to the Dutch famine. *Diabetes Care* 2006;29(8):1897–901.

38. Roseboom TJ, Painter RC, Van Abeelen AF, Veenendaal MV, De Rooij SR. Hungry in the womb: What are the consequences? Lessons from the Dutch famine. *Maturitas* 2011;70(2):141–5.

39. Song S. Mortality consequences of the 1959–1961 Great Leap Forward famine in China: Debilitation, selection, and mortality crossovers. *Soc Sci Med* 2010;71(3):551–8.

40. Brown AS, Susser ES. Prenatal nutritional deficiency and risk of adult schizophrenia. *Schizophr Bull* 2008;34(6):1054–63.

41. Song S. Does famine influence sex ratio at birth? Evidence from the 1959–1961 Great Leap Forward Famine in China. *Proc Biol Sci* 2012;279(1739):2883–90.

42. Kolominsky Y, Igumnov S, Drozdovitch V. The psychological development of children from Belarus exposed in the prenatal period to radiation from the Chernobyl atomic power plant. *J Child Psychol Psychiatry* 1999;40(2):299–305.

43. Stanner SA, Bulmer K, Andres C, Lantseva OE, Borodina V, Poteen VV, et al. Does malnutrition in utero determine diabetes and coronary heart disease in adulthood? Results from the Leningrad siege study, a cross sectional study. *BMJ* 1997;315(7119):1342–8.

44. Boersma G, Tamashiro, KL. Individual differences in the effects of prenatal stress exposure in rodents. *Neurobiol Stress* 2015;1:100–8.

45. Smith GC, Stenhouse EJ, Crossley JA, Aitken DA, Cameron AD, Connor JM. Early-pregnancy origins of low birth weight. *Nature* 2002;417(6892):916.

46. Cuckle HS. Screening for pre-eclampsia –lessons from aneuploidy screening. *Placenta* 2011;32 Suppl:S42–8.

47. Wright D, Akolekar R, Syngelaki A, Poon LC, Nicolaides KH. A competing risks model in early screening for preeclampsia. *Fetal Diagn Ther* 2012;32(3):171–8.

48. Baschat AA, Magder LS, Doyle LE, Atlas RO, Jenkins CB, Blitzer MG. Prediction of preeclampsia utilizing the first trimester screening examination. *Am J Obstet Gynecol* 2014;211(5):514 e1–7.

49. Stepan H, Herraiz I, Schlembach D, Verlohren S, Brennecke S, Chantraine F, et al. Implementation of the sFlt-1/PlGF ratio for prediction and diagnosis of pre-eclampsia in singleton pregnancy: Implications for clinical practice. *Ultrasound Obstet Gynecol* 2015;45(3):241–6.

50. Baschat AA. First-trimester screening for pre-eclampsia: Moving from personalized risk prediction to prevention. *Ultrasound Obstet Gynecol* 2015;45(2):119–29.

51. Scholten RR, Hopman MT, Sweep FC, Van de Vlugt MJ, Van Dijk AP, Oyen WJ, et al. Co-occurrence of cardiovascular and prothrombotic risk factors in women with a history of preeclampsia. *Obstet Gynecol* 2013;121(1):97–105.

52. McCowan LM, Thompson JM, Taylor RS, North RA, Poston L, Baker PN, et al. Clinical prediction in early pregnancy of infants small for gestational age by customised birthweight centiles: Findings from a healthy nulliparous cohort. *PloS One* 2013;8(8):e70917.

53. Scantlebury DC, Schwartz GL, Acquah LA, White WM, Moser M, Garovic VD. The treatment of hypertension during pregnancy: When should blood pressure medications be started? *Curr Cardiol Rep* 2013;15(11):412.

54. Ankumah NA, Cantu J, Jauk V, Biggio J, Hauth J, Andrews W, et al. Risk of adverse pregnancy outcomes in women with mild chronic hypertension before 20 weeks of gestation. *Obstet Gynecol* 2014;123(5):966–72.

55. Mosca L, Benjamin EJ, Berra K, Bezanson JL, Dolor RJ, Lloyd-Jones DM, et al. Effectiveness-based guidelines for the prevention of cardiovascular disease in women –2011 update: A guideline from the American Heart Association. *Circulation* 2011;123(11):1243–62.

56. The Diabetes Prevention Program (DPP): Description of lifestyle intervention. *Diabetes Care* 2002;25(12):2165–71.

57. Dodd JM, McLeod A, Windrim RC, Kingdom J. Antithrombotic therapy for improving maternal or infant health outcomes in women considered at risk of placental dysfunction. *Cochrane Database Syst Rev* 2013;7:CD006780.

58. Schramm AM, Clowse ME. Aspirin for prevention of preeclampsia in lupus pregnancy. *Autoimmune Dis* 2014;2014:920467.

59. Ruffatti A, Salvan E, Del Ross T, Gerosa M, Andreoli L, Maina A, et al. Treatment strategies and pregnancy outcomes in antiphospholipid syndrome patients with thrombosis and triple antiphospholipid positivity. A European multicentre retrospective study. *Thromb Haemost* 2014;112(4):727–35.

60. Clifton VL. Review: Sex and the human placenta: Mediating differential strategies of fetal growth and survival. *Placenta* 2010;31 Suppl:S33–9.

61. Bohrer J, Ehrenthal DB. Other adverse pregnancy outcomes and future chronic disease. *Semin Perinatol* 2015;39(4):259–63.

62. Smith GC, Pell JP, Walsh D. Pregnancy complications and maternal risk of ischaemic heart disease: A retrospective cohort study of 129,290 births. *Lancet* 2001;357(9273):2002–6.

63. Smith GD, Harding S, Rosato M. Relation between infants' birth weight and mothers' mortality: Prospective observational study. *BMJ* 2000;320(7238):839–40.

64. Bonamy AK, Parikh NI, Cnattingius S, Ludvigsson JF, Ingelsson E. Birth characteristics and subsequent risks of maternal cardiovascular disease: Effects of gestational age and fetal growth. *Circulation* 2011;124(25):2839–46.

65. Smith GD, Sterne J, Tynelius P, Lawlor DA, Rasmussen F. Birth weight of offspring and subsequent cardiovascular mortality of the parents. *Epidemiology* 2005;16(4):563–9.

66. Manor O, Koupil I. Birth weight of infants and mortality in their parents and grandparents: The Uppsala Birth Cohort Study. *Int J Epidemiol* 2010;39(5):1264–76.

67. Steffen KM, Cooper ME, Shi M, Caprau D, Simhan HN, Dagle JM, et al. Maternal and fetal variation in genes of cholesterol metabolism is associated with preterm delivery. *J Perinatol* 2007;27(11):672–80.

68. Melchiorre K, Sharma R, Thilaganathan B. Cardiovascular implications in preeclampsia: An overview. *Circulation* 2014;130(8):703–14.

69. Godfrey KM, Lillycrop KA, Burdge GC, Gluckman PD, Hanson MA. Non-imprinted epigenetics in fetal and postnatal development and growth. *Nestle Nutr Inst Workshop Ser* 2013;71:57–63.

70. Rikkonen K, Pesonen AK, Heinonen K, Lahti J, Kajantie E, Forsen T, et al. Infant growth and hostility in adult life. *Psychosom Med* 2008;70(3):306–13.

71. DiPietro JA, Caulfield LE, Irizarry RA, Chen P, Merialdi M, Zavaleta N. Prenatal development of intrafetal and maternal-fetal synchrony. *Behav Neurosci* 2006;120(3):687–701.

72. Chang MY, Chen CH, Huang KF. Effects of music therapy on psychological health of women during pregnancy. *J Clin Nurs* 2008;17(19):2580–7.

73. Nordentoft M, Lou HC, Hansen D, Nim J, Pryds O, Rubin P, et al. Intrauterine growth retardation and premature delivery: The influence of maternal smoking and psychosocial factors. *Am J Public Health* 1996;86(3):347–54.

74. Smits L, Krabbendam L, de Bie R, Essed G, Van Os J. Lower birth weight of Dutch neonates who were in utero at the time of the 9/11 attacks. *J Psychosom Res* 2006;61(5):715–7.

75. Khashan AS, McNamee R, Abel KM, Pedersen MG, Webb RT, Kenny LC, et al. Reduced infant birthweight consequent upon maternal exposure to severe life events. *Psychosom Med* 2008;70(6):688–94.

76. Hartwig IR, Pincus MK, Diemert A, Hecher K, Arck PC. Sex-specific effect of first-trimester maternal progesterone on birthweight. *Hum Reprod* 2013;28(1):77–86.

77. Dipietro JA. Maternal stress in pregnancy: Considerations for fetal development. *J Adolesc Health* 2012;51(2 Suppl):S3–8.

78. Crane JM, Keough M, Murphy P, Burrage L, Hutchens D. Effects of environmental tobacco smoke on perinatal outcomes: A retrospective cohort study. *BJOG* 2011;118(7):865–71.

79. Durmus B, Ay L, Hokken-Koelega AC, Raat H, Hofman A, Steegers EA, et al. Maternal smoking during pregnancy and subcutaneous fat mass in early

childhood. The Generation R Study. *Eur J Epidemiol* 2011;26(4):295–304.

80. Dior UP, Lawrence GM, Sitlani C, Enquobahrie D, Manor O, Siscovick DS, et al. Parental smoking during pregnancy and offspring cardio-metabolic risk factors at ages 17 and 32. *Atherosclerosis* 2014;235(2):430–7.

81. Abusalah A, Gavana M, Haidich AB, Smyrnakis E, Papadakis N, Papanikolaou A, et al. Low birth weight and prenatal exposure to indoor pollution from tobacco smoke and wood fuel smoke: A matched case-control study in Gaza Strip. *Matern Child Health J* 2012;16(8):1718–27.

82. Suter M, Ma J, Harris A, Patterson L, Brown KA, Shope C, et al. Maternal tobacco use modestly alters correlated epigenome-wide placental DNA methylation and gene expression. *Epigenetics* 2011;6(11):1284–94.

83. Czeizel AE. Human germinal mutagenic effects in relation to intentional and accidental exposure to toxic agents. *Environ Health Perspect* 1996;104 Suppl 3:615–17.

84. Romero R, Gotsch F, Pineles B, Kusanovic JP. Inflammation in pregnancy: Its roles in reproductive physiology, obstetrical complications, and fetal injury. *Nutr Rev* 2007;65(12 Pt 2):S194–202.

85. Velten M, Gorr MW, Youtz DJ, Velten C, Rogers LK, Wold LE. Adverse perinatal environment contributes to altered cardiac development and function. *Am J Physiol Heart Circ Physiol* 2014;306(9):H1334–40.

86. Chandrasiri UP, Chua CL, Umbers AJ, Chaluluka E, Glazier JD, Rogerson SJ, et al. Insight into the pathogenesis of fetal growth restriction in placental malaria: Decreased placental glucose transporter isoform 1 expression. *J Infect Dis* 2014;209(10):1663–7.

87. Persson E, Jansson T. Low birth weight is associated with elevated adult blood pressure in the chronically catheterized guinea-pig. *Acta Physiologica Scandinavica* 1992;145(2):195–6.

88. Holemans K, Gerber R, Meurrens K, De Clerck F, Poston L, Van Assche FA. Maternal food restriction in the second half of pregnancy affects vascular function but not blood pressure of rat female offspring. *Br J Nutr* 1999;81(1):73–9.

89. Zhao H, Wong RJ, Kalish FS, Nayak NR, Stevenson DK. Effect of heme oxygenase-1 deficiency on placental development. *Placenta* 2009;30(10):861–8.

90. Solano ME KM, O'Rourke GE, Horst AK, Modest K, Plösch T, Barikbin R, Remus CC, Berger RG, Jago V, Lydon JP, DeMayo FJ, Parker VJ, Hecher K, Karimi K, Arck PC. Progesterone and HMOX-1 promote fetal growth by CD8+T cell modulation. *J Clin Invest* 2015;125:1726–38.

91. Yachie A, Niida Y, Wada T, Igarashi N, Kaneda H, Toma T, et al. Oxidative stress causes enhanced endothelial cell injury in human heme oxygenase-1 deficiency. *J Clin Invest* 1999;103(1):129–35.

92. Brunton PJ, Russell JA, Douglas AJ. Adaptive responses of the maternal hypothalamic-pituitary-adrenal axis during pregnancy and lactation. *J Neuroendocrinol* 2008;20(6):764–76.

93. Robinson BG, Emanuel RL, Frim DM, Majzoub JA. Glucocorticoid stimulates expression of corticotropin-releasing hormone gene in human placenta. *Proc Natl Acad Sci U S A* 1988;85(14):5244–8.

94. Mastorakos G, Ilias I. Maternal and fetal hypothalamic-pituitary-adrenal axes during pregnancy and postpartum. *Ann N Y Acad Sci* 2003;997:136–49.

95. Reis FM, Fadalti M, Florio P, Petraglia F. Putative role of placental corticotropin-releasing factor in the mechanisms of human parturition. *J Soc Gynecol Investig* 1999;6(3):109–19.

96. Petraglia F, Potter E, Cameron VA, Sutton S, Behan DP, Woods RJ, et al. Corticotropin-releasing factor-binding protein is produced by human placenta and intrauterine tissues. *J Clin Endocrinol Metab* 1993;77(4):919–24.

97. Venihaki M, Carrigan A, Dikkes P, Majzoub JA. Circadian rise in maternal glucocorticoid prevents pulmonary dysplasia in fetal mice with adrenal insufficiency. *Proc Natl Acad Sci U S A* 2000;97(13):7336–41.

98. Michelsohn AM, Anderson DJ. Changes in competence determine the timing of two sequential glucocorticoid effects on sympathoadrenal progenitors. *Neuron* 1992;8(3):589–604.

99. Chapman K, Holmes M, Seckl J. 11beta-hydroxysteroid dehydrogenases: Intracellular gate-keepers of tissue glucocorticoid action. *Physiol Rev* 2013;93(3):1139–206.

100. Blasco MJ, Lopez Bernal A, Turnbull AC. 11 beta-Hydroxysteroid dehydrogenase activity of the human placenta during pregnancy. *Horm Metab Res* 1986;18(9):638–41.

101. Schoof E, Girstl M, Frobenius W, Kirschbaum M, Repp R, Knerr I, et al. Course of placental 11beta-hydroxysteroid dehydrogenase type 2 and 15-hydroxyprostaglandin dehydrogenase mRNA expression during human gestation. *Eur J Endocrinol* 2001;145(2):187–92.

102. Sacedon R, Vicente A, Varas A, Jimenez E, Munoz JJ, Zapata AG. Early maturation of T-cell progenitors in the absence of glucocorticoids. *Blood* 1999;94(8):2819–26.

103. Frost JM, Moore GE. The importance of imprinting in the human placenta. *PLoS Genet* 2010;6(7):e1001015.

104. Berger SL, Kouzarides T, Shiekhattar R, Shilatifard A. An operational definition of epigenetics. *Genes Dev* 2009;23(7):781–3.

105. Ordovas JM, Smith CE. Epigenetics and cardiovascular disease. *Nat Rev Cardiol* 2010;7(9):510–19.

106. Morgan HD, Santos F, Green K, Dean W, Reik W. Epigenetic reprogramming in mammals. *Hum Mol Genet* 2005;14 Spec No 1:R47–58.

107. Santos F, Dean W. Epigenetic reprogramming during early development in mammals. *Reproduction* 2004;127(6):643–51.

108. Drake AJ, McPherson RC, Godfrey KM, Cooper C, Lillycrop KA, Hanson MA, et al. An unbalanced maternal diet in pregnancy associates with offspring epigenetic changes in genes controlling glucocorticoid action and foetal growth. *Clin Endocrinol* 2012;77(6):808–15.

109. Odom LN, Taylor HS. Environmental induction of the fetal epigenome. *Expert Rev Obstet Gynecol* 2010;5(6):657–64.

110. Gluckman PD, Hanson MA, Bateson P, Beedle AS, Law CM, Bhutta ZA, et al. Towards a new developmental synthesis: Adaptive developmental plasticity and human disease. *Lancet* 2009;373(9675):1654–7.

111. Montenegro D, Romero R, Kim SS, Tarca AL, Draghici S, Kusanovic JP, et al. Expression patterns of microRNAs in the chorioamniotic membranes: A role for microRNAs in human pregnancy and parturition. *J Pathol* 2009;217(1):113–21.

112. Gluckman PD, Hanson MA, Cooper C, Thornburg KL. Effect of in utero and early-life conditions on adult health and disease. *N Engl J Med* 2008;359(1):61–73.

113. Gabory A, Roseboom TJ, Moore T, Moore LG, Junien C. Placental contribution to the origins of sexual dimorphism in health and diseases: Sex chromosomes and epigenetics. *Biol Sex Differ* 2013;4(1):5.

114. Hanson MA, Gluckman PD. Developmental origins of health and disease – global public health implications. *Best Pract Res Clin Obstet Gynaecol* 2015;29(1):24–31.

28

Fetal Growth Restriction: Recurrence Risks and Counseling

Jan Derks and Steven Koenen[1]

Introduction

Knowledge of the recurrence risk of FGR is essential to determine antenatal care in subsequent pregnancies and possible treatment strategies. Furthermore, delivering an infant that is SGA, especially when born very prematurely, has a huge impact on the life of parents and their psychosocial well-being. Singer and colleagues demonstrated that women delivering a high-risk VLBW infant (high risk defined as chronic lung disease and birth weight <1500 g) not only had a significantly higher incidence of psychosocial distress during the neonatal period, but also at 2-year follow-up [1,2]. The severity of maternal depression scores was inversely related to the child developmental outcome. Kusters and colleagues also showed in a Dutch national cohort study that preterm birth had a profound impact on psychosocial well-being in families even after 19 years, especially when the infant of the index pregnancy was handicapped. In these cases, divorce rates were higher, more financial problems were observed, and more negative effects were noted regarding work and social activities [3]. Although data are lacking for women who experienced an FGR pregnancy specifically, it is known from women who had a first pregnancy that was complicated by early-onset preeclampsia (45% infants with neonatal birth weight <10th centile) that 15.1% did not wish to achieve a future pregnancy. In 33% of these cases, fear of delivering another premature infant was the main reason, even though the outcome in women experiencing a second pregnancy is generally favorable [4,5]. Therefore adequate counseling of women regarding recurrence risk in a future pregnancy is of the utmost importance.

Counseling on recurrent (r)FGR typically comprises information on the etiology of the disease, risk of recurrence in subsequent pregnancy, and possible therapeutic options for prevention of recurrence.

FGR Recurrence Risk

The incidence of rFGR has been well described in a number of studies showing a median recurrence risk of 21%, range [18%–28.7%] [6–12], and are consistent over time (Table 28.1). Recurrence risks differ among studies, partly because of a large heterogeneity in study populations. Furthermore, the definition of FGR differs, including small-for-gestational age neonates, and various cut-off points were used for birth weight percentile.

Visser and colleagues [14] showed in 1986, in women with early fetal growth retardation leading to intrauterine death between 25 and 34 weeks, or to delivery before 34 weeks, that the recurrence risk of growth restriction in the subsequent pregnancy was up to 50% for women with an hypertensive disorder in this population, including intrauterine death.

Bakketeig and colleagues were the first to publish reliable recurrence rates in 1986 when they studied a nationwide Norwegian cohort from their Medical Birth Registry. They were able to link successive pregnancy outcome in a mother and investigated three matched singleton pregnancies. They could not study only the recurrence risk for SGA in a second pregnancy, but also in a third pregnancy if two previous pregnancies had been complicated by SGA. Between 1967 and 1976, 2,862 women were included with an SGA (<10th percentile) neonate in the first pregnancy without fetal congenital abnormalities in any of the studied pregnancies. They showed a 28.7% (n = 820) recurrence rate in the second pregnancy and a 44.4% (n = 364) recurrence rate in the third pregnancy among women with two previous SGA pregnancies [12]. This

[1] The authors would like to thank Afra Zaal and Monique Sterrenburg for their help with the literature search and writing of this chapter.

Table 28.1 Overview of recurrence rates in second and third pregnancies after a first pregnancy with an SGA infant. HTD: with hypertensive disease in first pregnancy; no HTD: without hypertensive disease in first pregnancy

Study author	Pregnancy	Year	N	Recurrence (%)	HTD (%)	No HTD (%)
Bakketeig [12]	2	1986	2,862	28.7	-	-
	3		820	44.4	-	-
Patterson [7]	2	1986	1,189	20.1	-	-
Kuno [11]	2	1995	95	26.3	-	-
Bakewell [9]	2	1997	10,701	21	-	-
Saemundsson [6]	2	2009	196	18.2	-	-
Evers [13]	2	2011	22	27.3	-	27.3
Voskamp [10]	2	2013	12,943	23.1	23.7	21
Hinkle [8]	2	2014	2,393	20.2	-	-

study was hampered by two major problems: first, dating of the pregnancy was less reliable at the time as it was solely based on LMP since first trimester CRL measurement was not available throughout the study period. Second, children born before 28 weeks GA and after 46 weeks GA were excluded, leading to selection bias. Furthermore, since their publication, it has become common practice to treat women with a history of preeclampsia and/or FGR with aspirin in a subsequent pregnancy. This could partially explain a lower recurrence rate in later studies as compared to their study. Nonetheless, their numbers have proven remarkably robust over time.

Evers and colleagues [13] were the first to separately study the recurrence rate of FGR in a small group of 22 women without concomitant maternal hypertension that were delivered before 34 weeks of gestation. Normotensive early-onset FGR prompting early delivery is a fairly uncommon condition. The authors not only provided detailed clinical data from the studied pregnancies, including ultrasound and Doppler measurements, they also displayed detailed information on the placental pathology in both index and subsequent pregnancies. In the subsequent pregnancy, six women (27.3%) had recurrent FGR (rFGR), four women developed a hypertensive disorder, and 11 women (54.4%) had an uneventful pregnancy. Although perinatal mortality was still high in the second pregnancy (13.6%), it was much lower than in the initial pregnancy (72%). Furthermore, in all clinical outcome parameters (e.g. gestational age at delivery, birth weight, Doppler findings), a vast improvement was seen. This was also reflected in the lower recurrence rates of different histopathological findings in the placenta. The study also demonstrates

the wide variety of different pathological findings in this specific subgroup, making it harder to provide these women with a general recurrence rate/percentage since different etiologies can have different recurrence rates.

The largest more recent study on SGA recurrence is by Voskamp and colleagues [10]. In this national Dutch cohort study, all women with a structurally normal first and subsequent singleton pregnancy between 1999 and 2007 were included. SGA was defined as a birth weight < 5th percentile for gestation, and incidence and recurrence rates were specified for women with and without a hypertensive disorder (HTD) in their first pregnancy. In total, 259,481 women were included, of whom 12,943 (5%) had an SGA firstborn. The risk of SGA in the second pregnancy was higher in women with a previous SGA neonate (N = 2996, 23.1%) than for women with a previous neonate with a normal weight (N = 8482, 3.4%; Figure 28.1).

Although the authors demonstrated a higher SGA recurrence rate in women with HTD in the first pregnancy, this finding did not seem clinically relevant since the absolute difference was fairly small between women with (23.7%) and without HTD (21%) in the index pregnancy. Furthermore, they also showed that in women without HTD, the increased recurrence risk was independent of the gestational age at delivery in the index pregnancy; whereas in women with HTD, this recurrence risk was increased only when the women with the index delivery delivered at >32 weeks' gestation.

Whether the severity of FGR was related to recurrence was investigated in two separate cohorts. A Hispanic cohort from the United States of matched singleton-singleton liveborns without anomalies and

Table 28.2 Birth weight percentiles in two consecutive pregnancies (table 1 by Patterson et al. [7], reprint with permission)

		Child 2 (No. of patients)			Row total (%)
		>10%	≤10%, >2.5%	≤2.5%	
Child 1 (No. of patients) (% of row total)	>10%	7,718 (91.8)	540 (6.4)	149 (1.8)	8,407 (87.6)
	≤10%, >2.5%	751 (81.9)	130 (14.2)	36 (3.9)	917 (9.6)
	≤2.5%	199 (73.2)	51 (18.8)	22 (8)	272 (2.8)
Column total (%)		8,668 (90.3)	721 (7.5)	207 (2.2)	9,596

χ2 = 194.74, P <0.0001

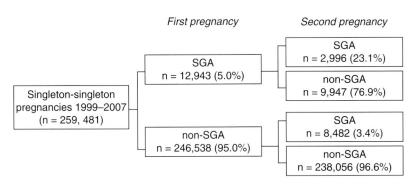

Figure 28.1 The flow diagram shows the incidence of SGA in the first and second singleton pregnancies in The Netherlands. Original Figure by Voskamp et al. [10], reprint with permission.

born at a gestational age greater than or equal to 26 weeks showed a 20.1% recurrence rate in the second pregnancy of 1,189 first pregnancies with a SGA neonate (≤10th percentile) [7]. Interestingly, they showed a significant increase in the prevalence and the degree of SGA as index pregnancy birth weight decreased (p<0.0001; see Table 28.2). The risk for delivering an SGA infant (≤10th percentile) in the second pregnancy was 19.7% for women who delivered a child in the first pregnancy with a birth weight between the 2.5th and 10th percentiles, versus 26.8% for women who delivered a child in the first pregnancy with a birth weight below the 2.5th percentile. A Japanese cohort study of 95 SGA first pregnancies showed an overall recurrence rate of 26.3% [11] and no recurrence-associated features were revealed. Although their data suggest that more severe FGR in the initial pregnancy is related to a higher recurrence rate in the subsequent pregnancy, they did not show a statistically significant difference. This was probably due to the small sample size.

Risk Factors

Specific risk factors for recurrent SGA among women with previous SGA were investigated in an American cohort of matched singleton pregnancies without structural abnormalities. They described 2,393 women with a SGA (<10th percentile) neonate in the first pregnancy. In total, 484 (20.2%) of these women delivered an SGA newborn in the following pregnancy. In this study, smoking, short stature, maternal weight (gain), and hypertensive disorders were shown to be involved in incident as well as recurrent FGR [8]. A previous large American cohort study in Missouri of 182,285 linked singleton live births between 1978 and 1990 described 10,701 women who delivered an infant with a low birth weight (<2,500 grams) in the first pregnancy and showed a recurrence rate of 21%. Furthermore they demonstrated that smoking, short inter-pregnancy interval, and maternal age were risk factors for low birth weight recurrence [9].

Uterine Artery and Umbilical Artery Doppler

The predictive value of uterine artery and umbilical artery Doppler in the first pregnancy for FGR recurrence was described in a Swedish cohort [6]. This cohort included 196 women with a suspected FGR (by ultrasound measurements) and a structurally normal first and subsequent singleton pregnancy. For the purpose of this chapter, we recalculated the results for the 132 women who delivered an SGA neonate (birth weight <3rd percentile). Of those, 24 women (18.2%) delivered an SGA newborn in the following pregnancy. The SGA recurrence rate was higher in the 33 women with an abnormal uterine artery Doppler (PI>2SD) in the first pregnancy (n = 12, 36.4%) than in the 99 women with a normal Doppler (n = 12, 12%). The higher recurrence rate in women with an abnormal Doppler in the first pregnancy probably reflects underlying vascular pathology leading to inadequate trophoblast invasion and subsequent placental insufficiency. Although numbers are small, this is an interesting finding, and might be a useful tool in future research regarding preventative treatment strategies.

Placental Histopathology

Although the overall recurrence rate of FGR is around 20%, there are some specific placental histopathological disorders not based on vascular pathology that carry a specific risk for recurrence of FGR. They include placental disorders, such as villitis of unknown origin, distal villous hypoplasia, advanced villous maturation, and maternal floor infarction [13,15]. Although all those placental disorders have recurrence rates up to about 20% to 40%, exact numbers are hard to give due to the small numbers of patients in the described studies. Maternal floor infarction (also called massive perivillous fibrin deposition) is one of those rare placental disorders that often leads to severe early FGR or fetal death. The reported incidence ranges from 0.028% to 0.5% and it has a recurrence rate as high as 39% in a subsequent pregnancy [16–18]. Placental histological characteristics are massive and diffuse fibrin depositions along the decidua basalis and the perivillous space of the basal plate [18]. Those fibrin depositions interfere with perfusion and exchange of oxygen and nutrients, resulting in early chronic placental insufficiency. Although the mechanisms responsible for these massive perivillous fibrin depositions are not entirely understood, a study by Romero and colleagues [19] found associations with plasma cell deciduitis, specific anti-HLA antibodies in maternal blood against fetal antigens, and evidence of antibody-mediated complement activation. These findings support the concept of fetal rejection by the mother, comparable to "graft versus host" rejection [19], leading to high recurrence rates in subsequent

pregnancies. Understanding of this underlying histopathological entity might lead to treatment options in the future.

Aspirin Treatment in a Subsequent Pregnancy

There is evidence that aspirin in a dosage of 60–150 mg has a beneficial effect in a high-risk population on reducing FGR by 20% and increasing birth weight by an average of 130 grams. However, specific data on the effect of aspirin on the FGR recurrence rate in women with a previous FGR pregnancy are lacking or insufficient. These issues should be addressed when counseling the patient. If the treatment option is chosen, aspirin administration should be started before 16 weeks. There is no significant effect on perinatal mortality, intracranial bleeding, or placental abruption [20].

Conclusion

The overall recurrence rate for FGR in a subsequent pregnancy is approximately 21%. The recurrence risk is related to the severity of the FGR in the initial pregnancy; the more severe the FGR, the higher the recurrence risk. However, the recurrence risk is also dependent on the underlying (histo)pathological mechanism. Treatment with aspirin in a high-risk population might reduce the recurrence risk when started before 16 weeks.

Key Points

- The recurrence risk of FGR in a subsequent pregnancy is approximately 21% in a second pregnancy and 44% in a third pregnancy.
- The recurrence risk is inversely related to the severity of the FGR in the initial pregnancy.
- The recurrence risk is dependent on the underlying histopathological mechanisms.
- Treatment with aspirin in a high-risk population reduces the risk of FGR with 20% when started before 16 weeks.

References

1. Singer LT, Davillier M, Bruening P, Hawkins S, Yamashita TS. Social support, psychological distress, and parenting strains in mothers of

very low birthweight infants. *Fam Relat* 1996 Jul 1;45(3):343–50.

2. Singer LT, Salvator A, Guo S, Collin M, Lilien L, Baley J. Maternal psychological distress and parenting stress after the birth of a very low-birth-weight infant. *JAMA* 1999 Mar 3;281(9):799–805.

3. Kusters CD, Van der Pal SM, Van Steenbrugge GJ, Den Ouden LS, Kollee LA. [The impact of a premature birth on the family; consequences are experienced even after 19 years]. *Ned Tijdschr Geneeskd* 2013;157(25):A5449.

4. Schaaf JM, Mol BW, bu-Hanna A, Ravelli AC. Trends in preterm birth: Singleton and multiple pregnancies in the Netherlands, 2000–2007. *BJOG* 2011 Sep;118(10):1196–204.

5. Van Rijn BB, Hoeks LB, Bots ML, Franx A, Bruinse HW. Outcomes of subsequent pregnancy after first pregnancy with early-onset preeclampsia. *Am J Obstet Gynecol* 2006 Sep;195(3):723–8.

6. Saemundsson Y, Svantesson H, Gudmundsson S. Abnormal uterine artery Doppler in pregnancies suspected of a SGA fetus is related to increased risk of recurrence during next pregnancy. *Acta Obstet Gynecol Scand* 2009;88(7):814–17.

7. Patterson RM, Gibbs CE, Wood RC. Birth weight percentile and perinatal outcome: Recurrence of intrauterine growth retardation. *Obstet Gynecol* 1986 Oct;68(4):464–8.

8. Hinkle SN, Albert PS, Mendola P, Sjaarda LA, Boghossian NS, Yeung E, et al. Differences in risk factors for incident and recurrent small-for-gestational-age birthweight: A hospital-based cohort study. *BJOG* 2014 Aug;121(9):1080–8.

9. Bakewell JM, Stockbauer JW, Schramm WF. Factors associated with repetition of low birthweight: Missouri longitudinal study. *Paediatr Perinat Epidemiol* 1997 Jan;11 Suppl 1:119–29.

10. Voskamp BJ, Kazemier BM, Ravelli AC, Schaaf J, Mol BW, Pajkrt E. Recurrence of small-for-gestational-age pregnancy: Analysis of first and subsequent singleton pregnancies in The Netherlands. *Am J Obstet Gynecol* 2013 May;208(5):374–6.

11. Kuno N, Itakura A, Kurauchi O, Mizutani S, Kazeto S, Tomoda Y. Decrease in severity of intrauterine growth retardation in subsequent pregnancies. *Int J Gynaecol Obstet* 1995 Dec;51(3):219–24.

12. Bakketeig LS, Bjerkedal T, Hoffman HJ. Small-for-gestational age births in successive pregnancy outcomes: Results from a longitudinal study of births in Norway. *Early Hum Dev* 1986 Dec;14(3–4):187–200.

13. Evers AC, Van Rijn BB, Van Rossum MM, Bruinse HW. Subsequent pregnancy outcome after first pregnancy with normotensive early-onset intrauterine growth restriction at <34 weeks of gestation. *Hypertens Pregnancy* 2011;30(1):37–44.

14. Visser GH, Huisman A, Saathof PW, Sinnige HA. Early fetal growth retardation: Obstetric background and recurrence rate. *Obstet Gynecol* 1986 Jan;67(1):40–3.

15. Kinzler WL, Kaminsky L. Fetal growth restriction and subsequent pregnancy risks. *Semin Perinatol* 2007 Jun;31(3):126–34.

16. Andres RL, Kuyper W, Resnik R, Piacquadio KM, Benirschke K. The association of maternal floor infarction of the placenta with adverse perinatal outcome. *Am J Obstet Gynecol* 1990 Sep;163(3):935–8.

17. Bane AL, Gillan JE. Massive perivillous fibrinoid causing recurrent placental failure. *BJOG* 2003 Mar;110(3):292–5.

18. Katzman PJ, Genest DR. Maternal floor infarction and massive perivillous fibrin deposition: Histological definitions, association with intrauterine fetal growth restriction, and risk of recurrence. *Pediatr Dev Pathol* 2002 Mar;5(2):159–64.

19. Romero R, Whitten A, Korzeniewski SJ, Than NG, Chaemsaithong P, Miranda J, et al. Maternal floor infarction/massive perivillous fibrin deposition: A manifestation of maternal antifetal rejection? *Am J Reprod Immunol* 2013 Oct;70(4):285–98.

20. Henderson JT, Whitlock EP, O'Conner E, Senger CA, Thompson JH, Rowland MG. *Low-Dose Aspirin for the Prevention of Morbidity and Mortality from Preeclampsia: A Systematic Evidence Review for the U.S. Preventive Services Task Force*. Rockville (MD): Agency for Healthcare Research and Quality (US): 2014 Apr Report No:14-05207-EF-1 2014 Apr.

Index